Smart
Biomaterial
DEVICES
Polymers in Biomedical Sciences

Smart Biomaterial DEVICES

Polymers in Biomedical Sciences

A.K. Bajpai
Jaya Bajpai
Rajesh Kumar Saini
Priyanka Agrawal
Atul Tiwari

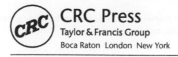

CRC Press
Taylor & Francis Group
Boca Raton London New York

CRC Press is an imprint of the
Taylor & Francis Group, an **informa** business

CRC Press
Taylor & Francis Group
6000 Broken Sound Parkway NW, Suite 300
Boca Raton, FL 33487-2742

First issued in paperback 2019

© 2017 by Taylor & Francis Group, LLC
CRC Press is an imprint of Taylor & Francis Group, an Informa business

No claim to original U.S. Government works

ISBN-13: 978-1-4987-0698-8 (hbk)
ISBN-13: 978-0-367-87189-5 (pbk)

Visit the Taylor & Francis Web site at
http://www.taylorandfrancis.com

and the CRC Press Web site at
http://www.crcpress.com

Table of Contents

Preface

Functional polymers are one of the most promising materials finding tremendous application in almost all the areas of science and technology, ranging from industrial to medical domains. With the emergence of new and newer synthetic strategies in chemical and allied sciences, specialty polymers of diversified structures have been designed with tailored properties and applications. The great ability to keep a precise control over the size, shape, molecular weight, functionalities, and physical and chemical properties of resulting polymers has enabled polymer scientists to fabricate materials of own choice, desired properties, and intended end uses. This book attempts to deliver a comprehensive account of various polymer-based materials that are being intensively used as biomaterials for various applications pertaining to human body.

This book consists of nine chapters that encompass almost entire range of applications of polymers in human body. Chapter 1 highlights the basic criteria of materials to be coined as biomaterials for dental, orthopedic, drug delivery, wound dressing, tissue engineering, ocular, and cardiovascular applications. Chapter 2 focuses on the use of polymers for dental applications. This chapter emphasizes the required mechanical properties of a polymer, which are essential for dental applications. It also gives an overview of different types of dental implants and various kinds of polymers being employed in dentistry. Chapter 3 is concerned with the use of polymer materials and nanocomposites that find applications as orthopedic materials. The chapter also covers metal- and ceramic-based hybrid materials, which are in current use in orthopedic surgery.

Chapter 4 describes the use of smart polymers in drug delivery applications. A variety of polymers and other macromolecular entities that have been used for designing smart drug delivery systems have also been discussed in this chapter. Chapter 5 focuses on the use of polymers as wound-dressing materials. This chapter also covers classification of wounds, type of wound dressings, naturally occurring polymers in wound dressing, etc. While Chapter 6 focuses on use of smart polymers in tissue-engineering applications and Chapter 7 pertains to ocular implants. Chapter 8 assesses the role of polymers in cardiovascular implantation and discusses how materials such as polymers, metals, and ceramics are currently being used for cardiovascular applications. Finally, Chapter 9 provides an authentic and conclusive information about the market scenario of biomaterial-based devises.

We are confident that this book will be useful for students and research scholars from different disciplines of science, engineering, and technology.

Authors

Anil Kumar Bajpai earned a PhD in chemistry in 1984. Dr. Bajpai joined Government Science College, Jabalpur, Madhya Pradesh, India in 1986, and since then he has been working as a professor in chemistry. While at service, he earned a DSc. The areas of his research interest include biomedical polymers synthesis, controlled drug delivery systems, nanostructure materials of pharmaceutical relevance, conducting polymer nanocomposites, water remediation using biopolymers nanoparticles, hydroxyapatite nanocomposites, etc. He has published more than 220 papers in reputed and high impact factor journals and contributed more than 15 chapters in encyclopedias of prestigious international publishers. Professor Bajpai has also supervised 40 students for their doctoral degree and successfully completed more than 10 major research projects funded by prime scientific and defense establishments of the government of India. He is associated with editorial boards of a few journals and serves as a regular reviewer of leading journals.

Jaya Bajpai, a postgraduate in chemistry at the University of Jabalpur (1982), earned a PhD at the same university in 1992. Dr. Bajpai has published more than 40 research papers in leading international journals and contributed several chapters as coauthor. Currently, she works as a professor of chemistry and actively engaged in research areas related to biomedical polymers, drug delivery systems, and nanomaterials.

Rajesh Kumar Saini is the coprincipal investigator in several major research projects and postdoctoral fellow in the Department of Chemistry, Government Model Science College, Jabalpur, Madhya Pradesh, India. He has worked as a faculty member in the Department of Chemistry, Shri Rawatpura Sarkar Institute of Technology, Jabalpur. Dr. Saini earned a PhD in 2008 in polymer chemistry and has published numerous research papers in reputed journals and written many book chapters and coauthored a book on the topic responsive drug delivery systems. His fields of interest are macroporous biomaterials, cryogels, and high-performance materials for biomedical applications.

Priyanka Agrawal earned a PhD in 2012 at the R. D. University, Jabalpur, Madhya Pradesh, India. His research areas include water remediation, adsorption studies, and nanoparticles synthesis of biopolymers in drug delivery and water remediation. She has published several papers in reputed journals. Dr. Agrawal has previously worked as an assistant professor of chemistry at the Hitkarini College of Engineering and Technology, Jabalpur, and she is currently working as a TIFAC (Technology Information, Forecasting and Assessment Council), women scientist trainee in Intellectual Property Rights at CSIR-URDIP (Council of Scientific and Industrial Research-Unit for Research and Development of Information Products), Pune, India.

Atul Tiwari currently serves as director, Research and Developments at Pantheon Chemicals in Phoenix, Arizona, USA. Previously, Dr. Tiwari was a research faculty member in the Department of Mechanical Engineering at the University of Hawaii, USA. He has achieved double subject majors in organic chemistry as well as in mechanical engineering. He earned a PhD in polymer materials science in 2003 along with earned Chartered Chemist and Chartered Scientist status from the Royal Society of Chemistry, UK. Dr. Tiwari is an active member of several professional bodies in the United Kingdom, the United States, and India. His area of research interest includes the development of smart materials, including silicones, graphene, and bio-inspired biomaterials for various industrial applications. Dr. Tiwari has the zeal to develop new materials and has received eight international patents on his inventions. He has published more than 80 research articles and 16 books. Most of his books are focused on newer developments in the area of materials science and engineering.

1 Smart Biomaterials in Biomedical Applications

1.1 INTRODUCTION

Time and time again humanity is faced with a unifying global crisis (widespread and insidious disease, harsh treatment of patients, etc.) that has inspired the researcher to create a biological molecular machine, so-called biomaterial, with tailored structures and properties that operate with the same efficiency and complexity as biological machines by uniting supramolecular chemistry, mechanostereochemistry, and nanotechnology, for the common good. Functional polymeric materials are essential components of a variety of biological and biomedical applications including drug delivery, tissue engineering, and medical imaging [1–4] as every day thousands of surgical procedures are performed to replace or repair tissue that has been damaged through disease or trauma. Despite the long history of biomedical engineering, polymers used in these applications have historically been polydisperse, with limited control over functionality and architecture [4,5]. In early stages of development, biomaterial selection focused on inertness and on mimicking the physical properties of the damaged tissue. Later development included design to illicit a specific biological response [6]. Meanwhile, polymer chemistry has experienced increased sophistication in terms of what can be controlled. "Smart" polymers with stimuli sensitivity, new architectures, and greater control over molecular weight (MW) and molecular weight distribution (MWD) have driven polymer research over the last 10–15 years [7–10]. In this context, it is logical that advanced synthetic techniques that can construct precision materials will lead to new applications and uses in biomedical engineering.

Biomaterials can be defined as any nonviable synthetic materials that become a part of the body either temporarily or permanently to replace, augment, or restore the function of a body tissue and are continuously or intermittently in contact with body fluids in a safe, reliably economically, and physiologically acceptable manner; they can be used for any period of time in contact with living tissue, to improve human health and they play a central role in extracorporeal devices, from contact lenses to kidney dialyzers, and are essential components of implants, from vascular grafts to cardiac pacemakers. A variety of devices and materials are used in the treatment of disease or injury. Common examples include suture needles, plates, teeth fillings, etc. However, this definition excludes surgical or dental instruments as they are exposed to body fluids, but do not replace or augment the function of a human tissue [11].

In the last decade, driven by the needs from engineering applications, various new materials such as metal and semiconductor nanocrystals, encoded nanoparticles (nanoparticles bearing biochemical information on their surfaces), functional nanoparticles (nanoparticles engineered to perform specific physical and/or chemical functions), functional magnetic nanostructures (nanoparticles where the release of drugs and/or biomolecules is triggered by the application of an external magnetic field), stimuli-responsive nanocarriers (designed to react on certain stimuli such as pH, temperature, redox potential, enzymes, light, and ultrasound), and so on have been developed for enhanced performance and/or new functions due to their optical, electrical, and magnetic properties, as they can be used to produce biologically relevant transformations [12,13].

Among them, stimuli-responsive polymer materials have gained much interest in recent years due to their ability to sense and react to environmental conditions or respond to a particular stimulus such as heat (thermo-responsive materials), stress/pressure (mechano-responsive materials), electrical current/voltage (electro-responsive materials), magnetic field (magneto-responsive materials), pH change/solvent/moisture (chemo-responsive materials), and light (photo-responsive materials) by means of altering their physical and/or chemical properties. Various smart materials have already existed, and are being researched extensively in biomaterials, bioinspired materials, functional nanomaterials, sensors, actuators, etc. [14].

1.2 SCAFFOLD REQUIREMENTS

Recently, numerous biomaterials have been used in biomedical devices in attempts to regenerate different tissues and organs in the body. The tissue response to an implant depends on a myriad of factors ranging from the chemical, physical, and biological properties of the materials to the shape and structure of the implant. Regardless of the tissue type, the ideal material or material combination should exhibit the following properties:

1. *Biocompatibility*: Biocompatibility can be defined as a dynamic two-way process that involves the time-dependent effects of the host on the material and the material on the host. The performance of a biomaterial should not be affected by the host and the host should not be

negatively affected by the implanted biomaterials. No clear, absolute definition of biocompatibility exists yet, mainly due to the fact that the biomaterial area is still evolving. It is the very first criterion of any polymeric device that is used in the regeneration of any type of tissue, that is, the chemical composition of device must be biocompatible to avoid adverse tissue reactions or must elicit a negligible immune reaction in order to prevent it, causing such a severe inflammatory response that it might reduce healing or cause rejection by the body after implantation.

2. *Biodegradability*: Biodegradation is an important property for biomaterials which refers to the process of break down into small molecular fragments by nature, that is, the rate of breakdown mediated by biological processes (e.g., the cleavage of hydrolytically or enzymatically sensitive bonds in the polymer leading to polymer erosion) inside the body that cause a gradual breakdown of the material [15]. The scaffolds that are used as implants must be biodegradable so as to allow cells to produce their own extracellular matrix [16]. Therefore, the implanted material should have appropriate permeability and processibility for the intended application acceptable. It should have acceptable shelf life to match the healing or regeneration process, should not evoke a sustained inflammatory or toxic response upon implantation in the body, as well as the degradation products should be nontoxic, and be able to get metabolized and cleared from the body. The chemical, physical, mechanical, and biological properties of a biodegradable material will vary with time, and degradation products can be produced that have different levels of tissue compatibility compared to the starting parent material.

3. *Mechanical properties*: The material should have appropriate mechanical properties consistent with the anatomical site into which it is to be implanted and, from a practical perspective, it must be strong enough to allow surgical handling during implantation for the indicated application and the variation in mechanical properties with degradation should be compatible with the healing or regeneration process. In attempting to engineer bone or cartilage tissues, the implanted scaffold must have sufficient acceptable strength to sustain cyclic loading endured by the joint, a low modulus to minimize bone resorption, high wear resistance to minimize wear-debris generation, as well as mechanical integrity to function from the time of implantation to the completion of the remodeling process [17]. In orthopedic applications, a patient's age must be considered for designing scaffold as the healing process rate differs in both young and elderly cases. In young individuals, fractures normally heal within six month and acquire weight-bearing capacity in 6 months but complete mechanical integrity develop after 1 year. In elderly patients, the rate is very slow than young individual.

4. *Scaffold architecture*: The interaction between implanted materials and blood depends on the composition of device and blood, device geometry (surface topography and high surface area provide additional available sites for protein adsorption, thereby enhancing the cell/material interaction), surface charge (anionic or cationic can influence plasma protein adsorption on the device surface), ratio of hydrophilicity and hydrophobicity (hydrophilic surfaces tend to adsorb fewer amounts of proteins than hydrophobic ones due to strong attraction between water molecules and the polymeric material), and local condition of flow of blood. The hemocompatibility of materials can be improved by surface modification, that is, by creating a surface that shows minimum nonspecific interactions with biological materials such as proteins and blood cells [18–20]. Therefore, the scaffold architecture is also one important factor that must be accounted for before manufacturing implantable materials. Materials must have an interconnected pore structure and high porosity. Its pores must be large enough to allow cells to migrate into the structure, where they eventually bound to the ligands within the scaffold, but are small enough to establish a sufficiently high specific surface, leading to a minimal ligand density to allow efficient binding of a the critical number of cells to the scaffold. They ensure cellular penetration and adequate diffusion of nutrients to cells within the construct and to the extracellular matrix formed by these cells as well as to allow the diffusion of waste products out of the scaffold, and the products of scaffold degradation should be able to exit the body without interference with other organs and surrounding tissues [21–26].

5. *Manufacturing technology*: The main objective of manufacturing technology must be to develop cost effective and clinically viable implant materials [27]. It must be scalable, efficiently developed and delivered, and made available to the clinician.

6. *Choice of materials*: The final criterion for scaffolds in tissue engineering, and the one on which all of the criteria listed above are dependent, is the choice of biomaterial from which the scaffold should be fabricated.

1.3 TYPES OF SMART POLYMERIC MATERIALS

Polymers such as proteins, polysaccharides, and nucleic acids are present as basic components in living organic systems that respond to its environment from the molecular to the macroscopic level due to their ability to adopt conformations according to the conditions in their surrounding environment, because response to stimulus is a basic process of living systems for maintaining normal function as well as fighting disease [28]. Similar adaptive behavior can be imparted to synthetic (co)polymers by incorporating multiple copies of functional groups such that their utility goes beyond providing structural support to allow active participation in a dynamic sense [29]. These examples have inspired scientists to fabricate "smart" materials that respond to light, pH, temperature, mechanical stress, or molecular stimuli. In the rapidly changing scientific world, scientists and engineers are designing biomolecule mimic materials as opportunities for treating and curing disease, and are leading to a variety of approaches for relieving suffering and prolonging life [30]. In recent years, the importance of smart polymers has increased significantly in the area of biotechnology, medicine, and engineering because of their response to internal and external stimuli as well as their shape, surface characteristics, solubility, viscoelasticity, transparency, conductivity, etc. can be controlled by modifying the structure and organization of the polymer chains [31]. Due to their own special physical or chemical properties and applications in various areas, these polymers are coined as "stimuli-responsive polymers" [32] or "smart polymers (SP)" [33,34] or "intelligent polymers" [35] or "environmentally sensitive" polymers [36] (Figure 1.1).

Smart materials can be classified into different ways on the basis of types of polymers, external stimuli, and their given response (Figure 1.2). Some important types of smart polymeric materials have been discussed in the following sections.

1.3.1 Classification on the Basis of Physical Form

Smart polymers can be classified into three categories such as linear free chains in solution, covalently cross-linked gels and reversible or physical gels, and chain-adsorbed or surface-grafted according to their physical forms (Figure 1.3).

1. *Linear free chains in solution*: In an aqueous solution, if the macromolecular chains are linear and solubilized, the solution will change from monophasic to biphasic due to polymer precipitation and the polymer undergoes a reversible collapse after an external stimulus is applied. This polymer phase transition is controlled by a delicate balance under hydrophobic and hydrophilic conditions and can be achieved either due to the reduction in the number of hydrogen bonds that the polymer forms with water or because of the neutralization of the electric charges that are present on the polymeric network. For example, aqueous solutions of thermo-responsive polymers show phase transition at temperature above their lower critical solution temperature (LCST) that is the temperature at which the phase transition occurs, also called demixtion denoted as T_d or the critical point (CP). Soluble pH (such as Eudragit S-100 [copolymer of methylmethacrylate and methacrylic acid] and the natural polymer, chitosan [deacetylated chitin]) and temperature-responsive polymers (poly-N-isopropylacrylamide) that overcome transition at physiological conditions (37°C and/or physiological pH) have been proposed as minimally invasive injectable systems for implant or scaffold useful for the drug delivery system (DDS) or tissue engineering applications [37,38].

2. *Covalently cross-linked gels and reversible or physical gels*: They can be either microscopic or macroscopic networks that are highly swollen material whose swelling behavior is controlled by environmental conditions. They do not dissolve in an aqueous environment due to the presence of extensive infinite crosslinking between polymeric networks. The gel-phase transition of such polymeric networks between a collapsed and an expanded state occurs due to chain reorganization under external stimuli. These phenomena are reversed when the stimulus is reversed, although the rate of reversion often is slower when the polymer has to redissolve or the gel has to reswell in an aqueous medium. Such systems are very useful in pulse DDSs [36].

3. *Chain-adsorbed or surface-grafted form*: These types of polymers either reversibly swell or collapse on the surface under external stimuli due to the conversion of the interface from hydrophilic to hydrophobic and vice versa. They may show other types of transitions in comparison to soluble

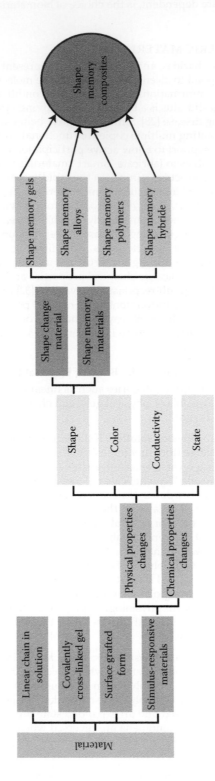

Figure 1.1 Location of various types of SMMs within the world of materials.

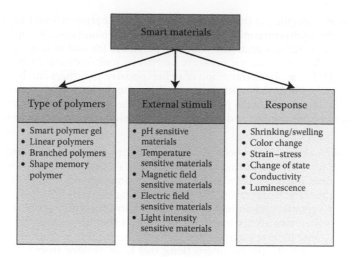

Figure 1.2 Schematic representation of classification of smart materials.

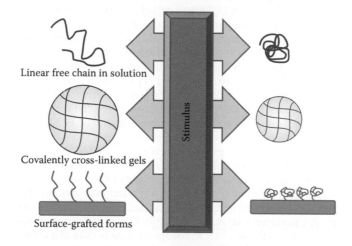

Figure 1.3 Different physical forms of stimuli-responsive polymers.

polymers due to change in surface hydrophobicity attributable to changing temperature, and can easily be exploited to allow the separation of substances that interact differently with the hydrophobic matrix.

The three forms of smart polymers as mentioned above can be easily conjugated with biomolecules such as proteins and oligopeptides, sugars and polysaccharides, single- and double-stranded oligonucleotides and DNA plasmids, simple lipids and phospholipids, and other recognition ligands and synthetic drug molecules, which are capable of responding to biological, physical, and chemical stimuli for widening their potential applications in many biomedical fields [39–42].

1.3.2 Classification on the Basis of External Stimulus

1. *pH-sensitive polymers*: pH-sensitive polymers show transition in phase in response to changes in environmental pH because they contain a large number of ionizable groups such as pendant acidic or basic groups that either accept or release protons in environmental pH. Those with weak acidic pendant groups in their polymer chain show high swelling in the basic medium due to the ionization of acidic groups that is not possible in the acidic medium due to the common ion effect. However, the polymers that contain a large number of weakly basic groups show a reverse response in the basic medium [43–45]. It is noticed that pH-sensitive polymers

show ionization at a specific pH that is called the pK_a value between 3 and 10 and that causes an alternation of the hydrodynamic volume of the polymer chains due to rapid change in the net charge of pendant groups, and, consequently, polymers transition from the collapsed state to the expanded state by the osmotic pressure exerted by mobile counter ions neutralizing the network charges [46]. The phase transition of pH-responsive polymers can be modulated either by selecting the ionizable moiety with a pK_a matching the desired pH range or by introducing more hydrophobic moieties into the polymer backbone because it becomes dominating when ionizable groups become neutral and electrostatic repulsion forces disappear within the polymer network.

2. *Temperature-sensitive polymers*: Physiologically, temperature plays an important role in a biological system, for example, during fever the cause of elevation of body temperature is the presence of pyrogens and an elevated concentration of prostaglandin E2 within certain areas of the brain that alters the firing rate of thermo-regulating neurons [47,48]. Thermo-responsive polymers are very versatile and an important class of stimuli-responsive 3D cross-linked polymer networks that have ability to exhibit substantial chemical, physical, or mechanical changes in response to temperature changes and their thermo-sensitivity dependence of hydrogen bonding and hydrophobic interactions, that is, originated from interactions between hydrophobic segments results in the polymer chain aggregation of physical crosslinking [49]. Polymers that become soluble upon heating have a so-called upper critical solution temperature (UCST) and called positive thermo-sensitive polymers. Those polymers that become insoluble in solutions upon heating possess an LCST and called negative thermo-sensitive polymers. Due to their response to small change in temperature, they are applied in various biomedical applications because change of temperature is not only relatively easy to control, but also easily applicable both in vitro and in vivo. It is observed that the phase transition of temperature-responsive polymers is controlled by the entropy-driven process because when polymers are dissolved in organic solvents, there is usually a negligible or small positive enthalpy of mixing or dilution that opposes the process, but the large positive gain in entropy drives it. This unusual behavior causes polymer phase separation when the temperature is raised to a critical value, called the "lower critical solution temperature" or LCST. However, the major thermodynamic force is the release of structured, bound water from the hydrophobic groups along the polymer backbone, as these groups interact with each other at phase separation [50]. At lower temperatures, hydrophobic polymer chains contain more water molecules in their vicinity due to hydrogen bonds that lower the free energy of mixing considerably. As a result, the polymer chains dissolve or swell in water, but when temperature is raised to a higher range, the hydrogen bonds weaken and the system tries to minimize the contact between water and hydrophobic surfaces, that is, the hydrophobic interaction increases and polymers show that the transition from the swollen to collapsed state occurs at a critical temperature [51]. Interpenetrating polymer networks (IPNs) are a unique type of polymer structure that is able to exhibit a relatively sharp transition with temperature without requiring the use of highly ordered block copolymers or polymers with very monodisperse molecular weights, because they form secondary hydrogen bonding complexes and show rapid swelling transition with temperature, termed the "zipper effect," which makes these polymers an ideal system for on/off-controlled release applications. Under certain conditions, this effect can also be reversed, as illustrated in Figure 1.4, which would allow these polymers to be used in pulsatile release applications as well [52,53].

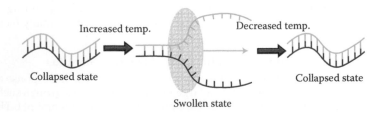

Figure 1.4 An illustration of the hydrogen bonding mechanism that controls swelling and deswelling with temperature in certain interpenetrating polymers networks referred to as the "Zipper Effect."

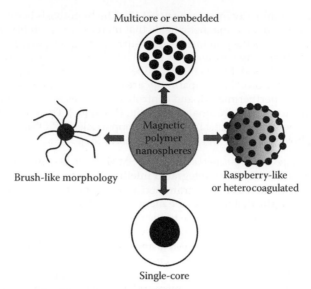

Multicore or embedded

Brush-like morphology

Raspberry-like
or heterocoagulated

Single-core

Figure 1.5 Schematic representation of different composite magnetic polymer nanospheres.

3. *Magnetically responsive polymers*: It is an established fact that magnetism and magnetic materials have a strong role to play in health care and biological applications [54–56]. In recent years, magnetic polymer composites or nanoparticles have gain much interest among scientists and researchers as diagnostic and therapeutic agents and have been widely used in drug delivery, cell labeling, magnetic resonance imaging (MRI), cell separation, magnetic hyperthermia, and as magnetic sensors for metabolites due to their relatively low toxicity (Figure 1.5) [57–59]. Magnetic polymer nanoparticles or composites contain magnetic material inside a polymer matrix and are typically made from iron oxides (magnetite (Fe_3O_4) or maghemite (γ-Fe_2O_3) core has high magnetic transition temperatures and has high saturation magnetization of about 80–95 emu/g) with diameters of 1–100 nm classified by size as oral or large superparamagnetic iron oxide (SPIO) agents (ferumoxsil, 300 nm, approved for clinical application), standard SPIO or SSIPO agents (ferumoxide, 80–150 nm, approved for clinical application), ultra-small SPIO or USPIO agents (ferumoxtran, 20–40 nm, approved for clinical application), and monocrystalline iron oxide nanoparticle or MION agents (5–10 nm, experimental) [60,61].

When an external magnetic field is applied on magnetic polymeric nanocomposites, a translational force will be exerted on the particle/drug complex, which guides the magnetic particle/ drug complex to a specific area of the body, and then the functionality of the particles will allow them to target-specific cells or tissues or targeted sites and release concentrated drugs at well-defined sites (Figure 1.6). Magnetic release has many advantages such as decreasing the amount of unnecessary damage to a healthy tissue, increasing the efficacy of the drug, and

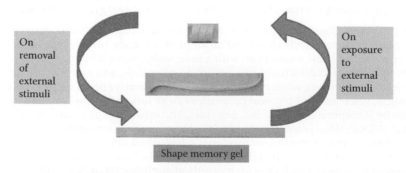

On removal of external stimuli

On exposure to external stimuli

Shape memory gel

Figure 1.6 Representation of bending of shape memory gel on application and removal of external stimuli.

treating ailments in a minimally invasive way [62,63]. The hypothesis behind it is that magnetic particles produce heat under AC magnetic fields that increase the mobility of the polymeric chain and as a result loosens the polymer strands surrounding the particles at temperatures above the glass transition temperature (T_g) of that particular polymer, allowing the encapsulated constituent to be released. In this regard, superparamagnetic nanoparticles exhibiting higher magnetization and good biocompatibility are of particular interest as magnetic drug targeting carriers for hyperthermia [64] and controlled drug release [65] and as contrast-enhancement agents in magnetic resonance imaging (MRI) [66]. The pharmacokinetics and biodistribution of superparamagnetic iron oxide nanoparticles (SPIONs) are highly dependent on their size, morphology, charge, and surface chemistry [67].

4. *Stimulus-responsive shape memory materials (SMMs)*: SMMs have become a very hot topic in recent years as materials for an ideal integrated intelligent system because they can sense and then generate reactive motion as preprogrammed and are able to recover their original shape, after being quasi-plastically distorted (shape memory effect, i.e., the subsequent recovery of the original, permanent shape in response to the application of a specific stimulus). At present, there are many types of SMMs that have been developed for various engineering applications. Among them, shape memory polymers (SMPs) and shape memory alloys (SMAs) have prime position. William J. Buehler of the US Naval Ordnance Laboratory synthesized shape-retaining alloy Nitinol (Nickel Titanium, Naval Ordnance Laboratory) and explained its behavior on the basis of the concept of a "metal with a memory" that plays an important role in various biomedical applications in orthopedics, orthodontics, and cardiovascular surgery. The shape memory effect of an SMA can be activated by applying a static or an alternating magnetic field (magneto-responsive or ferromagnetic SMAs) or by heating (thermo-responsive SMAs). In both cases, the driving force for the shape memory effect is reversible martensitic transformation. Presently, Cu-based (mainly CuAlNi and CuZnAl), NiTi-based, and Fe-based (e.g., FeMnSi, FeNiC, and FeNiCoTi) SMAs are widely applied in various engineering applications [68,69].

However, the application of SMAs is restricted in many fields due to their limited variation in mechanical properties, nonbiodegradable, demand temperatures of several hundred degrees Celsius for change, and the programming of these materials is time-consuming [70–72]. To overcome these problems, SMPs have been developed by scientist for various biomedical applications with shape memory properties. It should be noted that, SMPs can be deformed and fixed into a temporary shape only on exposure to an external stimulus and have the ability to recover the original, permanent shape when external stimulus is removed (Figure 1.6). SMAs follow reversible martensitic transformation, while SMPs follow the dual-segment/domain mechanism under right stimuli. It should be pointed out that, gels mostly show the shape memory effect due to swelling effect and/or electrical charge, and can be used to develop novel functional materials [73–75].

SMPs show the shape memory effect due to their stable polymer network (formed by molecule entanglement, crystalline phase, chemical crosslinking, or interpenetrated network) and a reversible switching transition (crystallization/melting transition, vitrification/glass transition, liquid crystal, anisotropic/isotropic transition, reversible molecule crosslinking, and supramolecular association/disassociation) result from the structure and morphology of the polymer coupled with the processing and programming technology. During the deformation of SMPs, strain energy captured in the SMM by a reversible morphology changes, which is used into exerting force, enabling the transduction of the stored latent energy to mechanical work [76].

5. *Conducting polymers*: Conducting polymers (CPs) are a class of polymeric materials that are polyconjugated polymers electrodeposited on an inert substrate and the resulting film adheres mainly due to hydrophobic interactions with a unique electronic structure which is responsible for their electrical conductivity, low ionization potentials, and high electron affinity that resemble to those of metals, while retaining properties of conventional organic polymers and their chemical, electrical, and physical properties can be tailored to the specific needs of their application by incorporating antibodies, enzymes, and other biological moieties [77–80].

Among various stimuli-responsive materials, there has been considerable interest in CPs because of their special properties such as large active strain and stress, moderate response time, high power/weight ratio, and excellent life cycle. The biocompatible nature of CPs also makes them as promising candidates for biomedical applications such as artificial muscles, neural interface, and sensors and drug delivery (Figure 1.7) [81–84]. One of the major drawbacks of CPs is their poor mechanical strength. However, this drawback can be overcome by

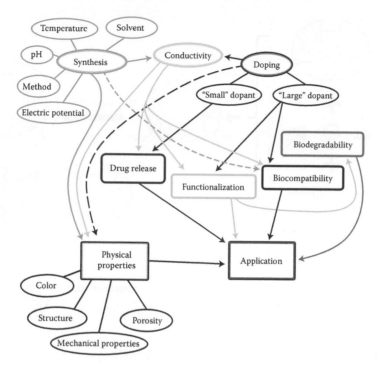

Figure 1.7 Schematic representation of various aspects of conducting polymers.

making composites, hybrid materials, and interpenetrating networks with other polymers, carbon nanotubes, etc. [85–87].

Recently, CPs included polyaniline, poly(phenylenevinylene), polypyrrole, and polythiophene which are used in many biomedical applications because they have unique electronic structure (π-bonds are partially localized due to a phenomenon called the Peierls distortion) which is responsible for their electrical conductivity, low ionization potentials, and high electron affinity. However, their conductivity can be improved by the doping process in which the excitation across the π–π* band gap creates self-localized excitations (polarons, bipolarons, and solitons) of conjugated polymers with localized electronic states in the gap region [88]. The choice of dopant defines the properties of the polymer and allows its functionalization for a specific application [80,89].

6. *Molecularly imprinted gels*: The design of a precise macromolecular chemical architecture that can recognize target molecules from an ensemble of closely related molecules, that is, molecular recognition is an elegant simple fundamental biological mechanism ubiquitous in nature which is driven largely by noncovalent forces, including ionic interactions, hydrogen bonding, van der Waals forces, π interactions, and entropic considerations such as the hydrophobic effect, and that was described by Emil Fischer as the "lock and key model" the result of intermolecular interactions between complementary functional groups on the lock or receptor (protein/enzyme) and the desired key or substrate (analyte), over a century ago, has a large number of potential applications [90]. Recently, intelligent-imprinted gels have been prepared that memorize their binding conformation and can be switched on and off by external stimuli that modify their swelling behavior [91]. It should be pointed that, systems based on natural recognition elements and enzyme amplification have many success in the biosensor field. However, they suffer from many inherent disadvantages including poor chemical, physical, and long-term stability; batch-to-batch variability; skilled-labor intensive; as well as relatively high cost [92,93]. Therefore, scientists and researchers have attempted to synthesize alternative synthetic receptor systems that can overcome these weaknesses by investigating the molecularly imprinting technique that has yielded proof of concept, harnessing nature's fundamentals to yield recognition receptor mimics from the miniaturized basics, borrowing on the ground rules, but conveniently avoiding the complexity, fragility, instability, costs and ethics of animal-based

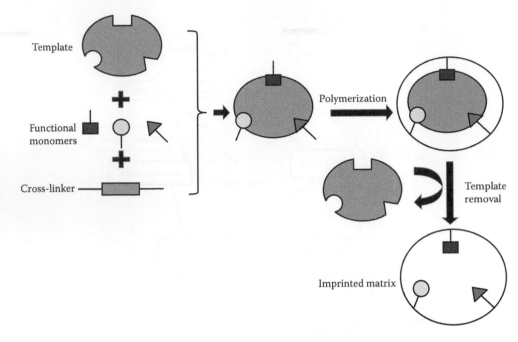

Figure 1.8 Schematic representation of a molecular imprinting process.

bio-affinity matrices, and has been successfully applied to small molecule templates in the areas of separations, artificial enzymes, chemical sensors, and pharmaceuticals [94].

Molecular imprinting is a promising viable synthetic approach to design robust molecular recognition materials able to mimic natural recognition entities, such as antibodies and biological receptors, in which a polymer network is formed between the template molecule and functional monomers or functional oligomers (or polymers) with specific recognition to interact with the desired template molecule either by covalent, noncovalent chemistry (self-assembly), or both. Briefly, functional monomers are chosen and then polymerized in the presence of the desired template (the polymerization reaction occurs in the presence of a crosslinking monomer and an appropriate solvent that controls the overall polymer morphology and macroporous structure); the template is subsequently removed; and the product is a heteropolymer matrix with binding sites specific to the template molecule of interest (Figure 1.8) [91].

Complexes formed in a solution by interactions between the template molecule (here black figure) and one or more functional monomer(s), become fixed during polymerization with a cross-linker. Polymeric recognition sites are formed, complementary to the template in size, shape, and position of the functional group.

1.3.3 Advance Functional Nanocarriers

Nanotechnology offers an unprecedented opportunity in rationalizing the delivery of drugs and genes to solid tumors following systemic administration [95]. Examples of nanotechnology applied in pharmaceutical product development include polymer-based nanoparticles (polymer-based nanostructure materials, whether nanoparticles or nanocomposites), lipid-based nanoparticles (liposomes, nanoemulsions, and solid-lipid nanoparticles), self-assembling nanostructures such as micelles and dendrimers-based nanostructures are gaining tremendous importance in a wide variety of applications in medical, pharmaceutical, and related fields, for example, wound dressings, contact lenses, artificial organs, and DDSs (Figure 1.9).

The delivery of a drug at a predetermined rate over a specified time to a selected target organ has been the ideal requisite in drug delivery technology and pharmacokinetics. Moreover, the need for carriers that exhibit the oscillatory behavior of the releasing bioactive agent has also emerged as a significant problem of drug design and formulation in recent years. The traditional methods of drug administration in conventional forms, such as pills and subcutaneous or intravenous injection, are still the predominant routes for drug administration. But pills and

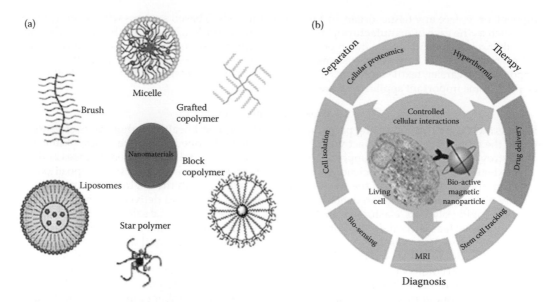

Figure 1.9 (a) Schematic representation of types of nanomaterial and (b) application of magnetic nanoparticles in various fields.

injections offer limited control over the rate of drug release into the body; usually, they are associated with an immediate release of the drug. Consequently, to achieve therapeutic levels that extend over time, the initial concentration of the drug in the body must be high, causing peaks that gradually diminish over time to an ineffective level. In this mode of delivery, the duration of the therapeutic effect depends on the frequency of dose administration and the half-life of the drug. This peak-and-valley delivery is known to cause toxicity in certain cases, most frequently with chemotherapy for cancer. Thus, the design of a DDS with optimum performance in specific circumstances poses challenges. Every biological level of organization presents a unique set of barriers to the delivery of therapeutic agents. These barriers include target-specific localization, enhanced clearance, selectivity and permeability of biological membranes, metabolizing enzymes, and endosomal/lysosomal degradation. Considering these barriers, the traditional focus of DDSs has been the optimization of pharmacokinetics and biodistribution [96]. As biological and drug delivery research has progressed, comprehensive strategies such as the use of multifunctional delivery systems have emerged. Through a synergistic effect, multifunctional carriers are capable of overcoming distinct physiological barriers and delivering therapeutic payload(s) and/or image contrast-enhancement agents to target sites in the body.

Majority of biomaterials that are currently in use are mostly derived from homo and copolymers of 2-hydroxyethyl methacrylate (HEMA), polyurethanes, etc. [97,98] which also suffer from the problems of low biocompatibility and mechanical strength. In recent years, bioceramics have also been introduced for specific applications [99] which exhibit remarkably good mechanical strength; however, their high cost and low biocompatibility restrict their wide acceptance. It is, therefore, desirous to synthesize pH-responsive polymeric materials that could not only display good biocompatibility but must also have high mechanical strength, and, foremost, must be of acceptable cost to the common community. Since smart materials have a specific mode of operability and are prone to typical experimental conditions, there is large scope for synthetic polymer chemistry to design multiresponsive delivery systems.

1.4 BIOMEDICAL APPLICATIONS OF SMART POLYMERIC MATERIALS

Living organisms involve many natural polymers such as protein, carbohydrate, and nucleic acids, etc. in biological systems for performing important structural and physiological roles. These natural polymers show response with change with environment and perform particular role in biochemical process. In the past 20 years, with the advances in polymer chemistry and materials science, combined with the knowledge of biology, polymer scientist has created the smart polymeric biomaterials ("materials intended to interface with biological systems to evaluate, treat, augment, or replace any tissue, organ, or function of the body") based systems with several advantages such as the ease of manufacturing, the ease of administration, biodegradability and the ability to alter release profiles of the incorporated agents, which imparts very promising applications in the biomedical field as delivery systems of therapeutic agents, tissue engineering, cell culture supports, gene carrier, textile engineering, radioactive wastage, protein purification, and oil recovery [100]. Some important applications are discussed here.

1.4.1 Dental Applications

Humans have used tooth-cleaning preparations to maintain oral health for thousands of years. Within the mouth, the metabolic activity of bacteria that are trapped by plaque (a film of mucus) can destroy both the tooth and supporting gum tissues by bacterially controlled diseases and can cause extensive tooth loss. The science of dental materials involves a study of the composition and properties of materials and the way in which they interact with the environment in which they are placed. Today, in human dentistry, a wide range of drugs and delivery methods, smart materials (rigid polymers, elastomers, metals, alloys, ceramics, inorganic salts, and composite materials), as well as clinical dental implant therapy (entirely and segments of teeth either can be replaced or restored) are available for the treatment and prevention of oral diseases. These materials have to work under a most hazardous environment, that is, temperature variations (0°C up to 70°C), wide variations in acidity or alkalinity (pH 2–pH 11) and high stresses. Current trends in clinical dental implant therapy include use of endosseous dental implant surfaces embellished with nanoscale topographies. Over the last few decades, a large number of metals and applied materials have been developed with significant improvement in various properties in a wide range of medical applications (Figure 1.10). A thorough review of these materials can be found in Chapter 2.

1.4.2 Orthopedic Applications

Currently, millions of patients are suffering from osteoarthritis, rheumatoid arthritis, and cartilage defects; occur due to various reasons including degenerative, surgical, and traumatic processes,

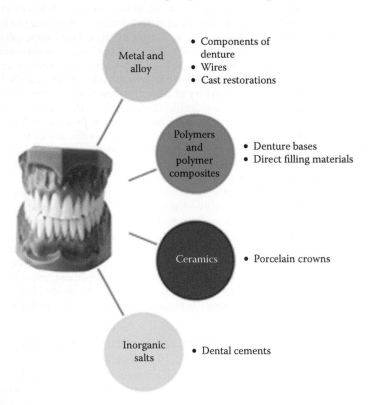

Figure 1.10 Diagram indicating the wide variety of materials used in dentistry and some of their applications.

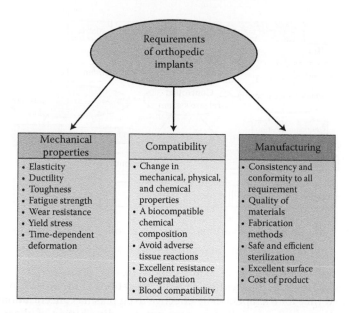

Figure 1.11 Schematic representations of requirements in orthopedic implants.

which significantly affect the structure of freely movable (synovial) joints, such as the hip, knee, shoulder, ankle, and elbow. According to a report, every year over 450,000 bone grafts and approximately 250,000 knee arthroplasty procedures performed in the United States alone. Bone and cartilage repair or regeneration is a common yet complex cascade of biological molecular events regulated by numerous hormones, cytokines and growth factors that provide signals at local injury sites allowing progenitors and inflammatory cells to migrate and trigger healing processes. For treatment of bone or cartilage defect, autologous transplants and allografts have been widely used in orthopedic surgery [101,102]. However, these methods suffer from various problems such as autologous transplants needs secondary surgery to procure donor bone from the patient's own body, possible morbidity, and limited quantity of donor tissue and allografts has the inherent problems of possible transmission of donor pathogens, immunogenic responses, and high risks of infection [103].

Over the last few decades, a large number of metals and applied materials have been developed but traditional metallic bone implants are dense and often suffer from the problems of adverse reaction, biomechanical mismatch and lack of adequate space for new bone tissue to grow into the implant. These problems of traditional metallic bone implants can be reduced by using biodegradable materials-based implants because they have many advantages such as transfer stress over time to the damaged area as it heals, allowing of the tissues, and there is no need of a second surgery to remove the implanted devices. Recently, scientific advancements have been made to fabricate bone tissue engineering substitutes which are biomimetic materials (natural and synthetic polymers, inorganic materials, and their composites formulated into porous scaffolds, nanofibrous membranes, microparticles, and hydrogels) that utilize combination of cells, biodegradable scaffolds, and bioactive molecules to recapitulate natural processes of tissue regeneration and development, and can be considered as another choice for treating bone defects, and have been heralded as an alternative strategy to regenerate bone [104,105]. However, the research on devices for load-bearing bone repair and implantable medical devices still has a long way to go. Chapter 3 deals with the materials and performance associated with orthopedic implants. Figure 1.11 lists the various material requirements that must be met for successful total joint replacement.

1.4.3 Drug Delivery Applications

Drug delivery technologies (the method or process of administering a pharmaceutical compound to achieve a therapeutic effect in humans or animals) are an important area within biomedicine [106]. Humans have always attempted to improve their health from acute disease or chronic illnesses by ingesting or administering drugs. Traditional methods of drug delivery include tablets,

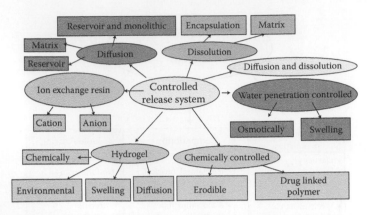

Figure 1.12 Schematic depiction of various types of controlled release system.

injections, suspensions, cream, ointments, liquids, and aerosols. Nowadays, these conventional DDSs are widely used. However, they suffer from the limitations of minimal synchronization between the required time for therapeutically effective drug plasma concentrations, not provide ideal pharmacokinetic profiles especially for drugs, not even distribution of pharmaceuticals throughout the body; lack of drug specific affinity toward a pathological site; the necessity of a large total dose of drug to achieve high local concentration; nonspecific toxicity, narrow therapeutic windows, and other adverse side-effects due to high drug doses [107]. The concept of controlled drug delivery (permeation regulated transfer of an active material from a reservoir to a targeted surface to maintain a predetermined concentration level for specified period of time) has arisen from the need to direct therapeutic agent to specific biological targets, and deliver the optimum dose of drug at a rate required by the body during the treatment period [108]. Drug–polymer systems may also be useful in protecting the drug from biological degradation prior to its release. The development of these devices starts with the use of nonbiodegradable polymers, which rely on the diffusion process, and subsequently progresses to the use of biodegradable polymers, in which swelling and erosion take place.

Recently, responsive DDSs have been developed by several research groups in which the amount of drug released can be affected according to physiological needs. These responsive DDSs can be classified as pulsed or externally regulated (work under external stimuli such as magnetic, ultrasonic, thermal, and electric) or self-regulated DDSs (utilize several approaches as rate-control mechanisms: pH-sensitive polymers, enzyme-substrate reactions, pH-sensitive drug solubility, competitive binding and metal concentration-dependent hydrolysis, and the release rate is controlled by feedback information, without any external intervention).

Delivery systems in which the drug release rates can be activated by an external stimulus are still largely experimental. On the basis of the physical or chemical characteristics of polymer, drug release mechanisms from a polymer matrix may be categorized in accordance to three main processes swelling, diffusion, and erosion [109]. Figure 1.12 shows various types of controlled DDSs. They are described in Chapter 4 in detail.

1.4.4 Wound Dressing Applications

A wound is a defect or a break in the skin, resulting from disruption of normal anatomic structure and function of skin due to physical, radiation, electricity, corrosive chemicals, and thermal sources or thermal damage or medical or physiological condition [110]. Wound healing is a natural dynamic complex biological process for regenerating damaged and/or lost tissues, involving ordered cascade of events including phases of hemostasis, inflammation, proliferation, and maturation, which begins at the moment of injury and can continue for months to years [111,112]. In the past 30 years, scientists have developed numerous wound-dressing materials to promote wound healing [113]. The ideal dressing materials must have perform following functions including maintain moist condition (warm, moist environment encourages rapid healing), provide thermal insulation to prevent introduction of external stress, controls local temperature and pH, occludes dead space, permits atraumatic removal of excessive exudate from the wound surface, minimize the loss of energy, macerated, and free of infection, while fulfilling prerequisites, noncytotoxic, biocompatible, to produce rapid and cosmetically acceptable healing, to prevent or combat infection, to reduce pain, ease of application and removal, and proper adherence, in order to ensure that there will be no areas of nonadherence left to create fluid-filled pockets for bacterial proliferation, and cost-effective [114]. Chapter 5 discusses the characteristics and properties of synthetic materials used in wound healing.

1.4.5 Tissue Engineering Applications

Connective tissue is one of the most important tissues consist of different types of cells and extracellular matrix (ECM) that not only support most organs but also responsible for connection and protection of different tissues. The main components of ECM are fibrous proteins, collagen and elastin. Their mechanical properties undergo changes with ageing and that affects the functionality and properties of tissues and organs. Therefore, it is important to replace the destroyed tissues. Removal of the damaged part was the most common practice. However, it suffers from one important problem, that is, significant decrease in quality of life. Tissue engineering can overcome the limitations of the current surgical procedures, can be used to replace and/or regenerate the damaged body regions by combining engineering methodologies with knowledge stemming from the biological sciences. Polymeric biomaterials are used as substitutes for damaged tissue and for the stimulation of tissue regeneration. One class of polymeric biomaterials is bioresorbable polymers that degrade both in vitro and in vivo and are eliminated by metabolic pathways of the organism, and are used as a temporary support for tissue regeneration. It is known that biomaterials have to fulfill many conditions for qualifying for substituents for damaged tissues (Figure 1.13) [115,116]. At present, new materials (permanent or temporary materials) are designed to elicit an effective interaction with tissues, provoking physiological responses such as cell growth and/or differentiation at the site of implantation [117], are used to replace damaged tissue (joints, heart valves, and intraocular lenses) for an undetermined period of time as well as to retain their mechanical and physicochemical properties for prolonged periods of time [118].

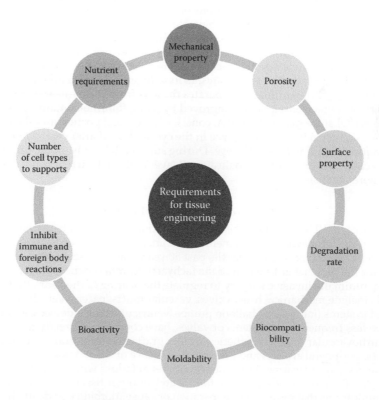

Figure 1.13 Illustration on materials, biological and medicinal properties required to obtain successful biomaterial for tissue engineering.

There are three ways in which materials have been shown to be useful in tissue engineering:

a. The materials are able to induce cellular migration or tissue regeneration.

b. The materials are used to encapsulate cells and act as an immunoisolation barrier.

c. The materials are used as a matrix to support cell growth and cell organization.

As a way to imitate natural tissues, one philosophy of tissue engineering involves the presence of a biodegradable scaffold onto which cells from appropriate sources are seeded. After a suitable incubation time, tissue-like structures are formed. The scaling-up of this procedure would involve mass production of scaffolds followed by storage, with cell seeding and culture conducted immediately prior to implantation. Another option would be to develop storage methods for premanufactured engineered tissue, although this has not proven to be very feasible in practice. In this context, a system, where scaffold production, seeding and storage can be synchronized, with the possibility of a single batch of product being able to produce scaffolds with tunable functional properties, would be desirable. As a way to imitate natural tissues, it is important to incorporate the effects of physical strains and stresses on cell behavior into their protocols because the in vitro conditions under which an engineered tissue is produced and the physiological environment with which it will interact after implantation are different. Thus, these stimuli might be used either to imitate the physiological environment or to replicate injury situations. Therefore, developing stimulus-responsive biomaterials with easy-to-tailor properties is a highly desired goal of the tissue engineering community. Recently, 3D matrices based on different structural characteristics or minimally invasive surgical methods have drawn attention for potential tissue engineering applications in the next generation [119–122] (see Chapter 6 for more details).

1.4.6 Ocular Applications

Several diseases of eye can lead to reduce eye vision, blindness, cloudiness of the eyes, etc. Diverse synthetic polymeric materials such as eyeglasses, contact lenses, and intraocular implants can be used to correct optical functions of eyes. These materials are in intimate contact with the tissues of eyes, so they must be biomaterials with good biocompatible nature. Soft contact lenses are made from slightly cross-linked hydrophilic polymeric hydrogels which are supple and fit snugly on the corneal surface, and are able to permeate oxygen to cornea due to hydrophilic nature. However, rigid contact lenses are made from are copolymers of methyl methacrylate with siloxane alkyl methacrylates, fit loosely on the cornea and move with the blink more or less freely over the tear film that separates the lens from the corneal surface. The oxygen permeability of contact lenses can be improved by using fluorine-containing contact lenses. Intraocularlenses (IOLs) are made of PMMA, consist of an optical portion and the haptics that support the optical portion in its proper place in the eye, and used after cataract extraction to replace the opaque crystalline lens of the eye. During surgery, IOL must not touch the corneal endothelium because it is an extremely delicate cell layer and can be irreversibly damaged (see Chapter 7 for more details).

1.4.7 Cardiovascular Applications

Valvular heart disease (VHD) is a major health problem that results in substantial morbidity and death worldwide. Unfortunately, the treatment of dysfunctional heart valves requires surgical or interventional repair or replacement. Over the past 50 years, cardiovascular devices complex electronic devices for the pacemaker function or the tachyarrhythmia function that are inserted into the chest using minimally invasive surgery to regulate the beating of the heart, that employ polymeric materials include mechanical heart valves, vascular grafts, pacemakers, blood oxygenators, and heart-assist systems (intra-aortic balloon pumps, ventricular-assist devices, and total artificial hearts) are used less frequently than stents or valves, have contributed greatly to the decrease in deaths from cardiovascular causes. Synthetic vascular grafts and stent grafts provide effective repair of stenotic peripheral arteries and aneurysmal disease of the thoracic and abdominal aorta as well as for hemodialysis treatment in patients with renal failure who lack suitable veins for arteriovenous (AV) fistulas. However, device failure and/or other tissue-biomaterial interactions may cause complications that necessitate reoperation or cause morbidity or death. In some cases, deleterious outcomes occur after many years of uneventful patient benefit [123] (see Chapter 8 for more details).

1.5 FUTURE CHALLENGES AND PROSPECTS

This chapter reviews some basic concepts of stimuli-responsive polymer-based smart materials (new generation materials surpassing the conventional structural and functional materials, which possess the ability to change their physical properties such as shape, stiffness, viscosity or damping in a specific manner in response to specific stimulus input, that is, pressure, temperature, electric and magnetic fields, chemicals, hydrostatic pressure or nuclear radiation). With the development of material science, many new, high-quality and cost-efficient materials have come into use in various field of engineering. In the last 10 decades, the materials became multifunctional and required the optimization of different characterization and properties. In spite of proven versatility of polymer materials in biomedical and pharmaceutical areas, there still remains a wide scope to further advance the field by adopting the following strategies:

1. Chemical modification of biopolymers may drastically alter their properties and impart desired characteristics that are indeed required for biomedical and pharmaceutical applications. For instance, the biopolymers may be made responsive to external stimuli so as to design targeted DDSs especially in treating complex diseases like cancers, tumors, etc.

2. The hybrid materials of naturally occurring polymers and synthetic counterparts may be designed to achieve desired porosity and morphology for tissue engineering applications, stem cell technology, etc.

3. Depending on the end use, such materials may be produced by choosing polymers of appropriate thermal and physicochemical properties that mimic soft or hard tissues. This may be accomplished by taking into consideration the hydrophilicity, hydrophobicity, glass transition temperature, rigidity of macromolecular chains, bulkiness of pendent groups, etc.

4. Greater proportion of naturally occurring polymers in the hybrid materials in comparison to the synthetic polymers may be economically more viable and this will reduce the cost of the biomedical and pharmaceutical devises.

REFERENCES

1. Langer R, Vacanti JP. Tissue engineering. *Science* 1993;260:920–926.

2. Duncan R. The dawning era of polymer therapeutics. *Nat Rev Drug Discov* 2003;2:347–360.

3. Langer R, Tirrell DA. Designing materials for biology and medicine. *Nature* 2004;428:487–492.

4. Anderson DG, Burdick JA, Langer R. Materials science—Smart biomaterials. *Science* 2004;305:1923–1924.

5. Hench LL, Polak JM. Third-generation biomedical materials. *Science* 2002;295:1014–1017.

6. Hench LL, Wilson J. Surface-active biomaterials. *Science* 1984;226:630–636.

7. Matyjaszewski K, Gnanou Y, Leibler L. *Macromolecular Engineering: From Precise Macromolecular Synthesis to Macroscopic Materials Properties and Applications.* Weinheim: Wiley-VCH; 2007. p. 2982.

8. Lutz JF, Badi N. Sequence control in polymer synthesis. *Chem Soc Rev* 2009;38:3383–3390.

9. Hartmann L, Borner HG. Precision polymers: Monodisperse, monomer-sequence-defined segments to target future demands of polymers in medicine. *Adv Mater* 2009;21:3425–3431.

10. Borner HG. Precision Polymers—Modern tools to understand and program macromolecular interactions. *Macromol Rapid Commun* 2011;32:115–126.

11. Agrawal CM. Reconstructing the human body using biomaterials. *JOM* 1998;Jan:31–35.

12. Alivisatos P. The use of nanocrystals in biological detection. *Nat Biotechnol* 2004;22:47–52.

13. Penn SG, He L, Natan MJ. Nanoparticles for bioanalysis. *Curr Opin Chem Biol* 2003;7:609–615.

14. Liu YJ, Lan X, Lu HB, Leng JS. Recent progresses in polymeric smart materials. *Int J Mod Phys B* 2010;24:2351–2356.

15. Andriano KP, Tabata Y, Ikada Y, Heller J. In vitro and in vivo comparison of bulk and surface hydrolysis in absorbable polymer scaffolds for tissue engineering. *J Biomed Mater Res* 1999;48:602–612.

16. Mikos AG, McIntire LV, Anderson JM, Babensee JE. Host response to tissue engineered devices. *Adv Drug Deliv Rev* 1998;33:111–139.

17. Hutmacher DW. Scaffolds in tissue engineering bone and cartilage. *Biomaterials* 2000 Dec;21(24):2529–2543.

18. Park YD, Tirelli N, Hubbell JA. Photopolymerized hyaluronic acid-based hydrogels and interpenetrating networks. *Biomaterials* 2003;24:893–900.

19. Patenaude M, Hoare T. Injectable, Mixed Natural-Synthetic Polymer Hydrogels with Modular Properties. *Biomacromolecules* 2012;13:369–378.

20. Peppas NA, Bures P, Leobandung W, Ichikawa H. Hydrogels in pharmaceutical formulations. *Eur J Pharm Biopharm* 2000;50:27–46.

21. Phelps EA, Garcia AJ. Update on therapeutic vascularization strategies. *Regen Med* 2009;4:65–80.

22. Ko HC, Milthorpe BK, McFarland CD. Engineering thick tissues—the vascularisation problem. *Eur Cell Mater* 2007;14:1–18.

23. Yannas IV, Lee E, Orgill DP, Skrabut EM, Murphy GF. Synthesis and characterization of a model extracellular matrix that induces partial regeneration of adult mammalian skin. *Proc Natl Acad Sci* 1989;86:933–937.

24. O'Brien FJ, Harley BA, Yannas IV, Gibson LJ. The effect of pore size on cell adhesion in collagen-GAG scaffolds. *Biomaterials* 2005;26:433–441.

25. Murphy CM, Haugh MG, O'Brien FI. The effect of mean pore size on cell. *Biomaterials* 2010;31:461–466.

26. Murphy CM, O'Brien FJ. Understanding the effect of mean pore size on cell activity in collagen-glycosaminoglycan scaffolds. *Cell Adh Migr* 2010;4:377–381.

27. Hollister SJ. Scaffold engineering: A bridge to where? *Biofabrication* 2009;1:012001.

28. Alarcón CH, Pennadam S, Alexander C. Stimuli responsive polymers for biomedical applications. *Chem Soc Rev* 2005;34(3):276–285.

29. Roy D, Cambre JN, Sumerlin BS. Future perspectives and recent advances in stimuli-responsive materials. *Prog Polym Sci* 2010;35(1–2):278–301.

30. Peppas NA, Langer R. New challenges in biomaterials. *Science* 1994;263:1715–1994.

31. Kumar A, Srivastava A, Galae IY, Mattiasson B. Smart polymers: physical forms and bioengineering applications. *Prog Polym Sci* 2007;32:1205–1237.

32. Jeong B, Gutowska A. Lessons from nature: Stimuli-responsive polymers and their biomedical applications. *Trends Biotechnol* 2002;20:305–311.

33. Hoffman AS, Stayton PS, Bulmus V, Chen G, Jinping C, Chueng Cl. Really smart bioconjugates of smart polymers and receptor proteins. *J Biomed Mater Res* 2000;52:577–586.

34. Galaev IYu, Mattiasson B. 'Smart' polymers and what they could do in biotechnology and medicine. *Trends Biotechnol* 2000;17:335–340.

35. Kikuchi A, Okano T. Intelligent thermoresponsive polymeric stationary phases for aqueous chromatography of biological compounds. *Prog Polym Sci* 2002;27:1165–1193.

36. Qiu Y, Park K. Environment-sensitive hydrogels for drug delivery. *Adv Drug Deliv Rev* 2001;53:321–339.

37. Packhaeuser CB, Schnieders J, Oster CG, Kissel T. *Eur J Pharm Biopharm* 2004;58(2): In situ forming parenteral drug delivery systems: An overview. 445–455.

38. Hatefi A, Amsden BJ. Biodegradable injectable in situ forming drug delivery systems. *Control Release* 2002;80(1):9–28.

39. Stayton PS, Hoffman AS. Immobilization of smart polymer–protein conjugates. In: Cass T, Ligler FS, editors. *Immobilized Biomolecules in Analysis*. Oxford: Oxford University Press; 1998. p. 135–147.

40. Monji, N, Hoffman, AS. A novel immunoassay system and bioseparation process based on thermal phase separating polymers. *Appl Biochem Biotechnol* 1987;14:107–120.

41. Lackey CA, Murthy N, Press OW, Tirrell DA, Hoffman AS, Stayton PS. Hemolytic activity of pH-responsive polymer-streptavidin bioconjugates. *Bioconjugate Chem* 1999;10:401–405.

42. Fong RB, Ding Z, Long CJ, Hoffman AS, Stayton PS. Thermoprecipitation of streptavidin via oligonucleotide-mediated self-assembly with poly(N-isopropylacrylamide). Bioconjugate Chem 1999;10:720–725.

43. Matzelle T, Reichelt R. Review: Hydro-, micro- and nanogels studied by complementary measurements based on SEM and SFM. *Acta Microsc* 2008;17:45–61.

44. Masteikova R, Chalupova Z, Sklubalova Z. Stimuli-sensitive hydrogels in controlled and sustained drug delivery. *Medicina (Kaunas)* 2003;39:19–24.

45. Zhang R, Tang M, Bowyer A, Eisenthal R, Hubble J. A novel pH- and ionic-strength-sensitive carboxy methyl dextran hydrogel. *Biomaterials* 2005;26:4677–4683.

46. Tonge SR, Tighe BJ. Responsive hydrophobically associating polymers: A review of structure and properties. *Adv Drug Deliv Rev* 2001;53(1):109–122.

47. Chaterji S, Kwon KI, Park K. Smart polymeric gels: Redefining the limits of biomedical devices. *Prog Polym Sci* 2007;32(8):1083–1122.

48. Aronoff DM, Neilson EG. Antipyretics: Mechanisms of action and clinical use in fever suppression. *Am J Med* 2001;111(4):304–315.

49. Demirel G. Adsorption of bovine serum albumine onto poly (N-t-butylacrylamide-co-acrylamide/maleic acid) Hydrogels. *J Polym Res* 2007;14(1):23–30.

50. Hoffman AS. Applications of thermally reversible polymers and hydrogels in therapeutics and diagnostics. *J Control Release* 1987;6(1):297–305.

51. Baltes T, Garret-Flaudy F, Freitag R. Investigation of the LCST of polyacrylamides as a function of molecular parameters and the solvent composition. *J Polym Sci A Polym Chem* 1999;37(15):2977–2989.

52. Kikuchi A, Okano T. Pulsatile drug release control using hydrogels. *Adv Drug Deliv Rev* 2002;54:53–77.

53. Shibayama M, Tanaka T. Volume phase transition and related phenomena of polymer gels. *Adv Polym Sci* 1993;109:1–62.

54. Blakemore RP, Frankel RB. Magnetic Navigation in Bacteria. *Sci Am* 1981;245(6):58–65.

55. Bahadur D, Giri J. Biomaterials and magnetism. *Sadhana* 2003;28(3–4):639–656.

56. Mykhaylyk O, Cherchenko A, Ilkin A, Dudchenko N, Ruditsa V, Novoseletz M, Zozulya Y. Glial brain tumor targeting of magnetite nanoparticles in rats. *J Magn Magn Mater* 2001;225(1):241–247.

57. Pankhurst QA, Connolly J, Jones S, Dobson J. Applications of magnetic nanoparticles in biomedicine. *J Phys D Appl Phys* 2003;36(13):R167–R172.

58. Suzuki M, Shinkai M, Honda H, Kobayashi T. Anticancer effect and immune induction by hyperthermia of malignant melanoma using magnetite cationic liposomes. *Melanoma Res* 2003;13(2):129–135.

59. Grimm J, Perez JM, Josephson L, Weissleder R. Novel nanosensors for rapid analysis of telomerase activity. *Cancer Res* 2004;64(2):639–643.

60. Hans M, Lowman A. Biodegradable nanoparticles for drug delivery and targeting. *Curr Opin Solid State Mater Sci* 2002;6(4):319–327.

61. Corot C, Robert P, Idee JM, Port M. Recent advances in iron oxide nanocrystal technology for medical imaging. *Adv Drug Deliv Rev* 2006;58(14):1471–1504.

62. Kumar CS, Leuschner C, Doomes EE, Henry L, Juban M, Hormes J. Efficacy of lytic peptide-bound magnetite nanoparticles in destroying breast cancer cells. *J Nanosci Nanotechnol* 2004;4(3):245–249.

63. Kim KS, Park JK. Magnetic force-based multiplexed immunoassay using superparamagnetic nanoparticles in microfluidic channel. *Lab Chip* 2005;5(6):657–664.

64. Jordan A, Scholz R, Wust P, Hling HF, Felix R. Magnetic Fluid Hyperthermia (MFH): Cancer treatment with AC magnetic field induced excitation of biocompatible superparamagnetic nanoparticles. *J Magn Magn Mater* 1999;201(1):413–419.

65. Detlef MS, Thomas SR. Thermosensitive magnetic polymer particles as contactless controllable drug carriers. *J Magn Magn Mater* 2006;302(1):267–271.

66. Wang SH, Shi X, Van Antwerp M, Cao Z, Swanson SD, Bi X, Baker JR. Dendrimer-functionalized iron oxide nanoparticles for specific targeting and imaging of cancer cells. *Adv Funct Mater* 2007;17(16):3043–3050.

67. Sledge G, Miller K. Exploiting the hallmarks of cancer: The future conquest of breast cancer. *Eur J Cancer* 2003;39(12):1668–1675.

68. Dong JW, Xie JQ, Lu J, Adelmann C, Palmstrom CJ, Cui J, Pan Q, Shield TW, James RD, McKernan S. Shape memory and ferromagnetic shape memory effects in single-crystal Ni2MnGa thin films. *J Appl Phys* 2004;95(5):2593–600.

69. Soderberg O, Aaltio I, Ge Y, Heczko O, Hannula SP. Ni-Mn-Ga multifunctional compounds. *Mater Sci Eng A – Struct Mater Prop Microstruct Process* 2008;481:80–85.

70. Wiese KG. Osmotically induced tissue expansion with hydrogels: A new dimension in tissue expansion. A preliminary report. *J Craniomaxillofac Surg* 1993;21:309–313.

71. Kauffman GB, Mayo I. The Story of Nitinol: The Serendipitous Discovery of the Memory Metal and Its Applications. *Chem Educator* 1996;2:1–21.

72. Yahia L, Manceur A, Chaffraix P. Bioperformance of shape memory alloy single crystals. *Biomed Mater Eng* 2006;16:101–118.

73. Lendlein A, Kelch S. Shape-memory polymers as stimuli-sensitive implant materials. *Clin Hemorheol Microcirc* 2005;32:105–116.

74. Lendlein A, Langer R. Biodegradable, elastic shape-memory polymers for potential biomedical applications. *Science* 2002;296:1673–1676.

75. Lendlein A, Schmidt AM, Langer R. AB-polymer networks based on oligo(ε-caprolactone) segments showing shape-memory properties. *Proc Natl Acad Sci USA* 2001;98:842–847.

76. Koerner H, Price G, Pearce NA, Alexander M, Vaia RA. Remotely actuated polymer nanocomposites–stress-recovery of carbon-nanotube-filled thermoplastic elastomers. *Nat Mater* 2004;3:115–120.

77. Lakard B, Ploux L, Anselme K, Lallemand F, Lakard S, Nardin M et al. *Bioelectrochemistry* 2009;75:148–157.

78. Rivers TJ, Hudson TW, Schmidt CE. Synthesis of a Novel, Biodegradable Electrically Conducting Polymer for Biomedical Applications Authors. *Adv Funct Mater* 2002;12:33–37.

79. Wallace GG, Smyth M, Zhao H. Conducting electroactive polymer-based biosensors. *Trends Analyt Chem* 1999;18:245–251.

80. Kim DH, Richardson-Burns SM, Hendricks JL, Sequera C, Martin DC. Effect of immobilized nerve growth factor on conductive polymers: Electrical properties and cellular response. *Adv Funct Mater* 2007;17:79–86.

81. Abidian MR, Kim DH, Martin DC. Conducting-polymer nanotubes for controlled drug release. *Adv Mater* 2006;18:405–409.

82. Abidian MR, Martin DC. Multifunctional nanobiomaterials for neural interfaces. *Adv Funct Mater* 2009;19:573–585.

83. Abidian MR, Ludwig KA, Marzullo TC, Martin DC, Kipke DR. Interfacing conducting polymer nanotubes with the central nervous system: Chronic neural recording using poly(3,4-ethylenedioxythiophene) nanotubes A. *Adv Mater* 2009;21:3764–3770.

84. Forzani ES, Zhang HQ, Nagahara LA, Amlani I, Tsui R, Tao NJ. Conducting Polymer Nanojunction Sensor for Glucose Detection. *Nano Lett* 2004;4:1785–1788.

85. Lin YH, Cui XL, Bontha J. Electrically Controlled Anion Exchange Based on Polypyrrole and Carbon Nanotubes Nanocomposite for Perchlorate Removal. *Environ Sci Technol* 2006;40:4004–4009.

86. Ammam M, Fransaer J. Highly sensitive and selective glutamate microbiosensor based on cast polyurethane/AC-electrophoresis deposited multiwalled carbon nanotubes and then glutamate oxidase/electrosynthesized polypyrrole/Pt electrode. *Biosens Bioelectron* 2010;25:1597–1602.

87. Hosseini SH, Entezami AA. Conducting polymer blends of polypyrrole with polyvinyl acetate, polystyrene, and polyvinyl chloride based toxic gas sensors authors. *J Appl Polym Sci* 2003;90:49–62.

88. Heeger AJ. Nobel Lecture: Semiconducting and metallic polymers: The fourth generation of polymeric materials. *Rev Mod Phys* 2001;73(3):681–700.

89. Guimard NK, Gomez N, Schmidt CE. Conducting polymers in biomedical engineering. *Prog Polym Sci* 2007;32:876–921.

90. Chen BN, Piletsky S, Turner APF. Design of "keys". *Comb Chem High Throughput Screen* 2002;5(6):409–427.

91. Byrne ME, Park K, Peppas NA. Molecular imprinting within hydrogels. *Adv Drug Deliv Rev* 2002;54:149–161.

92. Sapsford KE, Bradburne C, Detehanty JB, Medintz IL. Sensors for detecting biological agents. *Mater Today* 2008;11(3):38–49.

93. Haupt K, Mosbach K. Molecularly imprinted polymers and their use in biomimetic sensors. *Chem Rev* 2000;100(7):2495–504.

94. Cormack PAG, Mosbach K. Molecular imprinting: Recent developments and the road ahead. *React Funct Polym* 1999;41(1–3):115–124.

95. Nie S, Xing Y, Kim GJ, Simons JW. Nanotechnology applications in cancer. *Annu Rev Biomed Eng* 2007;9:257–288.

96. Bajpai AK, Shukla S, Saini R, Tiwari A. *Stimuli Responsive Drug Delivery Systems: From Introduction to Application.* UK: Smitheres Rapra Publications, ISBN 978-1-84735-416-7, 2010, p. 370.

97. Clayton AB, Chirila TV, Lou X. Hydrophilic sponges based on 2-hydroxyethyl methacrylate. V. effect of crosslinking agent reactivity on mechanical properties. *Polymer Int* 1997;201–207.

98. Cohn D, Aronhime M, Alido B. Poly(urethane)-cross-linked poly(HEMA) hydrogels. *J Macromol Sci Pure Appl Chem A* 1992;29(10):841–851.

99. Honiger J, Couturier C, Goldschmidt P, Maillet F, Kazatchkine MP, Laroche L. New anionic polyelectrolyte hydrogel for corneal surgery. *J Biomed Mater Res* 1997;37:548–553.

100. Yuk SH, Cho SH, Lee SH. pH/temperature responsive polymer composed of poly((N,N-dimethylamino)ethyl methacrylate-co-ethylacrylamide). *Macromolecules* 1997;30: 6856–6859.

101. Laurencin CT, Khan Y, Kofron M, El-Amin S, Botchwey E, Yu X, Cooper Jr. JA. The ABJS Nicolas Andry Award: Tissue engineering of bone and ligament: A 15-year perspective. *Clin Orthop Relat Res* 2006;447:221–236.

102. Hunziker EB. Articular cartilage repair: Basic science and clinical progress. A review of the current status and prospects. *Osteoarthr Cartil* 2002;10:432–463.

103. Carano RA, Filvaroff EH. Angiogenesis and bone repair. *Drug Discov Today* 2003;8:980–989.

104. El-Ghannam A. Bone reconstruction: From bioceramics to tissue engineering. *Expert Rev Med Devices* 2005;2:87–101.

105. Schmidmaier G, Lucke M, Schwabe P, Raschke M, Haas NP, Wildemann B. Collective review: Bioactive implants coated with poly(D, L-lactide) and growth factors IGF-I, TGF-beta1, or BMP-2 for stimulation of fracture healing. *J Long-Term Eff Med Implants* 2006;16:61–69.

106. Cregg PJ, Murphy K, Mardinoglu A. Inclusion of interactions in mathematical modelling of implant assisted magnetic drug targeting. *Appl Math Model* 2012;36:1–34.

107. Shen ZY, Ma GH, Dobashi T, Maki Y, Su ZG. Preparation and characterization of thermoresponsive albumin nanospheres. *Int J Pharm* 2008;346:133–142.

108. Dinauer N, Balthasar S, Weber C, Kreuter J, Langer K, Briesen H. Selective targeting of antibody-conjugated nanoparticles to leukemic cells and primary T-lymphocytes. *Biomaterials* 2005;26:5898–5906.

109. Leong KW, Langer R. Polymeric controlled drug delivery. *Adv Drug Deli Rev* 1987;1:199–233.

110. Lazarus GS, Cooper DM, Knighton DR, Margolis DJ, Percoraro ER, Rodeheaver G, Robson MC. Definitions and guidelines for assessment of wounds and evaluation of healing. *Arch Dermatol* 1994;130:489–493.

111. Falabella A, Kirsner R. Wound Healing (Basic and Clinical Dermatology). Boca Raton, Florida: Taylor & Francis; 2005.

112. Enoch S, Leaper DJ. Basic science of wound healing. *Surgery (Oxford)* 2005;23:37–42.

113. Paddle-Ledinek JE, Nasa Z, Cleland HJ. Effect of different wound dressings on cell viability and proliferation. *Plast Reconstr Surg* 2006;117(Suppl):110S–118S.

114. Quinn KJ, Courtney JM, Evans JH, Gaylor JDS, Reid WH. Principles of burn dressings. *Biomaterials* 1985;6:369–377.

115. Wisniewska JS, Sionkowska A, Kaminska A, Kaznica A, Jachimiak R, Drewa T. Surface characterization of collagen/elastin based biomaterials for tissue regeneration. *Appl Surf Sci* 2009;255:8286–8292.

116. Mikos AG, Herring SW, Ochareon P, Elisseeff J, Lu HH, Kandel R, Schoen FJ et al. Engineering complex tissues. *Tissue Eng* 2006;12(12):3307–3339.

117. Place ES, Evans ND, Stevens MM. Complexity in biomaterials for tissue engineering. *Nat Mater* 2009;8:457–470.

118. Törmälä P, Pohjonen T, Rokkanen P. Bioabsorbable polymers: Materials technology and surgical applications. *Proc Instn Mech Eng Part H – J Eng Med* 1998;212:101–111.

119. Hutmacher DW. Scaffolds in tissue engineering bone and cartilage. *Biomaterials* 2000;21:2529–2543.

120. Peter SJ, Miller MJ, Yasko AW, Yaszemski MJ, Mikos AG. Polymer concepts in tissue engineering. *J Biomed Mater Res (Appl Biomater)* 1998;43:422–427.

121. Nam YS, Yoon JJ, Park TG. A novel fabrication method of macroporous biodegradable polymer scaffolds using gas foaming salt as a porogen additive. *J Biomed Mater Res (Appl Biomater)* 2000;53:1–7.

122. Ma Z, Kotaki M, Inai R, Ramakrishna S. Potential of nanofiber matrix as tissue-engineering scaffolds. *Tissue Eng* 2005;11:101–109.

123. Jana S, Tefft BJ, Spoon DB, Simari RD. Scaffolds for tissue engineering of cardiac valves. *Acta Biomater* 2014;10:2877–2893.

2 Polymers in Dental Applications

2.1 INTRODUCTION

Over the past half century, extensive research has been done on the synthesis of biomaterial (materials intended to interface with biological systems to evaluate, treat, augment, or replace any tissue, organ, or function of the body)-based medical implants for treatment of millions of patients every year. To date, tens of millions of individuals have had the quality of their lives enhanced for as long as 25 years by the use of these man-made implants [1,2]. However, the first generation biomaterials did not fulfill medical need. The shortcomings of first generation biomaterials are driving force behind our ultimate goal of developing a synthetic entity that would entirely substitute and regenerate a damaged tissue or organ. Today, researchers are creating synthetics with the appropriate and full responsiveness toward biological milieu, that is, smart systems, that are able to control the behavior of adhered or encapsulated cells by releasing bioactive molecules into the local environment, or through extracellular protein/peptide mimetics built into the delivery substrates, could heal over the long term on the basis of biological mechanisms occurring in tissues and organs, and at biomaterial interfaces at the molecular, cellular, and macroscopic levels. Now, the biomaterials' field is shifting toward biologically active systems in order to improve their performance and to expand their use [3,4].

Teeth are the hardest materials in our body, that are mainly consist of partly organic and partly inorganic material. The inorganic component mainly consists of hydroxyapatite ($Ca_5 (PO_4)_3(OH)$) (HA). The outer layer of your teeth is called enamel which consists of approximately 92% HA. Enamel is a ceramic material. The bulk inner part of tooth covered with enamel, is made of a composite material containing a mixture of HA, collagen, water, and salts, is called dentin. Teeth function in one of the most inhospitable environments, that is, they are subject to larger temperature variations (0–70°C), pH range (2–11), and large mechanical stresses during chewing in the human body. When teeth are exposed to carbohydrate-containing food materials such as milk, some soft drinks, ice cream, cakes, and even some fruits, vegetables and juices, they start to decay because bacteria that live in the mouth form a white film on the teeth called plaque for their reproduction. Then bacteria produce acids by interacting with deposits (sugary and starchy foods) left on your teeth and erode and dissolve the HA present on the enamel surface of the tooth and create holes (cavities) (Figure 2.1). When cavities grow very large and destroy the nerve and blood vessels inside the tooth, then they begin to cause pain. Therefore, it is important that any cavities in our tooth are filled as soon as possible.

According to the National Institutes of Health, there are more than 100 million people missing teeth, and the need for implant dentistry is stronger than ever. Medical implants have undoubtedly made an indelible mark on our world in the last century. Despite that, however, most medical devices have been constructed using a significantly restricted number of conventional metallic, ceramic, polymeric, and composite biomaterials. It is critical for the dental team to be familiar with the implant procedures available [5]. The science of dental materials involves a study of the composition and properties of materials and the way in which they interact with the environment in which they are placed. The selection of materials for any given application can thus be undertaken with confidence and sound judgments.

2.2 PHYSICAL AND MECHANICAL REQUIREMENTS FOR MEDICAL DEVICE MATERIALS

Biomaterials are the man-made metallic, ceramic, or polymeric materials used for intracorporeal applications such as hard-tissue or soft-tissue augmentation, or replacement to repair cavities or replace broken teeth in the human body. In considering the parameters of materials for intracorporeal applications, several factors are of major importance. It is generally agreed that the material must meet the following requirements:

- Be biocompatible, nontoxic, and noncarcinogenic, cause little or no foreign-body reaction, and be chemically stable and corrosion resistant.

- Be able to endure large and variable stresses in the highly corrosive environment of the human body.

- Be able to be fabricated into intricate shapes and sizes.

In restorative dentistry, high compressive biting forces are combined with large temperature changes which initiate the corrosive attack on the chemical structure of the tooth, which may in

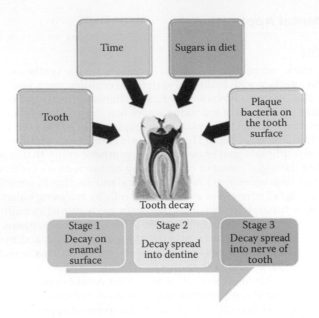

Figure 2.1 Schematic representation of cause of tooth decay and its various stages.

turn degrade the implant and/or cause release of ions that may adversely affect the body and acidity, producing a challenging environment. The biomaterials which are used as structural purpose in dental implant, must possess the great mechanical loading capacity demands.

2.2.1 Physical Properties

A denture polymer should possess adequate resilience and strength to biting, chewing, impact forces, and excessive wear under mastication. It should be stable under all conditions of service, including thermal and loading shocks [6,7]. It should also have reasonable specific gravity for certain special applications, making it lighter in weight.

2.2.2 Mechanical Properties

For dental materials that experience very highpoint forces in the mouth, creep, and compressive yield strengths are important. Important mechanical properties of polymeric materials include tensile strength, creep strength, modulus, and fatigue strength. Ceramics offer excellent compressive yield, and thus are often used for such applications. Tension and bending or tension fatigue are not primary strength attributes for study in ceramics, because tensile loads cause relatively rapid nonductile crack propagation. Wear resistance is also an important criterion for all biomaterials. Excessive wear can lead to premature mechanical failure of the replacement component. Mechanical properties of implants increase considerably with an increase in number average molecular weight, and become constant after a definite weight of materials used [8,9].

2.2.3 Esthetic Properties

The resin should exhibit sufficient translucency and transparency (hue, chroma, and value) to match the adjacent structures and tissues [6,7]. It should be capable of being pigmented or tinted to camouflage the surroundings. Once fabricated, it should maintain the appearance and color and not change subsequently.

2.2.4 Chemical Stability

The biomaterial should be chemically stable and not deteriorate inside the oral cavity by inducing some chemical reaction or an adverse event. It should preferably polymerize to completion, without leaching any residual monomers [6,7]. The most frequent cause of failure of dental implants is the loss of bone around the implant. Implants are in many ways similar to the roots of natural teeth. It is, therefore, unsurprising that when bone loss occurs around implants, it is largely due to the response of the peri-implant tissues to plaque [10], and may be exacerbated by metabolic disorders, smoking [11], the use of an inappropriate type of implant (too long or too wide), and poorly designed prostheses over the implant(s) which do not distribute occlusal loads evenly [12–14]. Presently, various diagnostic analyses have been suggested to define implant stability. Primary implant stability can be measured by either a destructive or a nondestructive method. Histomorphologic research, tensional test, push-out/pull-out test, and removal torque test are classified as destructive methods. Nondestructive methods include percussion test, radiography, cutting torque test while placing implants, Periotest® (SiemensAG, Benshein, Germany), and resonance frequency analysis [15].

2.2.5 Rheometric Properties

The flow behavior in polymers involves elastic and plastic deformation (viscous flow) and elastic recovery when stresses are released, as reported by Nielsen [16]. Molecular weight, chain length, number of cross linkages, temperature, and applied force greatly determine the typical behavior. Plastic flow is irreversible and causes permanent polymer deformation, compared to elastic recovery in certain polymers, when applied stress is removed. Biopolymers exhibit complex combined elastic—plastic deformation called as visco-elastic recovery.

2.2.6 Thermal Properties

Polymers normally show a large variation in their properties with respect to temperature. At sufficiently low temperatures, amorphous polymers are hard and glass-like, compared to softer and more flexible, when a critical temperature is reached, usually the glass transition temperature (T_g). At temperatures above T_g, the polymer chains display increased mobility, enabling the bulk material to flow. At temperatures below T_g, mobility is restricted and the polymer behaves like a glassy, elastic solid. The T_g of a polymer is determined by the chemical structure, molecular weight, and degree of chemical or physical crosslinking [17,18]. The T_g of a plastic is one of the very important set points in determining whether the polymer is thermosetting or thermoplastic, and hence our desired clinical properties are affected. T_g varies with the molecular weight, as described by Fox and Flory [8,9] and thus modifies the material properties.

$$T_g = T_g^{\,a} - K/Mn$$

where $T_g^{\,a}$ is the maximum glass transition temperature that can be achieved at a theoretical infinite molecular weight and K is an empirical parameter that is related to the free volume present in the polymer sample, and Mn number-average molecular weight.

2.2.7 Biocompatibility

When a synthetic material is placed within the human body, tissue reacts with the implant in a variety of ways depending not only on the bulk properties of the material, but also to their surface, chemical, and physical properties, which is responsible for recognition and interaction of the material with cells enzymes and other molecules through various immune system signaling processes. The mechanism of tissue interaction depends on the tissue response to the implant surface [19]. The biological compatibility of a material is a complex phenomenon, involving interactions from biology, patient risks, trials, clinical experience, and engineering expertise. Though ignored for several years, it is the fundamental requirement for any biological material today. Biocompatibility is the ability of a polymer material or a device to remain biologically inert during its functional period [20]. Toxicity is usually manifested by the release of several chemical constituents from the material, which induces an allergic response in terms of localized or generalized stomatitis/dermatitis, severe toxicological reactions, or carcinogenic/mutagenic effects. The selection criteria for implantable biomaterials for a given end use must be based on physicochemical properties, functions desired, nature of the physiological environment, adverse effect in case of failure, expected durability, and consideration relating to cost and ease of production. The dental resins should be nontoxic, nonirritating, and otherwise nondetrimental to oral tissues. To fulfill these requirements, they should be preferably insoluble in saliva and all other body fluids. They should not become insanitary or disagreeable in taste, odor, or smell and should be highly stable [1].

2.3 DENTAL IMPLANTS

Human skulls dating back to 600 AD show that man attempted to implant carved shells into the anterior mandible. However, the modern research in the dental field is said to have had its start since 1726, but this field gained interest in middle nineteenth-century when amalgam, porcelain, and gold foil materials were studied for research in dentistry. In 1919, National Bureau of Standard of USA Government set specification standards for the selection and grading of dental amalgam implants. Research associates investigated the properties of wrought and casting gold and accessory casting materials under the leadership of Dr. Wilmer Souder. In 1928, American Dental Association Research Commission worked for advances of dental implants such as inlay waxes, dental amalgam, casting gold, mercury, and silicate cement. Currently, it is also working for the advancement and specifications of dental materials [21].

Now the field of dental materials has gained much interest and new materials are investigated by scientist for the comfort of patients as well as to anchor dental implants into the alveolar bone, but to date have not been successful. Some of the materials are discussed below.

2.3.1 Osseointegrated Implant

The osseointegrated dental implants are those implants which are directly in contact with bone or direct bone-to-implant contact under load, with diameters from 3.3 to 6.0 mm and lengths from 6 to 16 mm, make in a variety of shapes, including hollow baskets, blades, tripods, needles, disks, truncated cones, cylinders, and screws. Currently, titanium (CP-Ti or Ti-6Al-4 V)-based implants are used (Figure 2.2) [22]. The physiochemical properties of implants affect the tissue reactions on the surface of implants. In osseointegrated dental implants, the abutment either connected to the implant with a screw, or it can be cemented, is used as connector which connects the implant and the prosthesis and makes contact with soft tissue. The prosthesis is attached to the abutment with a screw or cement. In order to improve the attachment of the bone cells to the implant surface, implants surface is coated with HA and titanium plasma spray. However, the coating has no long life, it separates from the implant once inserted in the alveolar bone.

They were introduced by Per-Ingvar Brånemark who developed a titanium chamber to study wound healing in the bone of a rabbit. He observed that the bone had fused (osseointegrated) to the titanium surface by strong bond that it could not be broken. The Brånemark system was introduced in the United States in 1982. These implants were machine surfaced to be a cylindrical screw [23,24].

Semenova et al. [25] analyzed the possibility of using ultrafine grain titanium in dentistry. They synthesized screw-shaped dental implants with pitch height of 0.5 mm, outer diameter of 3.3 mm, length of 8.0 mm, a square head, and inner threaded hole of 2.0 mm from ultrafine grain CP-Ti implants that showed the ultimate tensile strength as high as 1240 MPa while retaining a ductility of 11%.

People who are missing teeth have compromised chewing ability and speech, facial appearance, and self-confidence. Osseointegrated dental implants maintain facial muscles, aiding in improved mastication, muscle tone, the bone profile, and volume when chewing, by applying direct forces on the bone during mastication and provide a priceless, new, self-confidence to patients who can smile with confidence without worry of denture displacement or showing gaps when smiling.

2.3.2 Mini-Implants for Orthodontic Anchorage

Orthodontic mini-implants are temporary implants (diameter 1.2–2.0 mm) used to secure anchorage in contemporary orthodontic treatments, made from Ti-6Al-4 V alloy having superior strength (Figure 2.3). These were placed to support a denture or temporary prosthesis during the healing time following implant surgery (usually inserted and remain in place for 6–9 months, after which

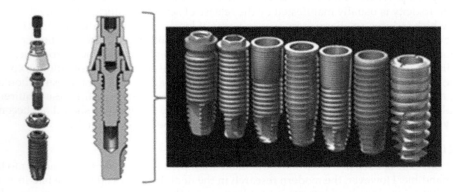

Figure 2.2 Components and shapes of osseointegrated dental implants.

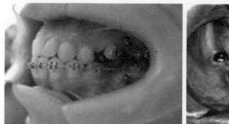
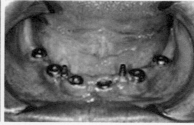

Figure 2.3 Types of mini orthodontic implants.

they are easily removed). The cost of a mini-implant is approximately one-fourth the cost of a regular implant making it more affordable for the patient. However, these implants suffer from two problems: lower corrosion resistance and deformation under orthodontic load. It is found that biomechanically the CP-Ti implants have significantly higher removal torque than the alloy implants [26–28].

2.3.3 Zygomatic Implants

Zygomatic implants made from CP-Ti, having a diameter equal to 4–5 and 30–53 mm length, penetrate the maxilla at the second premolar region as close to the alveolar crest; these are mostly used as posterior anchorage for implant-supported prostheses in patients for the treatment of the atrophic maxilla, posterior teeth are missing for an extended period of time, the sinus can pneumatize or drop down, and only a shell of bone remains between the sinus and oral cavity. It was initially conceived as a treatment for the victims of traumas or tumor resection where there was considerable loss of the maxillary structure [29–31]. By using zygomatic implants, the cost and need for bone grafting can be decreased.

2.3.4 Transosseous Implant

In 1968, the transosseous implant was introduced by Dr. Small. They were made from titanium, or a gold alloy, and inserted underneath the chin and transversed the mandible from the bottom to the top. They have a flat bone plate that was fixed under the skin against the inferior border of the mandible. Several threaded posts projected into the anterior mandible from the plate. Two to four of the posts went completely through the mucosa and into the oral cavity to help fixate the denture prosthesis. However, they suffer from problems such as frequent bone loss around the posts with bleeding on probing [32,33].

2.3.5 Endodontic Implants

The endosseous implant was introduced by Dr. Linkowin in 1966, also called as blade implants, that is, inserted intraorally in the bone by making a groove in the alveolar bone. One or more posts were attached to the fin-shaped plate, which anchored the restoration. They are used for the stabilization of preservation of natural teeth. Today, they are not used due to their lower success rate (under 50%), tendency to become loose, infected, and had to be removed [34,35] (Figure 2.4).

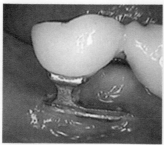
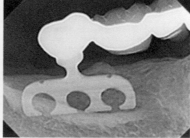

Figure 2.4 Endodontic implants design.

2.4 BENEFITS OF DENTAL IMPLANTS

Dental implants are considered "the standard of care" today to replace a missing tooth due to osseointegration and improved oral function. Dental implants not only maintain the bone profile and volume, but also give self-confidence to patients (Figure 2.5). The benefits of dental implants are as follows:

- Enhance the quality of life
- Work as natural teeth
- A dental implant most closely replicates natural tooth structure
- Preserve integrity of facial structure
- Dental implants do not decay or need root canal therapy
- Better health due to improved nutrients and proper digestion
- The mouth is restored as closely as natural state
- Convenience of hygiene
- Improved psychological health
- Adjacent tooth not compromising to replace missing tooth
- Improved smile
- Improved confidence
- Ideally esthetic teeth position

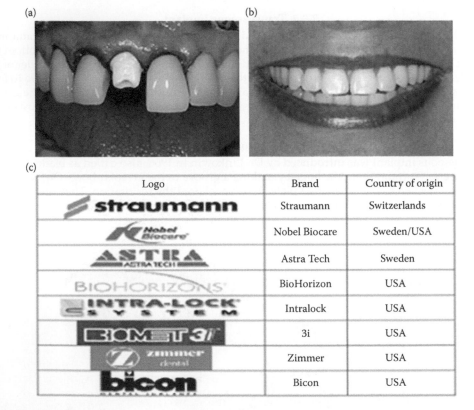

(a) (b) (c)

Logo	Brand	Country of origin
straumann	Straumann	Switzerlands
Nobel Biocare	Nobel Biocare	Sweden/USA
ASTRA TECH	Astra Tech	Sweden
BIOHORIZONS	BioHorizon	USA
INTRA-LOCK SYSTEM	Intralock	USA
BIOMET 3i	3i	USA
zimmer dental	Zimmer	USA
bicon	Bicon	USA

Figure 2.5 Schematically representation of (a) mouth without dental implants, (b) with dental implant, and (c) commercially available implants.

2.5 DISADVANTAGES OF DENTAL IMPLANTS

Dental implants have the following disadvantages:

- Length of treatment time

- Risk of fixture failure

- Failure to osseointegrate or bone loss while in function

- Require daily brushing and flossing or peri-implantitis can occur

- Gingival tissue infections occur shortly after surgery due to any one of the billions of bacteria in the oral cavity

- Need for multiple surgeries

- Mechanical complications include loosening of screws, fractured screws, and even fractured implants due to force overload

- Expensive

- Geriatric patients, patients with osteoporosis, and those receiving treatment for certain cancers have a higher incidence of implant failure due to decreased bone density

2.6 DENTURE MATERIALS

Dental materials for restorative dentistry include

- Amalgam alloys for direct fillings

- Noble metals and alloys for direct fillings, crowns and bridges, and porcelain fused to metal restorations

- Base metals and alloys for partial-denture frame work, porcelain–metal restorations, crowns and bridges, orthodontic wires and brackets, and implants

- Ceramics for implants, porcelain–metal restorations, crowns, inlays, and veneers, cements, and denture teeth

- Composites for replacing missing tooth structure and modifying tooth color and contour

- Polymers for denture bases, plastic teeth, cements, and other applications

2.6.1 Ceramics in Dentistry

Ceramics are also widely used in dentistry as restorative materials such as gold–porcelain crowns, glass or silica-filled resin composites, dentures, and so forth. In dental science, ceramics are referred to as nonmetallic, inorganic structures primarily containing compounds of oxygen with one or more metallic or semimetallic elements, offering the advantages of resistance to microbial attack, pH changes, solvent conditions, and temperature. They are usually sodium, potassium, calcium, magnesium, aluminum, silicon, phosphorus, zirconium, and titanium. Structurally, dental ceramics contain a crystal phase and a glass phase based on the silica structure, characterized by silica tetrahedra, containing central Si^{4+} ion with four O^- ions. It is not closely packed, having both covalent and ionic characteristics. The usual dental ceramic is glassy in nature, with short range crystallinity. Basically, the inorganic composition of teeth and bones are ceramics—HA. Hence ceramics like HA, wollastonite, etc., are used as bone graft materials. They have an entire plethora of synthetic techniques like wet chemical, sol–gel, hydrothermal methods, etc. Also they are added as bioactive filler particles to other inert materials like polymers or coated over metallic implants. These ceramics are collectively called as bioceramics. There are basically two kinds of bioceramics—inert (e.g., alumina) and bioactive (HA). They can be resorbable (tricalcium phosphate) or nonresorbable (zirconia) (Figure 2.6). The use of ceramics is encouraged by their biocompatibility, esthetics, durability, and easier customization. The specialty of ceramic teeth is the ability to mimic the natural tooth in color and translucency along with strength. Ceramics have excellent intraoral stability and wear resistance adding to their durability.

Basically, ceramics are used as indirect restorative materials such as crowns (a "Cap" placed on a tooth to protect it from fracture or sensitivity) and bridges (a fixed replacement of missing teeth, with support from adjacent teeth), inlays/onlays (an indirect filling placed on teeth), and

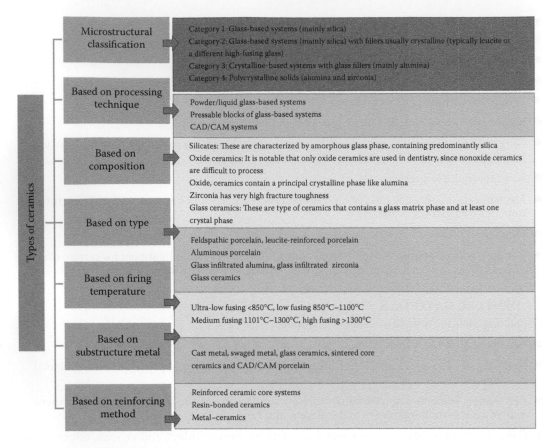

Figure 2.6 Classification of ceramics used in dental applications.

dental implants (basically a pillar/post placed into bone to act as a replacement to root of a tooth, on which a denture— fixed/removable—is placed). Recently, ceramic braces have been used in orthodontics. Ceramic teeth are manufactured in various shades, shapes, and sizes to be used in complete dentures [36].

2.6.2 Metals

Metals used as biomaterials must be either noble or corrosion resistant to the body environment. Metallic implants show many types of corrosions including general corrosion, pitting and crevice corrosion, stress-corrosion cracking, corrosion fatigue, and intergranular corrosion. For a material to be considered resistant to corrosion in the body, its general corrosion rate usually must be less than 0.01 mil/year (0.00025 mm/year). Besides orthopedics, there are other markets for metallic implants and devices, including oral and maxillofacial surgery (e.g., dental implants, craniofacial plates, and screws).

Presently, the principal metals such as stainless steels (205 GPa (30×10^6 psi)), cobalt-based alloys (240 GPa (35×10^6 psi)), pure titanium (CP-Ti), shape memory alloys (alloys based on the nickel–titanium binary system), zirconium alloys, and titanium-based alloys (lowest moduli (105–125 GPa, or $15–18 \times 10^6$ psi) are developed for biomedical application because of their biocompatibility, ability to bear significant loads, withstand fatigue loading, and undergo plastic deformation prior to failure as well as the discrepancy between the modulus of bone and that of the alloys used to support structural loads.

2.6.3 Polymeric Materials

Modern synthetic polymer chemistry has revolutionized the world of polymer materials. Among macromolecular systems of various chemical and architectural profiles, the polymers exhibiting the property of responsiveness to external signals have emerged as one of the most promising kind of materials in advanced materials science and owe versatile applications in biology and technology. Polymer-based materials offering the greatest versatility in properties and processing among all biomaterials are also used extensively in dentistry as composite (resin–ceramic) restorative materials, implants, dental cements, and denture bases and teeth. Polymers can be classified on the basis of their physical form (linear free chains in solution, covalently cross-linked gels and reversible or physical gels, chain adsorbed or surface-grafted form), different stimuli (temperature-, pH-, ionic strength-, light-, electric- and magnetic field-sensitive), and functionality and architecture (star polymers, brushes, dendrimers, polymeric micelles, block copolymer, and liposomes).

Polymeric materials have advantages over metallic implants because they can be selected on the basis of the conditions found in the body, taking into consideration that the circumstances under which polymers are most susceptible, including those of elevated temperature, electromagnetic radiation, and atmospheric oxygen, are not operative here as well as the isotonic saline solution that comprises the body's extracellular fluid is extremely hostile to metals but is not normally associated with the degradation of many synthetic high-molecular-weight polymers [37,38]. Mostly, aromatic dimethacrylate monomer, bisphenol A-glycidyl methacrylate (BIS-GMA), and diurethane dimethacrylates are used in dental applications.

2.6.3.1 Polymethyl Methacrylate

Dental clinicians are always looking for the ideal restorative material. This material should be tooth-colored, long-lasting, and strong; it should adhere to the tooth structure; and it should be able to be made directly within the preparation site: a direct, esthetic restorative material. The latter two factors may be the most desirable. Of all types of restorative materials, the polymeric classification best fulfills these requirements, as neither metals nor ceramics have successfully been able to be fabricated or placed in such a manner. The dental community, in its search for better, less expensive, easier-to-handle materials, is often quick to adapt a rising technology for new and different purposes. Before synthetic polymer systems were developed, many items classified as "plastic" materials were developed from natural resins or exudates and tissues from plants, animals, and insects. It was found that heating these materials would put them in a softened state, permitting them to be molded and shaped prior to their cooling. The first examples of such materials were horns and hoofs of animals [39]. With respect to insect exudates, the most notable are shellac products, which are still in use today [40]. These materials are derived from resins produced by tiny insects (*Coccus lacca*) that infest fig trees: literally Shell Lacca, from whence we derive the word "shellac" [41]. Early use of the product was as a protective coating and decorative finish for woods and metals. Later, the product was mixed with wood fillers to provide a moldable substance, and bulk products (primarily decorative cases) were produced.

In 1922, Dr. Herman Staudlinger synthesized styrene-copolymers-based thermoplastic polymers which display a physical change with heating, undergoing long-chain, segmental movement, and distortion [42]. Concurrent with the development of many of these synthetic materials was the proposal that they be used in dentistry. Of particular interest to the dental field is the development of acrylic chemistry. Acrylic acid and its derivatives were well known, even in the 1890s. Derivatives of acrylic monomers, methyl and ethyl acrylate, were made and also produced perfectly clear solid polymers. In 1927, Vernonite, a polymethyl methacrylate (PMMA), heat-processed material was used as a denture base, definitive restorative material for inlays, crowns, and fixed partial dentures. PMMA-based acrylic resins are the most commonly used polymeric materials (98% of all denture bases were constructed from methyl methacrylate polymers or copolymers) in denture dentistry as individual impression trays and orthodontic devices, in addition to dentures and artificial crowns (Figure 2.7). PMMA is prepared by free radical polymerization of methyl methacrylate. Heat polymerized PMMA and thicker areas of the denture show significantly fewer residual monomers [6,43–45]. The dimethacrylates (BIS-GMA) contains borosilicate or silicate glass powder as filler, used to cement cast restorations that have been etched to produce an increased irregular surface to a similarly etched enamel surface. But they suffer from problem of microleakage at the margin or tooth interface created by the polymerization shrinkage during setting [46].

2.6.3.2 Poly(Ortho Esters)

Poly(ortho esters) (POE) are hydrophobic and bioerodible polymers that have been investigated for pharmaceutical use since the early 1970s (Figure 2.8). Among various generations of POE, the third (POE III) and fourth (POE IV) are promising viscous and injectable materials which have been

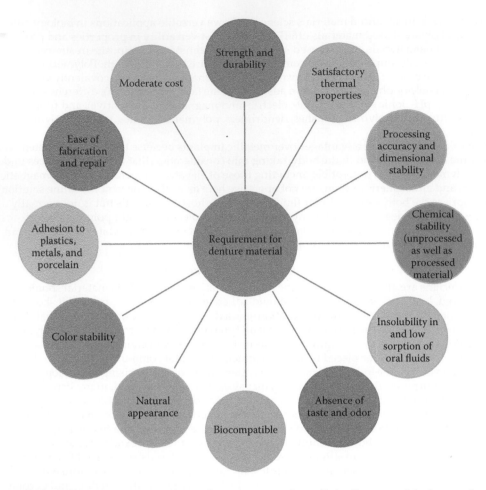

Figure 2.7 Schematic representations of requirements for a clinically acceptable denture base material.

investigated in numerous biomedical applications due to their excellent biocompatibility, and ability to undergo an erosion process confined to the polymer–water interface.

Periodontal disease (changes in the morphology of gingival tissues, bleeding upon probing as well as periodontal pocket formation provides an ideal environment for the growth and proliferation of anaerobic pathogenic bacteria) is a general term which encompasses several pathological conditions affecting the tooth-supporting structures. These conditions are characterized by a destruction of the period on a TAL ligament, a resorption of the alveolar bone and the tooth surface [47]. The aim of current periodontal therapy is to remove the bacterial deposits from the tooth surface and to shift the pathogenic microbiota to one compatible with periodontal health. As an adjunct therapy to mechanical treatment of refractory periodontitis, antimicrobial agents may be valuable. Many polymer-based systems have been studied for various antibiotic deliveries and evaluated in vitro or in vivo for the treatment of periodontal diseases [48]. Biodegradable polymer, that is, poly(ortho esters)-based antibiotic drug delivery systems are desirable to have a bioerodible drug delivery system that can maintain an effective drug release rate in the periodontal pocket while simultaneously eroding throughout the duration of treatment, over several days.

2.6.3.3 Dental Restorative Composites

The composition of resin-based dental composites has evolved significantly since the materials were first introduced to dentistry more than 50 years ago (Figure 2.9). Composite resin used for adhesive dental restoration has as main advantages the realization of minimum cavity preparation and superior esthetics, restorative materials, cavity liners, pit and fissure sealants, cores and buildups, inlays, onlays, crowns, provisional restorations, cements for single or multiple tooth

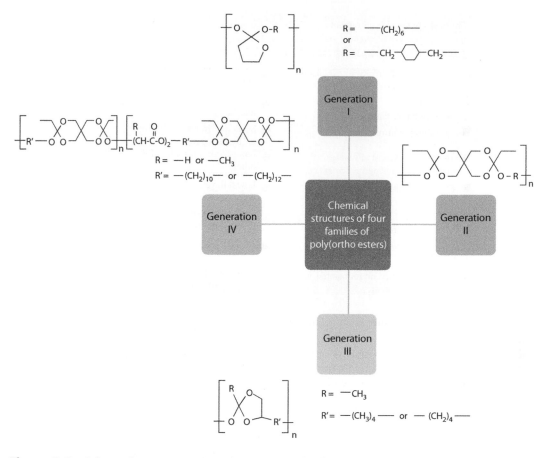

Figure 2.8 Schematic representation of generation of poly(ortho esters) with structure.

prostheses and orthodontic devices, endodontic sealers, and root canal posts [49]. Dental composites can be distinguished by differences in formulation tailored to their particular requirements as restoratives, sealants, cements, provisional materials, etc. The predominant base monomer used in commercial dental composites has been BIS-GMA, which due to its high viscosity is mixed with other dimethacrylates, such as TEGDMA, UDMA, or other monomers [50] (Figure 2.10). Restorative composites react by a mechanism of free radicals which are generated by the chemical

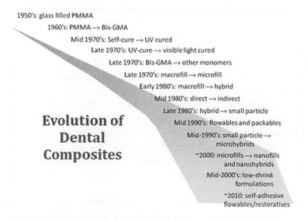

Figure 2.9 A perspective on the evolution of dental composites.

Physical/chemical requirements	Consequences for dental practices
■ Low volume shrinkage or expansion during polymerization	■ No marginal gap, easy processing of the filling composite
■ High rate of photopolymerization	■ Only a short curing time in necessary
■ Crosslinking properties	■ Sufficient mechanical properties of the restorative
■ Tg above 60°C and low water uptake of the formed polymer	■ Long-term durability of the filling
■ Excellent resistance to oral conditions	■ Low failure rate of the composite curing
■ Storage stability in the presence of dental fillers	■ Long term experienced fillers can be used for composite preparation
■ High light and coloration stability of the formed polymer	■ Long-term esthetics
■ Low oral toxicity, no mutagenic, and carcinogenic effect	■ Minimum toxicological risk for the patient and dentist

Figure 2.10 Basic requirements for monomers in restorative composites.

reaction of benzoyl peroxide with a tertiary amine, initiating the polymerization of methacrylic groups and forming a 3D polymer matrix. They are activated by visible light, initiating their polymerization process by absorbing visible light within a specific wavelength (450–500 nm) [51]. In the direct technique, the composite is cured directly on the tooth by means of a curing light; however, this technique presented some disadvantages. If light is not inserted correctly, layer sun cured can cause countless damage to restoration, especially with regard to mechanical properties [52]. Recently published investigations have shown that postcuring of dental resin restorative materials may improve properties such as flexural strength or wear resistance [53]. However, indirect application of composite resin can decrease the problems since the remaining tooth structure is reconstructed into a mold and the material is cured and postcured under controlled laboratory conditions.

Current research works are more focused on the polymeric matrix of the material, principally to develop systems with reduced polymerization shrinkage, and perhaps more importantly, reduced polymerization shrinkage stress, and to make them self-adhesive to the tooth structure. Several articles recently have reviewed the current technology of dental composites [54,55] and described future developments, such as self-repairing and stimuli-responsive materials [56].

Conventional dental composites had average particle sizes that far exceeded 1 μm, and typically had fillers close to or exceeding the diameter of a human hair (~50 μm). These "macrofill" materials were very strong, but difficult to polish and impossible to retain surface smoothness. To address the important issue of long-term esthetics, manufacturers began to formulate "microfill" composites, admittedly inappropriately named at the time, but probably done to emphasize the fact that the particles were "microscopic." Thus, the original "microfills" would have more accurately been called "nanofills," generally weak due to their relatively low filler content, and a compromise was needed to produce adequate strength by increasing the filler level by incorporating highly filled, prepolymerized resin fillers within the matrix to which additional "microfill" particles were added [57]. Years ago, novel organically modified ceramics (ORMOCERS) were developed and have been used in commercial products [58]. Similarly, the commercially available epoxy-based silorane system with good mechanical properties used in Filtek Silorane LS (3M ESPE) provides verified lower shrinkage than typical dimethacrylate-based resins, likely due to the epoxide curing reaction that involves the opening of an oxirane ring [59,60].

The latest trend has been toward the development of flowable composites containing adhesive monomers, such as Vertise Flow (Kerr) and Fusio Liquid Dentin (Pentron Clinical). These formulations are based on traditional methacrylate systems, but incorporating acidic monomers typically found in dentin bonding agents, such as glycerol phosphate dimethacrylate in Vertise Flow, which may be capable of generating adhesion through mechanical and possibly chemical interactions with the tooth structure. These materials are currently recommended for liners and small restorations, and are serving as the entry point for universal self-adhesive composites.

2.6.3.4 Polyethyl Methacrylate (PEMA) and Polybutyl Methacrylate (PBMA)

With respect to the diverse applications of polymers in denture science, higher molecular weight methacrylate polymers such as PEMA (T_g 65°C) and PBMA (T_g 30°C) have found uses as soft denture liners.

2.6.3.5 Future Polymers

Hydrogels formed by the crosslinking reaction of hydrophilic polymers with bridging agent, called a crosslinker, are capable of absorbing large amount of water, which is dependent on the type and concentration of the crosslinker. Hydrogel can be developed for soft tissue conditioners through hydrophilic and biocompatible polymers, primarily poly N-substituted methacrylamides, HEMA, etc. Polycarbonates formed by crosslinking bisphenol A with a di-substituted ketone group have high impact strength, compared to the traditional acrylic resins. Therefore, they can be used as denture base. Polyethylene-woven fibers, braided fibers, and unidirectional fibers [61–65] are under experimentation. Fiberflex based on Kevlar, developed by Dupont, is under consideration, as a unidirectional fiber reinforced denture material [66]. Glass-woven and braided fibers are also promoted for indirect system of fabrication by Swiss Dental Laboratories [67]. Fiberk or (glass unidirectional fibers) and Vectris (glass unidirectional fibers in mesh) are also under trial as future denture substitutes [68–73].

2.7 COMPLICATIONS IN IMPLANT DENTISTRY

Currently, the implant industry is greatly advanced and dental implants are rapidly becoming an alternative to traditional prostheses, and are one of the preferred treatment options for replacing missing teeth in both partially and completely edentulous ridges and have been introduced into the market. Although dental implants have improved the quality of life of many patients, a wide body of literature has reported their associated morbidity. Studies have also documented the association of complications with surgical implant procedures and prosthetic rehabilitation. Implant failures are categorized as primary (early), when the body is unable to establish osseointegration, or secondary (late), when the body is unable to maintain the achieved osseointegration and a breakdown process results [74]. Implant failures are also classified on the basis of the time of prosthesis placement; in this classification, early implant failure usually occurs before the prosthesis is placed, and late implant failure is associated with functional loading after the placement of the prosthesis.

The common complications are as follows:

- Systemic, environmental, and genetic risk factors associated with the failure of dental implants.

- Persistent pain after implant placement.

- Peri-implant diseases.

- Microbial species found around healthy and diseased implants.

- Mechanical complications and failures associated with implant-supported over dentures and implant-supported removable partial dentures.

- Malpositioning of implants can occur during implant surgery and may be the result of a number of factors, such as the quantity or quality of residual available bone, dental inclinations adjacent to the surgical implant site, and lack of previous prosthodontic planning.

- Injuries to the inferior alveolar nerve and, less frequently, the lingual nerve have been reported and are of concern when posterior mandibular implants are placed.

- Common pink-tissue esthetic failures and the less common white-tissue esthetic failures.

- Rough surfaced implants had significantly higher success rates compared with implants with more smooth surfaces.

- Shorter implants, a larger number of implants per patient, and a low number of implants per prosthesis were associated with a higher risk of implant failure.

2.8 CONCLUSIONS

With the success of dental implant treatment, new treatment protocols have been proposed. Immediate implant loading protocols provide patients with satisfactory results by reducing the time interval between implant surgery and prosthesis delivery. However, it is important that the practitioner carefully selects the patients before suggesting dental implant treatment. Although the aforementioned factors may influence implant failure, prosthetic design also can play an important role in affecting the implant outcome. The success of dental implants depends on the following factors.

1. Treatment-related factors that can be influenced by the implantologist (e.g., the implant design), including the macro and micro design. A small l diameter and short implants are good possible options for treating patients with limited bone volume.

2. Small diameter implants can be loaded immediately. However, controlling the amount of occlusal loading and ensuring primary stability of the immediately loaded implants are essential.

3. The effect of abutment design on the long-term success of implants is directly related to the loading protocol.

4. Clinicians should critically evaluate the patient's oral hygiene, compliance, motivation, and risk factors before suggesting dental implant treatment.

5. Host-related factors, operative-related factors, and implant-related factors may influence the outcome of implant treatment and should be thoroughly evaluated during treatment planning.

REFERENCES

1. Williams DF. *The Williams Dictionary of Biomaterials*. Liverpool: Liverpool University Press; 1999.

2. Hench LL, Polak JM. Third-generation biomedical materials. *Science* 2002;295:1014–1017.

3. Anderson DG, Levenberg S, Langer R. Nanoliter-scale synthesis of arrayed biomaterials and application to human embryonic stem cells. *Nat Biotechnol* 2004;22:863–866.

4. Lutolf MP, Hubbell JA. Synthetic biomaterials as instructive extracellular microenvironments for morphogenesis in tissue engineering. *Nat Biotechnol* 2005;23:47–55.

5. Fatiha El Feninat, Gaetan L, Michel F, Diego M. Shape memory materials in biomedical applications. *Adv Eng Mater* 2002;4(3):91–104.

6. Phillips RM. *Skinners Science of Dental Materials*. New York: W.B. Saunders; 1973, p. 162.

7. Maachi RL, Craig RG. Physical and mechanical properties of composite restorative materials. *J Am Dent Assoc* 1969;78:328.

8. Fox TG, Flory PJ. The glass transition. *J Appl Phys* 1950;21:581.

9. Fox TG, Flory PJ. The glass temperature and related properties of polystyrene—Influence of molecular weight. *J Polym Sci* 1954;14:315–319.

10. Allen PF, McMillan AS, Smith DG. Complications and maintenance requirements of implant-supported prostheses provided in a UK dental hospital. *Brit Dent J* 1997;182:298–302.

11. Martinelli E, Palmer RM, Wilson RF, Newton JT. Smoking behaviour and attitudes to periodontal health and quit smoking in patients with periodontal disease. *J Clin Periodontol* 2008;35:944–954.

12. Adell R. Clinical results of osseointegrated implants supporting fixed prostheses in edentulous jaws. *J Prosth Dent* 1983;50:251–254.

13. Albrektsson T, Sennerby L. State of the art in oral implants. *J Clin Periodontol*, 1991;18:474–481.

14. Kirsch A, Mentage PJ. The IMZ endo-osseous two phase implant system: A complete oral rehabilitation treatment concept. *J Oral Implantol* 1986;12:576–589; *J Polym Sci* 14:315.

15. Meredith N. Assessment of implant stability as a prognostic determinant. *Int J Prosthodont* 1998;11:491–501.

16. Nielsen LE. *Mechanical Properties of Polymers*. New York: Reinhold; 1962.

17. Young RJ, Lovell PA. *Introduction to Polymers*. London: Chapman and Hall; 1981, p. 456.

18. Ward IM. *Mechanical Properties of Solid Polymers*. New York: Wiley-Interscience; 1971, p. 492.

19. Heness G, Ben-Nissan B. *Innovative Bioceramics Mater. Forum* 2004;27:104–114.

20. Williams D, editor. *Biocompatibility of Clinical Implant Materials*. Boca Raton, Florida: CRC Press, Inc.; 1981, p. 235.

21. Souder WH, Peters CG. An investigation of the physical properties of dental materials. *Bur St Tech* Paper No. 157 1920; *Dent Cos* 1920;62:305.

22. Brånemark PI, Adell R, Albrektsson T, Lekholm U, Lundkvist S, Rockler B. Osseointegrated titanium fixtures in the treatment of edentulousness. *Biomaterials* 1983;4:25–28.

23. Branemark PI, Zarb GA, Albrektsson T. *Tissue-Integrated Prostheses: Osseointegration in Clinicaldentistry*. Chicago: Quintessence; 1985.

24. Biocare N. *The Story about an Invention That Makes People Smile*. Sweden: Nobel Biocare; 2005.

25. Elias CN, Lima JHC, Valiev R, Meyers MA. Biomedical applications of titanium and its alloys. *Overview Biological Materials Science* 2008;60:46–49.

26. Johansson CB, Han CH, Wennerberg A, Albrektsson T. Quantitative comparison of machined commercially pure Ti and Ti-6Al-4 V implant in rabbit. *J Oral Maxillofac Implants* 1998;13:315.

27. Mazor Z. Using transitional implants for immediate fixed temporary prostheses. [Interview]. *DentImplantol Update* 2000;11(4):29–31.

28. Singh K, Kumar D, Jaiswal RK, Bansal A. Temporary anchorage devices—Mini-implants. *Natl J Maxillofac Surg* 2010;1(1):30–34.

29. Parel SM, Brånemark PI, Ohrnell LO, Svensson B. Remote implant anchorage for the rehabilitation of maxillary defects. *J Prosthet Dent* 2001;86:377.

30. Duarte LR, Filho HN, Francischone CE, Peredo LG, Brånemark PI. The establishment of a protocol for the total rehabilitation of atrophic maxillae employing four zygomatic fixtures in an immediate loading system—A 30-month clinical and radiographic follow-up. *Clin Implant Dent Rel Res* 2007;9(4):186.

31. Sevetz EB Jr. Treatment of the severely atrophic fully edentulous maxilla: the zygoma implant option. *Atlas Oral Maxillofac Surg Clin North Am* 2006;14(1):121–136.

32. Small IA. The mandibular staple bone plate. Its use and advantages in reconstructive surgery. *Dent Clin North Am* 1986;30(2):175–187.

33. Small IA, Misiek D. A sixteen-year evaluation of the mandibular staple bone plate. *J Oral Maxillofac Surg* 1986;44(1):60–66.

34. Kapur KK. Veterans administration cooperative dental implant study–comparisons between fixed partial dentures supported by blade-vent implants and removable partial dentures. Part I: Methodology and comparisons between treatment groups at baseline. *J Prosthet Dent* 1987;58(4):499–512.

35. Kapur KK. Veterans administration cooperative dental implant study–comparisons between fixed partial dentures supported by blade-vent implants and removable partial dentures. Part II: Comparisons of success rates and periodontal health between two treatment modalities. *J Prosthet Dent* 1989;62(6):685–703.

36. Narasimha Raghavan R. 2012. Ceramics in dentistry, sintering of ceramics - new emerging techniques. In: Lakshmanan A, editors. ISBN: 978-953-51-0017-1, InTech, Available from: http://www.intechopen.com/books/sintering-of-ceramics-new-emerging-techniques/ceramics-in-dentistry.

37. Williams DF. *Biodegradation of Medical Polymers, Concise Encyclopedia of Medical and Dental Materials.* In: Williams DF, editor. Oxford, UK: Pergamon Press, the MIT Press; 1990, pp. 69–74.

38. Donachie M. Biomaterials, Metals Hand Book Desk Edition. (2nd ed.). In: Davis JR, editor. UK: ASM International; 1998. p. 702–709.

39. Rueggeberg FA. From vulcanite to vinyl, a history of resins in restorative dentistry. *J Prosthet Dent* 2002;87:364–369.

40. Fahey DE. A concise history of plastics: Plastics in nature. Available at: http://www.nswpmitb.com.au/historyofplastics.html. Accessed May 14, 2001.

41. The Plastics Historical Society. The Plastics Museum: Materials: Naturals: Shellac. Available at: http://www.plastics-museum.com/materials/naturals/shellac.htm. Accessed May 14, 2001.

42. Grossman LI. Denture base materials. In: *Dental Formulas and Aids to Dental Practice.* Philadelphia: Lea and Febiger; 1952, p. 318.

43. Trammsdorff E, Schildknecht CE. Polymerization in suspension. In: Schildknecht CE, editor. *Polymer Processes.* New York: Interscience; 1956, p. 69.

44. Fletcher AM, Purnaveja S, Amin WM, Ritchie GM, Moradians S, Dodd AW. The level of residual monomer in self curing denture base materials. *J Dent* 1983;62:118–120.

45. Tsuchiya H, Hoshino Y, Kato H, Takagi N. Flow injection analysis of formaldehyde leached from denture-base acrylic resins. *J Dent* 1993;21:240–243.

46. Simonsen R, Thompson VP, Barrack G. *Etched Cast Restorations: Clinical and Laboratory Techniques.* Hanover Park, IL: Quintessence Publishing; 1983.

47. Schwach-Abdellaoui K, Vivien-Castioni N, Gurny R. Local delivery of antimicrobial agents for the treatment of periodontal diseases. *Eur J Pharm Biopharm* 2000;50:83–99.

48. Tonetti M, Cugini MA, Goodson JM. Zero-order delivery with periodontal placement of tetracycline-loaded ethylene vinyl acetate fibers. *J Periodontol Res* 1990;25:243–249.

49. Sun-Hong M, Ferracane JL, In-Bog L. Effect of shrinkage strain, modulus, and instrument compliance on polymerization shrinkage stress light-cured composites during the initial curing stage. *Dent Mater* 2010;26:1024–1033.

50. Peutzfeldt A. Resin composites in dentistry: The monomer systems. *Eur J Oral Sci* 1997;105:97–116.

51. Hammouda IM. Effect of light method on wear and gardness of composite resin. *J Mech Biomed Mater* 2010;3:216–222.

52. Visvanathan A, Ilie N, Hickel R, Kunzelmann KH. The influence of curing times and light curing methods on the polymerization shrinkage stress of a shrinkage-optimized composite with hybrid-type prepolymer fillers. *Dent Mater* 2007;23:777–784.

53. Behr M, Rosentritt M, Hagenbuch K, Faltermeier A, Handel G. Electron beam irradiation of dental composites. *Dent Mater* 2005;21:804–810.

54. Klapdohr S, Moszner N. New inorganic components for dental filling composites. *Monatsh Chem* 2005;136:21–45.

55. Chen M-H. Update on dental nanocomposites. *J Dent Res* 2010;89:549–60.

56. Jandt KD, Sigusch BW. Future perspectives of resin-based dental materials. *Dent Mater* 2009;8:1001–1006.

57. Bayne SC, Heymann HO, Swift EJ Jr. Update on dental composite restorations. *J Am Dent Assoc* 1994;125:687–701.

58. Wolter H, Glaubitt W, Rose K. Multifunctional (meth) acrylatealkoxysilanes—a new type of reactive compounds. *Mat Res Soc Symp Proc* 1992;271:719–24.

59. Weinmann W, Thalacker C, Guggenberger R. Siloranes indental composites. *Dent Mater* 2005;21:68–74.

60. Ilie N, Hickel R. Silorane-based dental composite: Behavior and abilities. *Dent Mater J* 2006;25:445–454.

61. Eskitascioglu C, Eskitascioglu A, Belli S. Use of polyethylene ribbon to create a provisional fixed partial denture after immediate implant placement. *J Prosthet Dent* 2004;91:11–14.

62. Terry DA, Mcguire M. The perio aesthetic restorative approach for anterior reconstruction. *Pract Proced Aesthet Dent* 2002;14:363–369.

63. Culy G, Tyas MJ. Direct resin bonded fiber reinforced anterior bridges. *Aust Dent J* 1998;43:1–4.

64. Shuman IE. Replacement of tooth with a direct fiber reinforced direct bonded restoration. *Gen Dent* 2000;48:314–318.

65. Belli S, Ozer F. A simple method for single anterior tooth replacement. *J Adhes Dent* 2000;2:67–70.

66. Bae JM, Kim KN, Hattori M, Hasegawa K, Yoshinari M, Kawada E, Oda Yl. The flexural properties of fiber reinforced composites with light polymerized polymer matrix. *Int J Prosth* 2001;14:33–39.

67. Abel, MG. Alternative bridge design. *Oral Health* 1994;84:23–24.

68. Freilich MA, Meiers JC, Duncan JP, Eckrote KA, Goldberg AJ. Clinical evaluation of fiber rein forced fixed bridges. *J Am Dent Assoc* 2002;133:1524–1534.

69. Vallitu PK. Survival rates for resin bonded, glass fiber reinforced composite fixed partial dentures with a mean follow up of 42 months. *J Prosthet Dent* 2004;91:241–246.

70. Behr M, Rosentritt M, Handel G. Fiber reinforced composite crowns and FPDs. *Int J Prosthodont* 2003;16:239–243.

71. Bohlsen F, Kern M. Clinical outcome of glass fiber reinforced crowns and fixed partial dentures, a three year retrospective study. *Quintessence Int* 2003;34:493–496.

72. Monaco C, Ferrari M, Miceli GP, Scotti R. Clinical Evaluation of Fiber-Reinforced Composite Inlay FPDs. *Int Prosthodont* 2003;16:319–325.

73. Pfeiffer P, Grube L. In vitro resistance of reinforced interim fixed partial dentures. *J Prosthet Dent* 2003;89:170–174.

74. Heydenrijk K, Meijer HJ, van der Reijden WA, Raghoebar GM, Vissink A, Stegenga B. Microbiota around root-formendosseous implants: A review of the literature. *Int J Oral Maxillofac Implants* 2002;17(6):829–838.

3 Polymers in Orthopedic Devices

3.1 INTRODUCTION

Bone is a natural organic–inorganic complex and hierarchical tissue that combines high strength with special elastic properties and provides structural framework, protective shield for internal organs and marrow, mechanical strength, blood pH regulation, and maintenance of the calcium and phosphate levels for metabolic processes, and it provides stores of ions necessary for normal body functions [1]. Bone is also a living tissue, with about 15% of its weight being due to the cellular content (osteoblasts, osteocytes, bone lining cells, and osteoclasts) each with their own specific function, and an extracellular matrix. It basically consist of approximately 60% mineral (nanohydroxyapatite (HA,$Ca_{10}(PO_4)_6(OH_2)$)), 30% matrix (collagen, major structural protein of connective tissue), and 10% water by weight, and the ratios of hydroxyapatite-to-collagen-to-water volume and weight fraction depend on age and also species-specific [2–6]. The tensile strength of bone is due to collagen because of its highly aligned and very anisotropic structure. The mineral part of bone adopts a hexagonal geometry with the unit cell crystal dimensions being 9.42 Å in the a and b directions, and 6.88 Å along the c-axis. Bone can be classified as long, short, flat, irregular, and sesamoid. However, it consists of two parts: compact (cortical) bone, which makes outer layers of almost all the bones, 80%–90% mineralized with very few pores and void spaces, very strong, and capable of maintaining the mechanical and protective requirements of the skeleton; and cancellous or trabecular bone, found on the interior of most bones, 15%–25% mineralized, less dense, rich in bone marrow, blood vessels, and connective tissue (Figure 3.1).

Bone defects or fractures are increasing rapidly with age due to extra osseous factors such as the impaired reflex of the elderly, their reduced proprioceptive efficiency, reduced cushioning by fat, weakened musculature, by osseous factors such as the structural changes in the shape and size of the bone, and by deterioration of the condition of the bone material itself; it can also occur due to various reasons including degenerative, neoplasm, congenital defects, motor accident, osteoporosis, arthritis, surgical, and traumatic processes, which significantly compromise quality of life. Another cause may be trauma [1]. Currently, millions of patients are suffering from bone and cartilage defects such as osteoarthritis and rheumatoid arthritis that affect the structure of freely movable (synovial) joints, such as the hip, knee, shoulder, ankle, and elbow, cause considerable pain in such joints, particularly weight-bearing joints like the hip and knee, and the effects on ambulatory function are quite devastating [7,8]. Generally, two types of methods are commonly used as standard procedure for the treatment of bone or cartilage defect: autologous transplantation in which cortical bone is selected for strength and mechanical support, while cancellous bone autografts are used to promote lattice formation and rapid bone regeneration; and allograft or xenograft transplantation in which allogenic bone has been successfully used in osseous reconstruction. Autograft promotes bone formation over its surface by direct bone bonding (osteoconduction) and induces local stem cells to differentiate into bone cells (osteoinduction) without any associated immune response; while in autologous bone grafting fresh cortical or trabecular bone or a combination of both are transplanted from one site in the body, such as the iliac crest, to another within the same patient [9–11]. However, these methods suffer from many problems such as less immunocompatibility, need of a secondary surgery, high cost, possible morbidity, limited quantity of donor tissue, possible transmission of donor pathogens, immunogenic responses, and high risks of infection [12]. Therefore, it is highly desired to synthesize artificial organs and implants for replacement of injured and diseased hard tissues. Recently, researchers are trying to construct the artificial bone with a large number of synthetic materials (metals, metal alloys, collagen, carbon-based materials, polymers, ceramics, and composites) and synthesized as bioactive materials that open new possibilities for clinical application, mainly in orthopedics and dentistry. However, the materials that can be used in successful treatment of bone cartilage defect should exhibit the following properties: excellent biocompatibility; resistance to degradation; be structurally, functionally, and mechanically equal to healthy bone; acceptable strength; low modulus to minimize bone resorption; low cost and cell adhesion; cell proliferation and differentiation for bone tissue regeneration; and high wear resistance to minimize wear-debris generation [13]. Figure 3.2 describes some unassembled parts for total hip replacement and presents broad criteria for orthopedic implant materials.

3.2 MATERIALS USED IN ORTHOPEDIC APPLICATIONS

Bone graft materials represent one of the most common tissue transplants (i.e., allografts, autografts, and synthetic bone grafts substitutes), are quickly becoming a vital tool in reconstructive

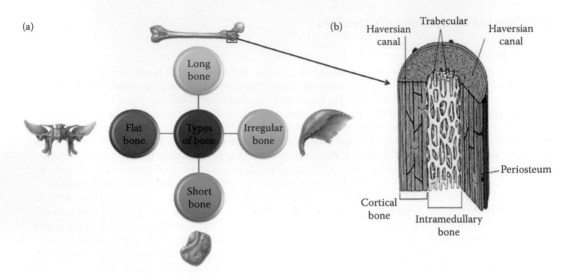

Figure 3.1 (a) A schematic representation of types of bone and (b) its internal structure.

orthopedic surgery, provide a structural substrate for these processes, and serve as a vehicle for direct antibiotic delivery [14]. Regeneration of bone defects caused by trauma, infection, tumors, or inherent genetic disorders leading to abnormal skeletal development is a clinical challenge. With the advancement of science, in last decade, a large number of metals and applied materials have been developed with properties similar to natural bone. Presently, more efforts are given to fabricate porous (provides necessary framework for the bone cells to grow into the pores and integrate with host tissue, known as osteointegration), high strength-to-weight ratio, lower elastic modulus, superior corrosion resistance, biocompatible materials that mimic the architecture and mechanical properties of natural bone because the traditional metallic bone implants are dense and often suffer from the problems of adverse reaction, biomechanical mismatch, and lack of adequate space for new bone tissue to grow into the implant [15].

Various types of synthetic substitutes have been developed in order to comply with biofunctionality and biocompatibility. They belong to the following main material classes:

1. Metals such as titanium, titanium alloys, stainless steel, and cobalt–chromium alloys

2. Ceramics such as aluminum oxide, carbon, calcium phosphates, and glass–ceramics

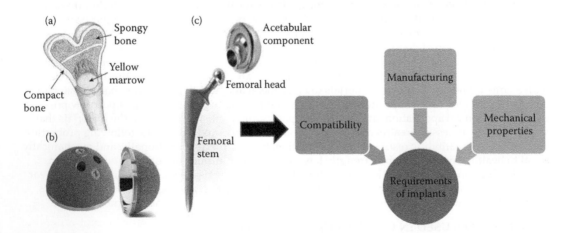

Figure 3.2 Some orthopedic implants: (a) knee joint (femur), (b) hip joint prosthesis, (c) acetabular cup, and basic requirements of implants for application.

3. Polymers such as silicon, poly(methyl methacrylate), polylactide (PLA), poly (urethane), and ultrahigh molecular weight polyethylene (UHMWPE)

4. Composites such as ceramic coating on metal implants or ceramic-reinforced polymers

The choice of one material above another will depend on the application and the type of function that needs replacement. Although numerous types of materials can be involved in this fast developing field, some of them are discussed here.

3.2.1 Metals

Human tissue consists of self-assembled protein, bone minerals, and trace amount of metal (Figure 3.3). The use of metallic materials for medical implants can be traced back to the nineteenth century that have played a predominant role as structural biomaterials in orthopedics as bone repair, typically internal fracture fixation of long bones [16]. Metallic implants have been used either as permanent prostheses (e.g., the total joint replacements, hip prosthesis, and dental implants), or as temporary implants (e.g., bone plates, pins, screws, and rods for the fixation of bone fractures).

Currently, stainless steel [17], cobalt–chrome alloys [18], titanium and its alloys [19] have been used to fabricate the implants. These implants are usually not integrated by the bone tissue or only after extended implantation periods. Improvement of implant integration in bone can either be accomplished by cement fixation, the use of a porous bead implant surface to allow bone ingrowth and thus mechanical fixation or the application of bioactive ceramic coatings. Despite the large number of metals and alloys produced in industry, only a few are biocompatible and capable of long-term success as an implant material because of many limitations, unfavorable corrosion properties, wear, encapsulation by dense fibrous tissues to develop improper stress distribution, and/or adverse tissue reactions [20] (Figure 3.4).

3.2.1.1 Essential Considerations in Design of Metallic Biomaterials

Biomaterials can be defined as a biocompatible substance either natural or synthetic (any instrument, apparatus, implement, machine, appliance, implant, in vitro reagent or calibrator, software, material), designed to be used in intimate contact with living tissue, to replace or assist part of an organ or tissue, or one or more of the specific purposes of diagnosis, prevention, monitoring, treatment, investigation, supporting or sustaining life, control of conception, and disinfection of medical devices [21]. It is essential that the implanted material does not cause any harmful effects and must serve safely and appropriately for a long period of time without rejection. Metallic implant should possess, but not limited to, the following essential characteristics:

1. Excellent biocompatibility (nontoxic elements or their alloying elements should be used)

2. High corrosion resistance (metal should be corrosion resistance because the environment inside the human body is physically and chemically different from ambient conditions, and corrosion may cause chronic allergy and toxic reactions in the host body, which are only diagnosed after a sufficiently long postimplantation period)

3. Suitable mechanical properties (strong and tough, biomaterials must be able to match with natural bone because of their ability to bear significant loads and undergo plastic deformation prior to failure)

4. High wear resistance (materials used for several types of mobile joints between long bones must be wear resistant)

5. Osseointegration (in the case of bone prosthetics), implant to have an appropriate surface to integrate well with surrounding bone. Surface chemistry, surface roughness, and surface topography are all factors that need to be considered for good osseointegration

3.2.1.2 Stainless Steels

Stainless steel (304, 316, and 316L stainless steel), the alloy of iron, chromium, and nickel can be categorized into two groups on the basis of chemical composition: the chromium, used in temporary devices following bone trauma, such as fracture plates, screws and hip nails, and in permanent implants such as total hip replacements, has great affinity for oxygen, which allows formation of an invisible chromium-rich oxide film (~2 nm thick) that is adhesive, promoting self-healing

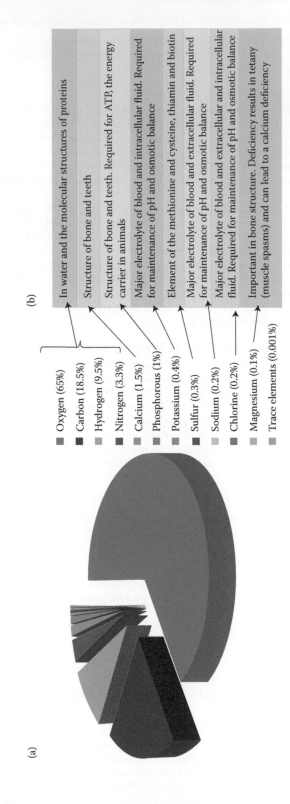

Figure 3.3 Schematic representation of weight percent of elements and their role in human body (a) elements in human body and (b) role in human body.

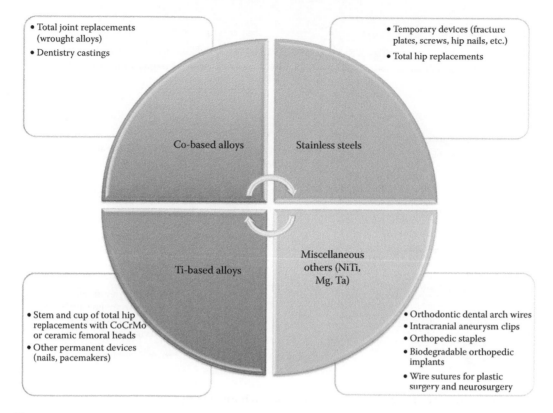

- Total joint replacements (wrought alloys)
- Dentistry castings

- Temporary devices (fracture plates, screws, hip nails, etc.)
- Total hip replacements

Co-based alloys

Stainless steels

Ti-based alloys

Miscellaneous others (NiTi, Mg, Ta)

- Stem and cup of total hip replacements with CoCrMo or ceramic femoral heads
- Other permanent devices (nails, pacemakers)

- Orthodontic dental arch wires
- Intracranial aneurysm clips
- Orthopedic staples
- Biodegradable orthopedic implants
- Wire sutures for plastic surgery and neurosurgery

Figure 3.4 Four categories of metallic biomaterials and their primary applications as implants.

in the presence of oxygen; and chromium–nickel stainless steel (resistance to specific corrosion mechanisms, has desired mechanical and physical properties). It contains a high percentage (11–30 wt%) of chromium (needed to prevent the formation of rust in unpolluted atmosphere), and varying amounts of nickel (increased corrosion resistance by the formation of protective oxide films on the surface of the alloys). Stainless steels can be further classified into four groups on the basis of characteristic microstructure of the alloys: martensitic, ferritic, austenitic, or duplex (austenitic plus ferritic). Except duplex type, other three have applications in medical field; for example, martensitic stainless steels used in dental and surgical instruments, ferrite stainless steels in medical devices, austenitic stainless steels applied in various nonimplantable medical devices where good corrosion resistance and moderate strength are required because of their availability, lower cost, excellent fabrication properties, accepted biocompatibility, and toughness. Their mechanical properties can be controlled over a wide range, for optimal strength and ductility [22]. Today, 316L stainless steels are widely used in a variety of surgical instruments and short-term implant devices due to cost savings. However, corrosion of stainless steel implants in body may be due to pitting, crevices, corrosion fatigue, fretting corrosion, stress corrosion cracking, and galvanic corrosion that can enhance level of iron, chromium, and nickel in body, which may cause many side effects (Figure 3.5).

3.2.1.3 Cobalt-Based Alloys

The cobalt–molybdenum, also called stellite, was developed by Haynes for use in aircraft engines, in 1930, first time used in medical devices or implants due to their higher strength at elevated temperatures and better corrosion resistance property [23–25]. In the 1940s, second alloy of cobalt called vitallium (CoCrMo alloy) was used in dental and orthopedics applications as permanent and short-term implants [22]. The cobalt–chromium alloy shows better corrosion resistance, demonstrating excellent performance in a chloride-rich environment and mechanical properties than stainless steel. In cobalt–chromium alloy, the excellent corrosion resistance and enhanced wear

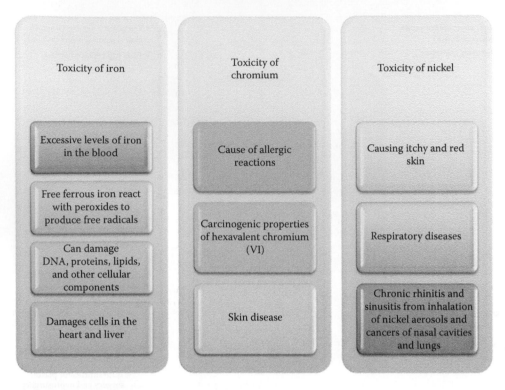

Figure 3.5 Toxicity of iron, chromium, and nickel in human body.

resistance arise due to spontaneous formation of a passive oxide (Cr_2O_3) layer within the human body environment [26–30].

Currently, cobalt–chromium-based alloys such as Co–28Cr–6Mo, Co–20Cr–15W–10Ni, Co–35Ni–20Cr–10Mo, Co–Ni–Cr–Mo–W–Fe, Co–28Cr–6Mo, Co–35Ni–20Cr–10Mo, Co–Cr–Ni–Mo–Fe, and Co–28Cr–6Mo have a high Young's modulus (220–230 GPa), which is much higher than that of cortical bone (20–30 GPa), are widely applied in many biomedical applications due to their enhance wear resistance, solid-solution strengthening, and corrosion resistance properties. However, Co–20Cr–15W–10Ni and Co–Ni–Cr–Mo–W–Fe alloys are not applied in permanent implants due to their unsatisfactory corrosion resistance and a high amount of toxic nickel release when used for permanent implantation. However, there is in general a local release of metallic particles, and in some individuals there is a hypersensitivity reaction that causes more severe damage to the tissues in the immediate vicinity of the prosthesis [31]. It was observed that the toxicity of cobalt alloy is reported after 4–5 years of implantation. The release of cobalt from implants may cause contact dermatitis, interstitial lung disease, painful muscle fatigue and cramping, dyspnea, inability to perform simple motor tasks, decline in cognitive function, memory difficulties, severe headaches, and anorexia [32–34]. ASTM F75, a cast Co–Cr–Mo alloy, is used in artificial hip joints due to its excellent wear resistance, and excellent tribological properties against plastic sockets, that is, in a metal-on-plastic joint [22]. ASTM F799 is a wrought version of F75 alloy, has superior in-fatigue strength imparted by the wrought microstructure and processed by hot forging rough billets to make the final shape. ASTM F90 is a wrought Co–Cr–W–Ni alloy having improved machinability and fabrication characteristics than F75 alloy [35]. Similarly, ASTM F562, a wrought Co–Ni–Cr–Mo alloy, possesses microstructure and excellent mechanical properties [36]. Currently ~20% of total hip replacements have stems and/or the hard-on-hard bearing system made out of wrought CoCrMo alloys. As for total knee and ankle replacements, the prostheses are almost exclusively made out of CoCrMo alloys with UHMWPE as a lining. The cobalt alloys contain Cr, Mo, Ni that also cause many problems when released into body due to corrosion of implants. These problems include irritation to the eyes and skin, accidental deaths, diarrhea, growth retardation, infertility, low birth weight and gout, with further effects on the lungs, kidneys and liver, fatigue, headaches, and joint pains [37–40].

3.2.1.4 Titanium Alloys Used as Orthopedic Implants

Titanium is a low-density element, nontoxic even in large doses, and undergoes an allotropic transformation from an HCP crystal structure (α phase) to a BCC crystal structure (β phase) at approximately 885°C. The high solubility of oxygen and nitrogen also makes titanium unique among metals and also creates problems not of concern to most other metals. For instance, heating titanium in air at high temperatures results not only in oxidation but also in solid-solution hardening of the surface due to the inward diffusion of oxygen (and nitrogen). Presently, titanium alloys are used as biomaterials in various biomedical devices and favored by most clinicians, surgeons, materials scientists, and medical device designers, because they are more inert and more biocompatible than stainless steels and cobalt alloys due to their lower modulus (about half of stainless steels and cobalt–molybdenum alloys), superior biocompatibility and enhanced corrosion resistance, ability to bond with bone, as well as not rejected by the body, and generally making good physical connections with the host bone. Titanium alloys can be categorized into α alloys (low strength and high ductility, ultimate tensile strength (UTS) and yield strength vary from 240 to 550 MPa, and from 170 to 480 MPa, respectively), near-α alloys (contain small additions of b stabilizers), α–β alloys (complex alloys, strengthened by solution treating and aging), and β alloys (second-generation titanium biomaterials, having a modulus closer to that of bone, excellent forgeability, and good cold formability), on the basis of their microstructure after processing [22]. The α–β alloy Ti–6Al–4V is the most widely used titanium alloy, accounting for approximately 45% of total titanium production. V, Al, Nb, Zr, Mo, Fe, and Ta are the most important elements, which are alloyed with titanium to improve its mechanical properties and corrosion resistance nature. Titanium is nontoxic in nature; however, other alloying elements such as vanadium cause problems such as carcinogenicity and various adverse effects on the respiratory system, blood parameters, liver, neurological system, and other organs [41,42]. Aluminum causes reduced skeletal mineralization (osteopenia) observed in infants, kidney disease, contact dermatitis, and digestive disorders [43,44]; niobium is a more toxic metal ion, along with cobalt, tested for their ability to induce DNA damage and causing immune cell death [45]. However, excellent biocompatibility and nonmutagenicity of titanium alloy makes them superior biomaterial, which is safe for humans and animals. However, the first-generation titanium alloy (Ti–6Al–4V [Ti64]) was not good for application in human body because it caused allergic reactions [46]. Thereafter in 1990, Mo, Ta, and Zr are used as alloying elements to synthesize second-generation titanium alloys (β-titanium alloys) that possess lower elastic moduli, good corrosion resistance, free from vanadium, and enhanced biocompatibility in comparison to Ti–6Al–4V and other α–β alloys. The Ti–Nb–Zr–Ta system (TNZT alloys) possesses the lowest elastic moduli of any metallic implant alloy developed to date [47–49].

Pure titanium (CP-Ti) (applied in making pacemaker cases, housings for ventricular-assist devices and implantable infusion drug pumps, dental implants, maxillofacial and craniofacial implants, and screws and staples for spinal surgery) and Ti–6Al–4V ELI (used in dental implants and parts for orthodontic surgery; replacement parts for hip, knee, shoulder, spine, elbow, and wrist joints; bone fixation devices such as nails, screws, and nuts; housing parts for pacemakers and artificial heart valves; surgical instruments and components in high-speed blood centrifuges) are the most commonly used titanium materials for implant applications [50–52]. Hip joint simulation testing has shown that the wear rates of UHMWPE is ~35% greater than Ti–6Al–4V, suggesting the mechanical instability of the metal oxide layer over the surface of Ti alloys as it breaks down by externally applied stresses, not able to heal immediately, leading to further loss of alloy material locally [50]. Some surface modifications are applied to increase wear resistance of titanium alloys, such as nitriding or plasma treatment. Methods such as physical vapor deposition coating (TiN, TiC), ion implantation (N^+), thermal treatments (nitriding and oxygen diffusion hardening), and laser alloying with TiC have been examined for improving wear [53].

3.2.1.5 Stainless Steels, Cobalt, and Titanium Alloys in Total Joint Replacement

In 1890, German surgeon Themistocles Gluck was the first who produced an ivory ball and socket joint, inserted into the knee of a 17-year-old girl and fixed it with bone with nickel-plated screws [54,55]. After that, many attempts were performed by various surgeons and scientists to prepare artificial hip joint with unique design changes, revolutionary surgical procedures, and innovative usage of new and existing materials [56]. Now, modern total hip replacements comprise primarily of three components: stem, head, and socket, which are synthesized from stainless steels (used by Philip Wiles in 1938), Co–Cr alloy (used by Austin Moore in the 1950s). However, the use of stainless steel has been limited due to its poor corrosion, fatigue and wear resistances, and heavy metal toxicity. Today, orthinox-, cobalt/chromium-, or titanium-based alloy, is being used. Cobalt–chromium-based alloys or ceramic materials (aluminum oxide or zirconium oxide) are used in making the ball portions, which are polished smooth to allow easy rotation within the acetabular socket, made of metal, UHMWPE, or a combination of polyethylene backed by metal. With the huge success of application in total hip replacements, cobalt alloys were soon used in other total joint replacements (TJR) for load-bearing sites, including knee and ankle joints [57]. Despite the huge success, failure of the femoral stem and loosening caused by wearing of acetabular components, due to fretting corrosion fatigue, remain major and serious postimplantation complications of all TJR [58].

3.2.2 Ceramics

In orthopedic applications, many ceramics such as calcium sulfate (plaster of Paris), metallic oxides (e.g., Al_2O_3, MgO are nearly bioinert in biological environments), calcium phosphate (e.g., hydroxyapatite [HA] bond to bone in bony sites), tricalcium phosphate (TCP), octacalcium phosphate (OCP), and glass ceramics (e.g., Bioglass, Ceravital) are widely used as bioceramics for hard tissue replacement since long. Hydroxyapatite $Ca_{10}(PO_4)_6(OH)_2$ (HAP) is chemically similar to the mineral component of bones and hard tissues in mammals and widely used in orthopedic and dental fields as a biomedical surface modifier due to its excellent biocompatibility and tissue bioactivity properties (support bone in growth and osseointegration), does not induce adverse local tissue reactions, immunogenicity, or systemic toxicity, increases the rate and longevity of implant fixation and osseointegration, as well as being the material most similar to the mineral component of the bone [59]. Furthermore, because this material is osteoconductive, it acts as a support for new bone formation within the pore sites [60], which are deliberately generated in the structure. However, HAP does not have sufficient tensile strength and is too brittle to be used in most load-bearing applications, as well as its mechanical properties depend on the preparation technique [60,61]. Therefore, HAP can be used in hard tissue replacement by coating it into metal core or by incorporating into polymers as composites [62,63].

3.2.3 Polymer Composites Materials

Many metals are widely used as bone substituents but their density and elastic modulus mismatch with nature bone. Therefore, scientists are trying to develop composite-based biomaterials as a bone substitute material using a synthetic polymer as a matrix and different ceramic material to replace body parts and restoration of human anatomical structures [64–67].

Polymer composites are widely used materials for treatment of bone and cartilage defects due to their unique properties such as avoiding the problem of stress shielding, biodegradability properties that eliminate the need for a second surgical procedure to remove the implants, and also the elimination of the ion release problem of metal implants. The mechanical and bioactivity, that is, bone-bonding ability of polymer composites can be improved by adding a secondary reinforcing phase, or fibers and mineral filler particles into polymer matrix.

3.2.3.1 Fiber-Reinforced Composites (FRC)

Fiber-reinforced composites (FRC) may be totally biodegradable, partially degradable, or nonbiodegradable and can be prepared by incorporation of carbon fiber, aramid (Kevelar), glass fiber into polymers like epoxy resin, polyether ether ketone (PEEK), polysulfone (PS), polymethyl methacrylate (PMMA), poly(lactide) PLA, poly(glycolide), polycaprolactone, etc. The introduction of fiber and filler not only affects its biodegradability but also their mechanical properties. For example, PEEK with 30% carbon fiber has an elastic modulus of 17 GPa and a flexural strength of 320 MPa [68,69]. However, the interfacial bonding strength between fibers and polymer matrix is usually weaker than the polymer matrix [70]. Therefore, the fatigue fractures usually occur at the interface of fiber and polymer. There is clearly a need for the improvement of the interface of fiber/polymer matrix to improve both the mechanical properties of the composites and the wet stability of the interfacial bond.

3.2.3.2 Filler-Reinforced Composites

Filler-reinforced composites contain bioactive fillers such as hydroxyapatite (HA), AW ceramic, or bioglass particles with polymers matrix that show fair mechanical (elastic modulus, fatigue behavior) characteristics, diminishing the creep of the composites, with the possibility to control the biodegradation rate, decreasing the temperature rise during the polymerization of bone cements, and fair biocompatibility and bioactivity during their applications in dental restorative resins and bone cement. HAP-reinforced polymer matrix showed bone apposition and thus creates a secure bond between the natural bone and the implant. The degradation of polymer implant will finally be replaced by bone tissue. The load thus can be gradually transferred to the newly formed bone [71,72].

3.2.4 Polymers

Replacing body parts, and specifically hard tissues, dates back centuries by the use of natural or synthetic materials. Presently, polymer-based hard tissue replacement matrix used for bone replacement purposes have gained much attention due to their biocompatibility, biodegradability (if the implant has to be eliminated after certain period), ability to bond with bone or to induce bone ingrowth, and desired mechanical properties (if the polymer is going to be used as load-bearing material) (Figure 3.6 and Table 3.1). The ideal polymer for an application would have the following properties:

- Does not evoke an inflammatory/toxic response, disproportionate
- Has beneficial effect
- Is metabolized in the body after fulfilling its purpose
- Leaving no trace
- Is easily processed into the final product form
- Has acceptable shelf-life
- Is easily sterilized

At present limited number of polymers such as UHMWPE, PMMA, PLA (tensile strength up to 72 MPa), polyglycolide (PGA) (tensile strength 57 MPa), and polyhydroxybutyrate have been used as very promising candidates for bone replacement (Table 3.2). Figure 3.7 shows synthesis of some polymers used in orthopedic applications. However, their mechanical properties are poorer than bone but there is possibility to improve their mechanical properties by either the modification of the structure of the polymer (includes crosslinking, copolymerization more than one type of monomer, using new type of monomers to synthesize new polymers) or by strengthening the polymer with fiber and/or filler.

The second important property of polymer is biodegradation, which makes them suitable for short-time bone replacement materials which can be improved by introducing ester bonds, imino bonds, etc. to the polymer structure. However, their mechanical properties are weaker than cortical bone. The third important criteria for polymers to be selected as the materials for bone defect treatment is the bone-bonding property. Presently, polyethylene glycol/polybutylene terephthalate (PEG/PBT) block copolymer (Polyactive™) has been identified as a "bone-bonding polymer"

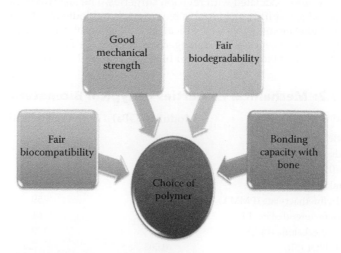

Figure 3.6 The criteria for selection of polymers for treatment of bone defects.

Table 3.1: Various Factors of Importance in Materials Selection for Orthopedic Applications

Factors	Description		
First level material properties	Chemical/biological characteristics	Physical characteristics	Mechanical/structural characteristics
	Chemical composition (bulk and surface)	Density	Elastic modulus
			Poisson's ratio
			Yield strength
			Tensile strength
			Compressive strength
Second level material properties	Adhesion	Surface topology (texture and roughness)	Hardness
			Shear modulus
			Shear strength
			Flexural modulus
			Flexural strength
Specific functional requirements (based on application)	Biofunctionality (nonthrombogenic, cell adhesion, etc.)	Form (solid, porous, coating, film, fiber, mesh, powder)	Stiffness or rigidity
	Bioinert (nontoxic, nonirritant, nonallergic, noncarcinogenic, etc.)	Geometry	Fracture toughness
		Coefficient of thermal expansion	Fatigue strength
	Bioactive	Electrical conductivity	Creep resistance
	Biostability (resistant to corrosion, hydrolysis, oxidation, etc.)	Color, esthetics	Friction and wear resistance
		Refractive index	Adhesion strength
		Opacity or translucency	Impact strength
	Biogradation		Proof stress
			Abrasion resistance
Processing and fabrication	Reproducibility, quality, sterilizability, packaging, secondary processability		

because the PEG segments of the material can create complex with calcium ions and thus cause calcification of the polymer, which is a prerequisite for the following bone-bonding to occur. This property of polymers can be improved by the introduction of certain functional groups, like the phosphinyl group, the carboxylic acid group, the sulfonate group, fluoride, to the polymer chain or the surface. Tretinnikov et al. [73] synthesized phosphate groups containing high-density polyethylene (HDPE) for bone substitute. They found that introduction of phosphate groups on the surface of HDPE initiated the formation of a firmly bonded carbonated apatite layer on the surface in physiologic solution when implanted in the rat femur.

Although significant advances have been made in medical techniques that reconstitute damaged organs or tissues as a result of an accident, trauma, or cancer, transplantation of organs or tissues is still a widely accepted therapy to treat patients. The major driving force being the long-term biocompatibility issues with many of the existing permanent implants and many levels of ethical and technical issues associated with revision surgeries. The last two decades of the twentieth century saw a paradigm shift from biostable biomaterials to biodegradable (hydrolytically and enzymatically degradable) biomaterials for medical and related applications because they could help the body to repair and regenerate the damaged tissues [74–76]. There are several reasons for the favorable consideration of biodegradable over biostable materials for orthopedic applications.

Table 3.2: Mechanical Properties of Typical Biomaterials

Material	Modulus (GPa)	Tensile Strength (MPa)
Polyethylene (PE)	0.88	35
Polyurethane (PU)	0.02	35
Polytetrafluoroethylene (PTFE)	0.5	27.5
Polyacetal (PA)	2.1	67
Polymethylmethacrylate (PMMA)	2.55	59
Polyethylene terepthalate (PET)	2.85	61
Polyetheretherketone (PEEK)	8.3	139
Silicone rubber (SR)	0.008	7.6
Polysulfone (PS)	2.65	75

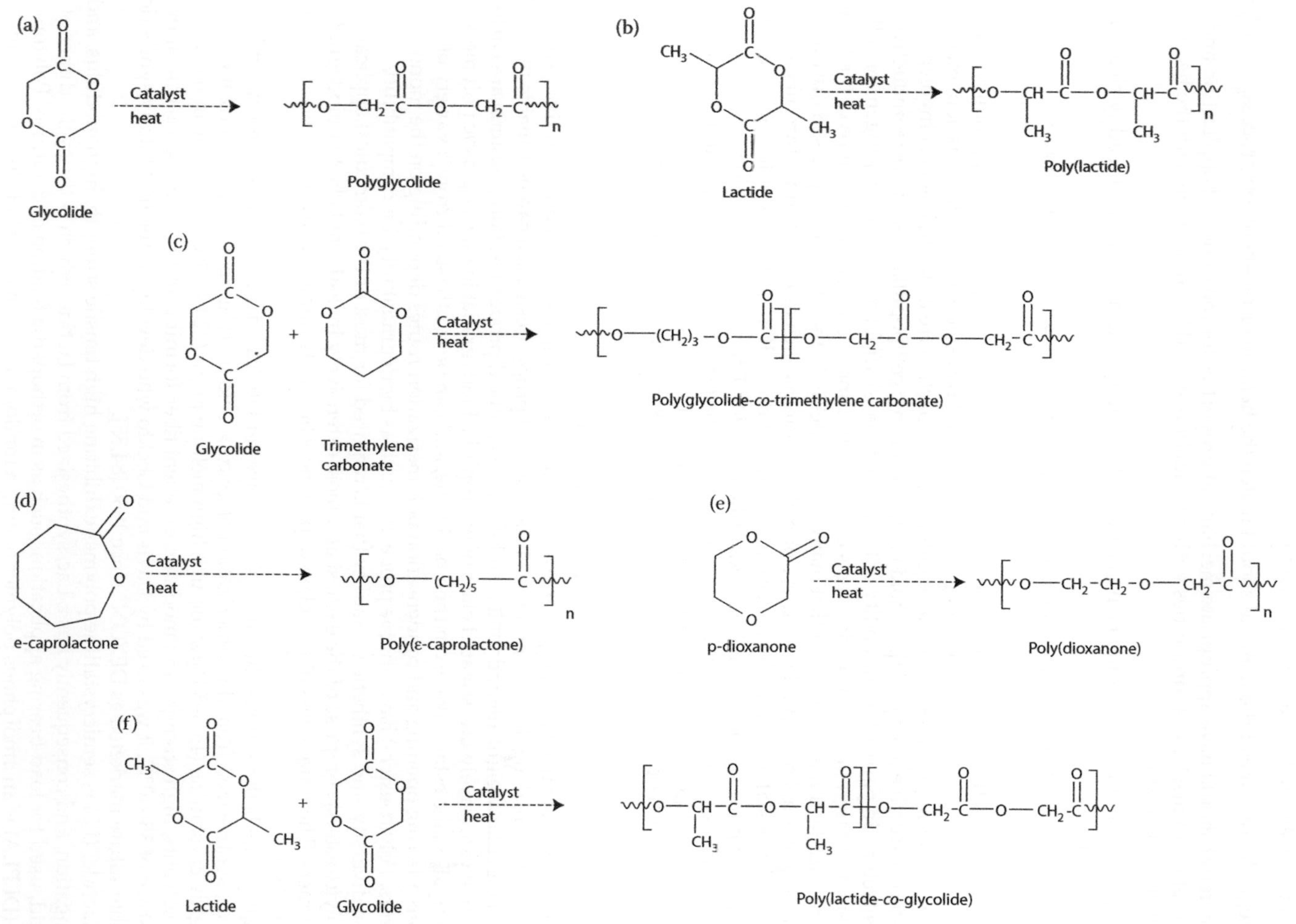

Figure 3.7 A schematic representation of synthesis route of various polymers (a) polyglycole, (b) poly(lactide), (c) poly(glycolide-*co*-trimethylene carbonate), (d) poly(ε-caprolactone), (e) poly(dioxanone), and (f) poly(lactide-*co*-glycolide).

Some of the important properties of a biodegradable biomaterial can be summarized as follows [77]:

1. The material should not evoke a sustained inflammatory or toxic response upon implantation in the body.

2. The material should have acceptable shelf-life.

3. The degradation time of the material should match the healing or regeneration process.

4. The material should have appropriate mechanical properties for the indicated application and the variation in mechanical properties with degradation should be compatible with the healing or regeneration process.

5. The degradation products should be nontoxic, and able to get metabolized and readily cleared from the body.

6. The material should have appropriate permeability and processability for the intended application.

Bone formation is the result of sequential events that begin with recruitment and proliferation of osteoprogenitor cells from surrounding tissues, followed by osteoblastic differentiation, matrix formation, and mineralization. A tissue engineering approach to treat skeletal defects involves the use of osteoconductive biomaterial scaffolds with osteogenic cell populations and osteoinductive bioactive factors. In particular, the ability of the biomaterial scaffold to allow osteoprogenitor cell attachment and migration in the early stages of wound healing is crucial for later steps of the bone formation cascade. It has been found that many glycoproteins in the ECM are expressed during new bone formation. For example, a variety of matrix proteins such as osteopontin, thrombospondin, and bone sialoprotein, which were important in bone cell migration, proliferation, matrix deposition, and mineralization, have been identified [78–80]. The integration of biomimetic scaffolds into bone tissue takes place at the material–tissue interface that is often determined by initial cell and substrate interactions [81]. Thus, it may be necessary to design biomimetic scaffolds modified with bone matrix proteins that serve as biological cues for cell–matrix interactions to promote bone growth [82].

3.2.4.1 Polyesters

Polyesters are widely used in indegradable bone fixation, soft tissue suture, bone void filler, soft tissue regeneration, drug delivery because of their special properties which can be tunable by varying molecular weight, degradability, and good mechanical properties. Poly(α-esters) are earliest and most extensively investigated class of hydrophilic biodegradable thermoplastic polymers containing aliphatic ester linkages in their backbone, and can be synthesized from a variety of monomers via ring opening and condensation polymerization routes depending on the monomeric units. Poly(α-esters) have unique properties such as biodegradability, biocompatibility, immense diversity, and synthetic versatility that is required for most of the biomedical applications. Poly(α-esters) comprise of the earliest and most extensively investigated class of biodegradable polymers. The uniqueness of this class of polymers lies in its immense diversity and synthetic versatility [83].

Poly(glycolide) is the simplest linear aliphatic polyester fabricated into a variety of forms and structures, synthesized from the dimerization of glycolic acid by ring-opening polymerization, have highly crystalline (45%–55%) structure, high melting point (220–225°C), insoluble in most organic solvents, high strength and modulus, excellent fiber-forming ability, and a glass transition temperature of 35–40°C. It was used by Davis and Geckto who developed the first totally synthetic absorbable suture marketed as DEXON® since 1960 [84,85].

Poly(lactide) (PL) is semicrystalline polymer exhibiting high tensile strength, high modulus, and low elongation, and consequently has a Lac, synthesized from lactide, which is the cyclic dimer of lactic acid, used for load-bearing applications such as in orthopedic fixation and sutures. Poly(DL-lactide) (DLPLA) is an amorphous polymer having a random distribution of both isomeric forms of lactic acid and suitable for drug delivery applications due to its noncrystalline organized structure, lower tensile strength, and higher elongation and much more rapid degradation time.

Poly(L-lactide) is another polyester compound, which has approximately 35% crystalline structure and slow degradation rate (requiring greater than 2 years to be completely absorbed), melting point of 175–178°C, and a glass transition temperature of 60–65°C [86–88]. The copolymers of L-lactide with glycolide or DL-lactide, that is, poly(lactide-*co*-glycolide) (PLG) have been widely used in orthopedic and drug delivery applications because copolymerization disrupt the L-lactide-crystallinity and accelerate the degradation process [85,89]. PLGA has been shown to undergo bulk erosion through hydrolysis of the ester bonds and the rate of degradation depends on a variety of parameters including the LA/GA ratio, molecular weight, and the shape and structure of the matrix. The Biologically Quiet™ line of products composed of 85/15 poly(DL-lactide-*co*-glycolide) are used as suture anchors and as screws and plates for craniomaxillo facial repair, respectively [90,91]. A composite PLGA–collagen matrix is currently in the market (CYTOPLAST Resorb®) as a guided tissue regeneration membrane. LUPRON DEPOT® is a drug delivery vehicle composed of PLGA used for the release of a gonadotropin-releasing hormone analog for prostate cancer and endometriosis.

Poly(ε-caprolactone) (PCL) is a semicrystalline polymer (m.p. 59–64°C, T_g 60°C), prepared from the ring-opening polymerization of ε-caprolactone, has a degradation time of the order of 2 years (undergoes hydrolytic degradation due to the presence of hydrolytically labile aliphatic ester linkages), having the ability to form miscible blends with wide range of polymers, low tensile strength (approximately 23 MPa), but an extremely high elongation at breakage (~700%). However, the copolymers of ε-caprolactone with DL-lactide show fast degradation [92]. Ethicon synthesized monofilament suture MONOCRYL® by block copolymerization of ε-caprolactone with glycolide has reduced stiffness compared to pure PGA [84,93,94]. PDS® is the first nontoxic clinically tested monofilament suture of poly(dioxanone) (a polyether-ester), synthesized by the ring-opening polymerization of *p*-dioxanone, has about 55% crystallinity (T_g ~10–0°C) [85]. It is also used as absorbable pin for fracture fixation market by Johnson and Johnson Orthopedics [90].

High-molecular-weight flexible poly(trimethylenecarbonate) (PTMC), also called polyglyconate, can be obtained by the ROP of trimethylene carbonate, is widely used in sutures(MAXON®), tacks, and screws (Acufex®), is copolymers of glycolide with trimethylene carbonate, has better flexibility than pure PGA, and absorbed in about 7 months [85]. BIOSYN® is the trade name of copolymer of TMC and *p*-dioxanone (terpolymer composed of glycolide, trimethylene carbonate, and dioxane), used in suture due to its high rate of degradation, and reduced stiffness compared to pure PGA fibers [90].

Poly(amino acids) are natural polymers but less used in biomedical field due to high crystallinity, insolubility, antigenicity of polymers with more than three amino acids, and very slow rate of degradation, making them inappropriate for use in vivo [95]. Poly(ester amide) derived from symmetrical bisamide-diols and succinyl chloride led to its investigation as a potential bioresorbable suture materials due to their good mechanical and thermal properties, as well as degradable in nature that take place by the hydrolytic cleavage of the ester bonds.

Polyanhydrides and the polyorthoesters are also used in biomedical applications as drug delivery carriers. Polyanhydrides are extensively investigated biodegradable surface-eroding polymers specifically designed and developed for drug delivery applications. Degradable, biocompatible polymers are synthesized by the dehydration of diacid molecules by melting polycondensation, and their degradation rate can be controlled by monomer selection. Gliadel® has been produced by Guilford, and approved by FDA for delivery of BCNU in the brain [85,96]. Alzamer® is poly(ortho esters)-based material produced by ALZA corporation and used as a hydrophobic, surface-eroding polymer designed specifically for drug delivery applications.

3.2.4.2 Polymethyl Methacrylate

Poly methyl methacrylate (PMMA)-based acrylic resins are nonbiodegradable polymers, prepared by free radical polymerization of methyl methacrylate, and most commonly used polymeric materials in denture dentistry as individual impression trays and orthodontic devices such as bone replacement, load-bearing sites, bone void filler (cement) fixation of hip prostheses, and vertebroplasty.

3.2.4.3 Poly(ethyleneglycol)

PEG is another polymer that is widely used in biomedical applications such as drug and cosmetic excipient, hard and soft tissue repair due to its hydrophilicity, ability to make injectable water gel, antithrombogenicity, degradability, and good biocompatibility. Although its application in bone tissue engineering is limited to minimal or no load-bearing areas, PEG is an excellent candidate to deliver growth factors with controlled release kinetics and minimal adverse effects on the activity and half-life.

3.2.4.4 Polyphosphazenes

Polyphosphazenes are inorganic–organic hybrid polymers with a backbone of alternating phosphorus and nitrogen atoms containing two organic side groups attached to each phosphorus atom, showing unprecedented functionality, synthetic flexibility, and adaptability, as the side groups play a crucial role in determining the properties for these polymers. This allows for the possibility of designing and developing polymers with highly controlled properties such as extent of crystallinity, solubility, appropriate thermal transitions, and hydrophobicity/hydrophilicity. Therefore, they have also been investigated as potential biodegradable biomaterials.

3.2.4.5 Natural Polymers

Natural polymers such as collagen, fibrin, alginate, silk, hyaluronic acid, and chitosan are used in bone tissue engineering due to their properties such as biocompatible, degradable, and readily solubilized in physiological fluids. However, they have several disadvantages such as immunogenicity, difficulty in processing, and a potential risk of transmitting animal-originated pathogens [97]. Collagen is the most abundant extracellular matrix (ECM) protein, is the main organic component that is originally secreted by osteoblasts, which can be fabricated as gels, nanofibers, porous scaffolds, and films, and actively investigated as favorable artificial microenvironment for bone ingrowth, as drug delivery carriers due to its biocompatibility [98–102]. However, it is mechanically weak and undergoes rapid degradation upon implantation. Therefore, optimization of degradation rate and molecular properties may be required by crosslinking of collagen with appropriate chemical reagents such as difunctional or multifunctional aldehydes, carbodiimides, hexamethylene-diisocyanate, polyepoxy compounds, and succinimidyl ester polyethyleneglycol, can also occur by thermal or high-energy irradiation, as well as by chemical modification. Several collagen-based gentamicin delivery vehicles are currently on the market worldwide (Sulmycin®-Implant, Collatamp®-G), showing a prolonged local delivery of antibiotics with very low systemic exposure. Duragen® is a suture-free, 3D collagen matrix graft developed for spinal dural repair and regeneration, currently undergoing late-stage clinical trial [103]. Collagraft® is a composite of fibrillar collagen, hydroxyapatite, and tricalcium phosphate, and has been FDA approved for use as a biodegradable synthetic bone graft substitute [104].

Fibrin, derived from blood clots, is enzymatically cross linked to form a gel as adhesive glue that showed bone healing property, and used as soft tissue healing, bone void filler [105]. Chitosan, deacetylated derivative of chitin and linear polysaccharide, has been formulated as a sponge, porous scaffold, and nanofiber, and combined with many growth factors to promote bone formation [106,107].

3.3 ADVANCE BIOMATERIALS

The main focus of research in implantology is the development of an optimal implant, which means that the choice of design, the implant length, as well as the implant surface will be carried out intensively and made according to the prerequisites of the individual case. Bone implants primarily refer to orthopedic prostheses like bone grafts, bone plates, fins, and fusion devices; orthopedic fixation devices such as interference screws in the ankle, knee, and hand areas, rods, and pins for fracture fixation, screws and plates for craniomaxillo facial repair; bone tissue engineering scaffolds as autografts or allografts for fractures and dental implants [108]. The fact that the design of implants has an influence on osseointegration is well known. Stability and osseointegration of an implant are also dependent on the prosthetic restoration. Despite short and mini-implants, it is nevertheless possible that implants cannot be immediately inserted due to lack of bone. In order to increase the natural bone, there is need for substitution materials. The interdisciplinary nature of this field has made it possible for researchers to incorporate principles from various allied areas like pharmaceutics, bioengineering, biotechnology, chemistry, electronics, biophysics, etc. to develop superior medical solutions, offering better prospects to the patient. In last decade, a great amount of research activity has been initiated to synthesize ideal bone substitute by employing principles of nanotechnology to healing fractures (Figure 3.8). Recently, Frician et al. fabricated scaffolds of cross-linked pullulan and dextran supplemented with nanohydroxyapatite (nHA) particles and in vitro studies revealed the expression of early and late bone-specific markers with human bone marrow stromal cells in a medium deprived of osteoinductive factors. Moreover this composite matrix induced a highly mineralized tissue in small and large animal models (goat and rats, respectively), new osteoid tissue formation in the defect region, and direct contact of bone tissue regeneration with the scaffold matrix attributed to the nanoscale HA [109]. Similarly, chitosan/nanohydroxyapatite/Cu–Zn alloy NP composite scaffolds with enhanced antibacterial activity

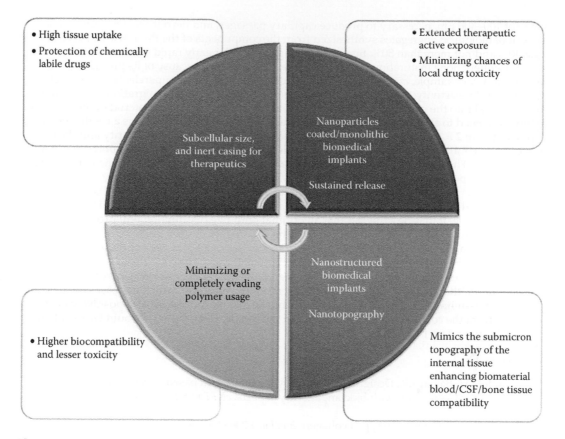

Figure 3.8 Advantages of nanoengineering on biomedical implants.

have been indicated as potential for bone tissue engineering [110]. The same group has also suggested the incorporation of nanosilica in composite scaffolds for this application [6]. The above-mentioned NP-based technologies for bone implants are noncomprehensive as they have been mentioned for representational purposes only. The scope is unlimited and research is ongoing.

Si_3N_4 and SiC are nonoxide ceramic materials, containing amorphous and partially crystalline grain boundary phases, which are used in under extreme thermal and mechanical conditions, possess high hardness, as well as unusually high strength and fracture toughness [21], which make them suitable for total joint replacement (TJR) applications because they have an increased ductility and resistance to high loads. Carbon-fiber reinforced (CFR) polyarylehterehterketone (PEEK), which is produced by injection molding with a certain amount of either pitch or polyacrylnitrile fibers, was rarely considered as candidate for a new bearing material following poor results with early CFR PE in 980. Nanocrystalline diamond (NCD) is another type of diamond-based material, which consists of sp3 diamond bonds and has grain sizes ranging from 3 to ~100 nm. It is interesting for a variety of applications, including use as a TJR bearing material. NCD coatings can be deposited up to a thickness of several microns from an activated gas phase containing carbon and hydrogen, for example, methane, using low-pressure CVD techniques at increased temperatures of 550–800°C. In the 1980s, nitrated titanium (TiN) was considered as the first ceramic coating for total hip and knee replacements. TiN, as well as titanium niobium nitride (TiNbN), titanium carbonate (TiC), and titanium carbon nitride (TiCN), are deposited by physical vapor deposition (PVD) or ion implantation. They are easily identifiable through their golden color and, compared with the metal substrate, exhibit an increase in hardness and a decrease in metal-ion release from the substrate [111].

3.4 MATERIAL PROPERTY REQUIREMENTS FOR BONE REPLACEMENT

The bone replacement materials must possess the porous nature because size is also an important factor in tissue or biological aggregate growth. Synthetic materials must contain pore sizes in the range of 100–400 μm, necessary to produce capillary passages, and permit the development or growth of biological aggregates synthesized from the components of the fluid, with a porosity of at least 40% and not more than 80%. Such morphology allows for early rapid cartilaginous ingrowth and subsequent bone maturation over the lifetime of the implant because of its physicomechanical qualities, for example, mechanical durability, corrosion resistance, superelasticity, and deformational cycloresistivity. Capillarity is advantageous in that it promotes migration of a desired fluid material into the network of passageways, and retention of the fluid material in the network without the need to apply external hydraulic forces. In general, the network has a coefficient of permeability of 2×10^{-13} to 2×10^{-5}, and the permeability is isotropic. The capillarity and the isotropic character are achieved when the network defining the porosity comprises pores of different pore sizes. The ideal implant material would also match Young's modulus of the parent bone. The size of the pores, the directional penetrability, and the coefficient of wettability for biological fluids as well as factors such as differential hydraulic pressure in the saturated and unsaturated porous materials determine the speed and adequacy of penetration of the biological fluid into the porous article. It may be expected that an optimal pore size distribution will provide permeability to the fluid and effective contact for bonding of components (e.g., cells, extra cellular matrix proteins) within the fluid to the interior pore surfaces of the article; the area of these surfaces depends on the pore sizes and the pore size distribution. If the pore size is decreased, the permeability changes unpredictably, since, on the one hand, the hydraulic resistance increases, while, on the other hand, the capillary effect appears at a certain low pore size, which increases the permeability. As for an implant, the material should be minimally biocompatible and positively bioactive. Also from the commercial aspect, the product of combustion synthesis would be acceptable machinability and/or formability [112,113].

REFERENCES

1. Bundela H, Bajpai AK. Designing of hydroxyapatite-gelatin based porous matrix as bone substitute: Correlation with biocompatibility aspects. *eXPRESS Polym Lett* 2008;2(3):201–213.

2. Lees S. Mineralization of type I collagen. *Biophys J* 2003;85:204–207.

3. Vuong J, Hellmich C. Bone fibrillogenesis and mineralization: Quantitative analysis and implications for tissue elasticity. *J Theor Biol* 2011;287:115–130.

4. Fritsch A, Hellmich C, Dormieux L. Ductile sliding between mineral crystals followed by rupture of collagen crosslinks (experimentally supported micromechanical explanation of bone strength). *J Theor Biol* 2009;260:230–252.

5. Biltz RM, Pellegrino ED. The chemical anatomy of bone. I. A comparative study of bone composition in sixteen vertebrates. *J Bone Joint Surg* 1969;51:456–466.

6. Sowjanya JA, Singh J, Mohita T, Sarvanan S, Moorthi A, Srinivasan N et al. Biocomposite scaffolds containing chitosan/alginate/nano-silica for bone tissue engineering. *Coll Surf B* 2013;109:294–300.

7. Laurencin CT, Khan Y, Kofron M, El-Amin S, Botchwey E, Yu X et al. The ABJS Nicolas Andry Award: Tissue engineering of bone and ligament: A 15-year perspective. *Clin Orthop Relat Res* 2006;447:221–236.

8. Hunziker EB. Articular cartilage repair: Basic science and clinical progress. A review of the current status and prospects. *Osteoarthr Cartil* 2002;10:432–463.

9. Zhang J, Liu W, Schnitzler V, Tancret F, Bouler JM. Calcium phosphate cements for bone substitution: Chemistry, handling and mechanical properties. *Acta Biomater* 2014;10:1035–1049.

10. Goulet JA, Senunas LE, DeSilva GL, Greenfield MLVH. Autogenous iliac crest bone graft. *Clin Orthop Relat Res* 1997;339:76–81.

11. Moore WR, Graves SE, Bain GI. Synthetic bone graft substitutes. *ANZ J Surg* 2001;71:354–361.

12. Allison DC, McIntyre JA, Ferro A, Brien E, Menendez LR. *Curr Orthop Pract* 2013;24:267–279, 210.1097/BCO.1090b1013e3182910f3182994

13. Langer R, Vacanti JP. Tissue Engineering. *Science* 1993;260:920–926.

14. Beaman FD, Bancroft LW, Peterson JJ, Kransdorf MJ. Bone graft materials and synthetic substitutes. *Radiol Clin North Am* 2006;44:451–461.

15. Nouri A, Hodgson PD, Wen C. Biomimetic porous titanium scaffolds for orthopedic and dental applications. In: Mukherjee A, editor. *Biomimetics Learning from Nature.* Croatia: InTech; 2010.

16. Park JB, Lakes RS. *Biomaterials: An Introduction.* New York: Springer; 2007.

17. Small IA, Misiek D. A sixteen-year evaluation of the mandibular staple bone plate. *J Oral Maxillof Surg* 1986;44:60–67.

18. Albrektsson T, Zarb G, Worthington P, Ericsson AS. The long-term efficacy of currently used dental implants: A review and proposed criteria of success. *Int J Oral Maxillof Impl* 1986;1:11–25.

19. Steflik DE, Sisk AL, Parr GR, Gardner LK, Hanes PJ, Lake FT et al. Osteogenesis at the dental implant interface: High-voltage electron microscopic and conventional transmission electron microscopic observations. *J Biomed Mater Res* 1993;27:791–800.

20. Hench LL, Ethridge EC. *Biomaterials: An Interfacial Approach.* New York: Academic Press; 1982.

21. Andreas F von Recum. *Handbook of Biomaterials Evaluation: Scientific, Technical and Clinical Testing of Implant Materials.* London, UK: Taylor & Francis; 1999. p. 719.

22. Metallic materials. In: Davies JR, editor. *Handbook of Materials for Medical Devices.* Ohio: ASM International, Materials Park; 2003. p. 21–50.

23. Sumita M, Hanawa T. Failure processes in biometallic materials. *Bioengineering* 2003;9:131–167.

24. Nakazawa K, Sumita M, Maruyama N. Fatigue and fretting fatigue of austenitic and ferritic stainless steels in pseudo-body fluid. *J Jpn Inst Met* 1999;63:1600–1608.

25. Nakazawa K, Sumita M, Maruyama N. Fatigue and fretting fatigue of austenitic and ferritic stainless steels in pseudo-body fluid. In: Wu XR, editor. *Fatigue'99: Proceedings of the 7th International Fatigue Congress,* Beijing, P.R. China, June 8–12, 1999, EMAS Publishing, vol. 2, p. 1359–1364.

26. Alvarado J. Biomechanics of hip and knee prostheses. In: *Applications of Engineering Mechanics in Medicine.* Mayaguez: GED—University of Puerto Rico; 2003.

27. Navarro M, Michiardi A, Castaño O, Planell JA. Biomaterials in orthopedics. *J R Soc Int* 2008;5:1137–1158.

28. Ramsden JJ, Allen DM, Stephenson DJ, Alcock JR, Peggs GN, Fuller G et al. *CIRP Ann Manuf Technol* 2007;56:687–711.

29. Öztürk O, Türkan U, Eroğlu AE. Metal ion release from nitrogen ion implanted CoCrMo orthopedic implant material. *Surf Coat Technol* 2006;200:5687–5697.

30. Vidal CV, Muñoz AI. Effect of thermal and applied potential on the electrochemical behaviour of CoCrMo biomedical alloy. *Electrochim Acta* 2009;54:1798–1809.

31. Jones DA, Lucas HK, Odriscoll M, Price CHG, Wibberley B. Cobalt toxicity after McKee hip arthroplasty. *J Bone Joint Surg Am* 1975;57:289–296.

32. Mao X, Wong AA, Crawford RW. Cobalt toxicity—An emerging clinical problem in patients with metal-on-metal hip prostheses? *Med J Aust* 2011;194:649–651.

33. Basketter DA, Angelini G, Ingber A, Kern PS, Menne T. Nickel, chromium and cobalt in consumer products: Revisiting safe levels in the new millennium. *Contact Dermatitis* 2003;49:1–7.

34. Lison D. Human toxicity of cobalt-containing dust and experimental studies on the mechanism of interstitial lung disease (hard metal disease). *Crit Rev Toxicol* 1996;26:585–616.

35. Brunski JB. Metals. In: Ratner BD, Hoffman AS, Schoen FJ, Lemons JE, editors. *Biomaterials Science: An Introduction to Materials in Medicine*. London: Academic Press; 1996. p. 37–50.

36. Davis JR et al., editors. *Cobalt-Based Alloys*. Materials Park, Ohio: ASM International; 2000.

37. Barceloux DG. Cobalt. *J Toxicol Clin Toxicol* 1999;37:231–237.

38. Liber K, Doig LE, White-Sobey SL. Toxicity of uranium, molybdenum, nickel, and arsenic to Hyalella azteca and Chironomus dilutus in water-only and spiked-sediment toxicity test. *Ecotoxicol Environ Saf* 2011;74:1171–1179.

39. Anke M, Seifert M, Arnhold W, Anke S, Schaefer U. The biological and toxicological importance of molybdenum in the environment and in the nutrition of plants, animals and man part V: Essentiality and toxicity of molybdenum. *Acta Aliment* 2010;39:12–26.

40. Vyskocil A, Viau C. Assessment of molybdenum toxicity in humans. *J Appl Toxicol* 1999;19:185–192.

41. Rhoads LS, Silkworth WT, Roppolo ML, Whittingham MS. Cytotoxicity of nanostructured vanadium oxide on human cells in vitro. *Toxicol In Vitro* 2010;24:292–296.

42. Ress NB, Chou BJ, Renne RA, Dill JA, Miller RA, Roycroft JH et al. Carcinogenicity of inhaled vanadium pentoxide in F344/N rats and B6C3F1 mice. *Toxicol Sci* 2003;74:287–296.

43. Kerr DNS, Ward MK, Ellis HA, Simpson W, Parkinson IS. Aluminium intoxication in renal disease. *Ciba Found Symp* 1992;169:123–141.

44. Darbre PD. Metalloestrogens: An emerging class of inorganic xenoestrogens with potential to add to the oestrogenic burden of the human breast. *J Appl Toxicol* 2006;26:191–197.

45. Caicedo M, Jacobs JJ, Reddy A, Hallab NJ. Analysis of metal ion-induced DNA damage, apoptosis, and necrosis in human (Jurkat) T-cells demonstrates Ni2+ and V3+ are more toxic than other metals: Al3+, Be2+, Co2+, Cr3+, Cu2+, Fe3+, Mo5+, Nb5+, Zr2. *J Biomed Mater Res A* 2008;86A:905–913.

46. Niinomi M. Recent research and development on titanium for biomedical applications in Japan. *J Miner Met Mater Soc* 1999;51:32–34.

47. Niinomi M. Biologically and mechanically biocompatible titanium alloys. *Mater Trans* 2008;49:2170–2178.

48. Niinomi M. Recent metallic materials for biomedical applications. *Metall Mater Trans A* 2002;33:477–486.

49. Niinomi M. Recent biocompatible metallic materials. In: Niinomi N, Okabe T, Taleff EM, Lesure DR, Lippard HE, editors. *Structural Biomaterials for the 21st Century, 2001, the 2001 TMS Annual Meeting in New Orleans*, LA, on February 11–12, p. 3–14.

50. Kirby RS, Heard SR, Miller P, Eardley I, Holmes S, Valve J. *J Urol* 1992;148:1192–1195.

51. Machara K, Doi K, Matsushita T, Susaki Y. Application of vanadium-free titanium alloys to artificial hip joints. *Mater Trans* 2002;43:2936–2942.

52. Akahori T, Niinomi M, Hisao H, Ogawa M, and Toda H. Improvement in fatigue characteristics of newly developed beta type titanium alloy for biomedical applications by thermomechanical treatments. *Materl Sci Eng C* 2005;25(3):278–254.

53. Long M, Rack HJ. Titanium alloys in total joint replacement—A materials science perspective.*Biomaterials* 1998;19:1621–1639.

54. Hughes S, McCarthy I. *Science Basic to Orthopaedics*. Philadelphia, PA: WB Saunders Company Ltd.; 1998.

55. Rang M. *Anthology of Orthopaedics*. London: Churchil Livingstone; 1966.

56. Pramanik S, Agarwal AK, Rai KN. Chronology of total hip joint replacement and materials. *Trends Biomater Artif Organs* 2005;19:15–26.

57. Luetjring G, Albrecht J, Sauer C, Krull T. The influence of soft, precipitate-free zones at grain boundaries in Ti and Al alloys on their fatigue and fracture behaviour. *Mater Sci Eng A* 2007;468:201–209.

58. Rostoker W, Chao EYS, Galante JO. *J Biomed Mater Res* 1978;12:635–651.

59. Janaki K, Elamathi S, Sangeetha D. Development and characterization of polymer ceramic composites for orthopedic applications. *Trends Biomater Artif Organs* 2008;22(3):169–178.

60. LeGeros RZ, Parsons JR, Daculsi G, Driessens F, Lee D, Liu ST et al. Significance of the porosity and physical chemistry of calcium phosphate ceramics. Biodegradation-bioresorption. *Ann NY Acad Sci* 1988;523:268–271.

61. Daculsi G, Hartmann DJ, Heughebaert M, Hamel L, Le Nihouannen JC. In vivo cell interactions with calcium phosphate bioceramics. *J Submicrosc Cytol Pathol* 1988;20:379–384.

62. Lemons JE. Hydroxyapatite coatings. *Clin Orthop* 1988;235:220–223.

63. Kamei S, Kato K, Tomita N, Tamai S, Ikada Y. Implantation of hydroxyapatite bonded polymer. *Trans 5th World Biomaterials Congress*, Toronto, II-52; 1996.

64. Vijayalakshmi U, Balamurugan A, Rajeswari S. Synthesis and characterization of porous silica gels for biomedical applications. *Trends Biomater Artif Organs* 2005;18:101–105.

65. Hench LL. Bioceramics: From concept to clinic. *J Am Ceram Soc* 1991;74:1487.

66. Tanner KE, Downer RA, Bonfield W. Clinical applications of hydroxyapatite reinforced materials. *Br Ceramic Trans* 1994;93:104.

67. Pal S, Roy S, Bag S. Hydroxyapatite coating over Alumina-ultra high molecular weight polyethylene composite biomaterials. *Trends Biomater Artif Organs* 2005;18:106–109.

68. Boeree NR, Dove J, Cooper JJ, Knowles J, Hastings GW. Development of a degradable composite for orthopaedic use: Mechanical evaluation of a hydroxyapatite–polyhydroxybutyrate composite material. *Biomaterials* 1993;14:793–796.

69. Bradley JS, Hastings GW, Johnson-Nurse C. Carbon-fibre reinforced epoxy as a high strength, low modulus material for internal fixation plates. *Biomaterials* 1980;1:38–40.

70. Pigott MR, Chua PS, Andeison P. The interface between glass and carbon fibers and thermo setting polymers. *Polym Comp* 1985;6:242–248.

71. Verheyen CCPM, de Wijn JR, van Blitterswijk CA, de Groot K. Evaluation of hydroxyapatite/ poly(L-lactide) composites: Mechanical behavior. *J Biomed Mater Res* 1992;26:1277–1296.

72. Verheyen CCPM, de Wijn JR, van Blitterswijk CA, de Groot K, Rozing PM. Hydroxyapatite/ poly(L-lactide composites: An animal study on push-out strengths and interface histology. *J Biomed Mater Res* 1993;27:433–444.

73. Tretinnikov ON, Kato K, Ikada Y. In vitro hydroxyapatite deposition onto a film surface-grafted with organophosphate polymer. *J Biomed Mater Res* 1994;28:1365–1373.

74. Shalaby SW, Burg KJL, editors. *Absorbable and Biodegradable Polymers (Advances in Polymeric Materials)*. Boca Raton, FL: CRC Press; 2003.

75. Domb AJ, Wiseman DM, editors. *Handbook of Biodegradable Polymers*. Boca Raton: CRC Press; 1998.

76. Piskin E. Biodegradable polymers as biomaterials. *J Biomat Sci Polym Ed* 1995;6:775–795.

77. Lloyd AW. Interfacial bioengineering to enhance surface biocompatibility. *Med Device Technol* 2002;13:18–21.

78. Robey PG, Young MF, Fisher LW, McClain TD. Thrombospondinis an osteoblast-derived component of mineralized extracellular matrix. *J Cell Biol* 1989;108:719–727.

79. Denhardt DT, Guo X. Osteopontin: A protein with diverse functions. *FASEB J* 1993;7:1475–1482.

80. Fisher LW, McBride OW, Termine JD, Young MF. Human bone sialo protein. Deduced protein sequence and chromosom allocalization. *J Biol Chem* 1990;265:2347–2351.

81. Puleo DA, Nanci A. Understanding and controlling the bone–implant interface. *Biomaterials* 1999;20:2311–2321.

82. Rebaron RG, Athanasiou KA. Extracellular matrix cell adhesion peptides: Functional applications in orthopedic materials. *Tissue Eng* 2000;6:82–103.

83. Kirschvink JL, Walker MM, Diebel CE. Magnetite-based magnetoreception. *Curr Opin Neurobiol* 2001;11:462–467.

84. Kohn J, Langer R. Bioresorbable and bioerodible materials. In: Ratner BD, Hoffman AS, Schoen FJ, Lemons JE, editors. *Biomaterials Science*. New York: Academic Press; 1996. p. 64–72.

85. Shalaby SW, Johnson RA. Synthetic absorbable polyesters. In: Shalaby SW, editor. *Biomedical Polymers: Designed to Degrade Systems*. New York: Hanser; 1994. p. 1–34.

86. Daniels AU, Chang MKO, Andriano KP, Heller J. Mechanical properties of biodegradable polymers and composites proposed for internal fixation of bone. *J Appl Biomater* 1990;1:57–78.

87. Agrawal CM, Niederauer GG, Micallef DM, Athanasiou KA. The use of PLA–PGA polymers in orthopedics. In: Wise DL, Trantolo DJ, Altobelli DE, Yaszemski MJ, Greser JD, Schwartz ER, editors. *Encyclopedic Handbook of Biomaterials and Bioengineering: Part A: Materials*, vol. 2. New York: Marcel Dekker; 1995. p. 1055–1089.

88. Bergsma JE, de Bruijn WC, Rozema FR, Bos RRM, Boering G. Late degradation tissue response to poly(L-lactide) bone plates and screws. *Biomaterials* 1995;16(1):25–31.

89. Gilding DK, Reed AM. Biodegradable polymers for use in surgery—polyglycolic/poly(lactic acid) homo- and copolymers: 1. *Polymer* 1979;20:1459–1464.

90. Barber FA. Resorbable fixation devices: A product guide. *Orthoped Special Ed* 1998;4:1111–1117.

91. Pietrzak WS, Verstynen BS, Sarver DR. Bioabsorbable fixation devices: Status for the cranio-maxillo faxial surgeon. *J Craniofaxial Surg* 1997;2:92–96.

92. Schindler A, Jeffcoat R, Kimmel GL, Pitt CG, Wall ME, Zwiedinger R. Biodegradable polymers for sustained drug delivery. *Contemp Topics Polym Sci* 1977;2:251–289.

93. Goupil D. Sutures. In: Ratner BD, Hoffman AS, Schoen FJ, Lemons JE, editors. *Biomaterials Science*. New York: Academic Press; 1996. p. 356–360.

94. Lewis OG, Fabisial W. Sutures. In: *Kirk-Othmer Encyclopedia of Chemical Technology* (4th ed.). New York: Wiley; 1997.

95. Nathan A, Kohn J. Amino acid derived polymers. In: Shalaby SW, editor. *Biomedical Polymers Designed to Degrade Systems*. New York: Hanser; 1994. p. 117–151.

96. Domb AJ, Amselem S, Langer R, Maniar M. Polyanhydrides as carriers of drugs. In: Shalaby SW, editor. *Biomedical Polymers Designed to Degrade Systems*. New York: Hanser; 1994. p. 69–96.

97. Seeherman H, Wozney JM. Delivery of bone morphogenetic proteins for orthopedic tissue regeneration. *Cytokine Growth Factor Rev* 2005;16:329–345.

98. Welch RD, Jones AL, Bucholz RW, Reinert CM, Tjia JS, Pierce WA, Wozney JM, Li XJ. Effect of recombinant human bone morphogenetic protein-2 on fracture healing in a goat tibial fracture model. *J Bone Miner Res* 1998;13:1483–1490.

99. Kandziora F, Bail H, Schmidmaier G, Schollmeier G, Scholz M, Knispel C et al. Bone morphogenetic protein-2 application by a poly(D,L-lactide)-coatedinterbody cage: In vivo results of a new carrier for growth factors. *J Neurosurg* 2002;97:40–48.

100. Toung JS, Ogle RC, Morgan RF, Lindsey WH. Repair of a rodent nasal critical-size osseous defect with osteoblast augmented collagen gel. *Laryngoscope* 1999;109:1580–1584.

101. Sanchez C, Arribart H, Guille MM. Biomimetism and bioinspiration as tools for the design of innovative materials and systems. *Nat Mater* 2005;4:277–288.

102. Arnander C, Westermark A, Veltheim R, Docherty-Skogh AC, Hilborn J, Engstrand T. Three-dimensional technology and bone morphogenetic protein in frontal bone reconstruction. *J Craniofac Surg* 2006;17:275–279.

103. Narotham PK, Jose S, Nathoo N, Taylon C, Vora Y. Collagen matrix (DuraGen) in dural repair: Analysis of a new modified technique. *Spine* 2004;29:2861–2867.

104. Duan X, McLaughlin C, Griffith M, Sheardown H. Biofunctionalization of collagen for improved biological response: Scaffolds for corneal tissue engineering. *Biomaterial* 2007;28:78–88.

105. Park YJ, Lee YM, Park SN, Sheen SY, Chung CP, Lee SJ. Platelet derived growth factor releasing chitosan sponge for periodontal bone regeneration. *Biomaterials* 2000;21:153–159.

106. Kim IS, Park JW, Kwon IC, Baik BS, Cho BC. Role of BMP, betaigh3, and chitosan in early bony consolidation in distraction osteogenesis in a dog model. *Plast Reconstr Surg* 2002;109:1966–1977.

107. Jiang T, Abdel-Fattah WI, Laurencin CT. In vitro evaluation of chitosan/poly(lactic acid-glycolic acid) sintered microsphere scaffolds for bone tissue engineering. *Biomaterials* 2006;27:4894–4903.

108. Arsiwala AM, Raval AJ, Patravale VB. Nanocoatings on implantable medicaldevices. *Pharm Pat Anal* 2013;2:499–512.

109. Frician JC, Schlaubitz S, Le Visage C, Arnault I, Derkaoui SM, Siadous R et al. A nano-hydroxyapatite-pullulan/dextranpolysaccharide composite macroporous material for bone tissue engineering. *Biomaterials* 2013;34:2947–2959.

110. Tripathi A, Saravanan S, Pattnaik S, Moorthi A, Patridge NC, Selvamurugan AN. Bio composite scaffolds containing chitosan/nano-hydroxyapatite/nano-copper–zinc for bone tissue engineering. *Int J Biol Macromol* 2012;50:294–299.

111. Sonntag R, Reinders J, Kretzer JP. What's next? Alternative materials for articulation in total joint replacement. *Acta Biomater* 2012;8:2434–2441.

112. Simiske SJ, Ayers RA, Bateman TA. Porous materials for bone engineering. In: Liu DM, Dixit V, editors. *Porous Materials for Tissue Engineering*. Uetikon-Auerich: Trans Tech Publications; 1997. p. 151.

113. Ayers RA, Bateman TA, Simske SJ, Porous NiTi as a material for bone engineering. In: LH Yahia, editor. *Shape Memory Implants*, Berlin: Springer-Verlag, 2000, pp. 73–88.

4 Smart Biomaterials in Drug Delivery Applications

4.1 INTRODUCTION

Drug delivery systems (DDSs) are the systems used for administration of a pharmaceutical compound in a controlled manner to achieve a therapeutic effect in humans or animals. DDS appeared during the mid-1960s as macrosystems while a group of researchers were circulating rabbit blood inside a silicon rubber arteriovenous shunt and discovered that if the tube was exposed to anesthetic gases outside, the rabbits fell asleep. Thus, the possibility of a "constant rate drug delivery device" was proposed by this group [1].

Drug delivery is a field of vital importance to medicine and healthcare. Controlled drug delivery improves bioavailability by preventing premature degradation and enhancing uptake, maintains drug concentration within the therapeutic window by controlling the drug release rate, and reduces side effects by targeting disease site and target cells. Since the first FDA approval of DDS, Liposomal amphotericin B, in 1990, more than 10 DDS are now commercially available to treat diverse diseases ranging from cancer to fungal infection and to muscular degeneration (Figure 4.1 and Table 4.1) [2].

DDS improve the administration and efficacy of pharmaceutical compounds including antibodies, peptides, vaccines, drugs, and enzymes, among others. Pharmaceutical particles include a variety of sizes and shapes, ranging from traditional tablets and granules to microparticles and nanoparticles. The relative sizes of commonly used pharmaceutical particles are shown in Figure 4.2. Tablets are most well-known and accepted formulations with a long history. Powders are processed and granules are made to make tablet formulations. Quite frequently, however, granules are used to make formulations different from traditional immediate-release tablets. Drug-containing granules can be mixed or coated with pharmaceutical polymers to render them with delayed-release or sustained-release properties. In fact, the first sustained-release DDS were made in 1952 by coating drug-containing cores with a polymer of varying thicknesses [3]. Microparticle and nanoparticle formulations are a more recent development in drug delivery. Research in drug delivery has focused not only on improving oral and injectable systems, but also on opening additional routes of administration including pulmonary [4], transdermal [5], ocular [6], and nasal routes [7]. Each route has its own advantages and limitations (Table 4.2 and Figure 4.3) [8,9]. Many novel DDS that make use of these routes are beginning to enter clinical trials and some have already reached the market. To accomplish successful clinical translation, DDS must, at minimum, be safe, perform their therapeutic function, offer convenient administration, and offer ease of manufacturing.

For more than a decade, nanoparticles have been used for developing formulations with special features, and the search on the nanoparticle-based DDS has dominated the literature. While significant advances have been made, the current nanoparticle-based formulations require drastic improvements to achieve their intended goals of developing unique delivery systems that others could not have achieved (Figure 4.4 and Table 4.3) [10].

4.2 CARRIER MATERIALS USED FOR DDS

Rapid progress in the application of nanotechnology for therapy and diagnosis has made a new field called "nanomedicine" and related subfields such as "pharmaceutical nanocarriers." Nanoscale aggregates called nanocarriers are available in various classes including nanoparticles made of metals, polymers, hydrogel, ceramic; lipid-based carriers such as liposomes niosomes and nanoburrs, etc. [12]. In this section, we describe the three main classes of nanomaterial—organic, inorganic, and hybrid (Figure 4.5a) and the ways they can be used to design pH-responsive nanosystems for delivery of therapeutic agents.

Examples of nanotechnology applied in pharmaceutical product development include polymer-based nanoparticles, lipid-based nanoparticles (liposomes, nanoemulsions, and solid-lipid nanoparticles), self-assembling nanostructures such as micelles and dendrimer-based nanostructures among others (Figure 4.5b). These engineered nanocarriers offer numerous advantages: small particle size, narrow size distribution, surface features for target-specific localization, protective insulation of drug molecules to enhance stability, opportunity to develop nanocarriers that respond to physiological stimuli, feasibility for delivery of multiple therapeutic agents in a single formulation, combination of imaging and drug therapy to monitor effects in real time, and the opportunity to combine drugs with energy (heat, light, and sound) delivery for synergistic therapeutic effects (Figure 4.5c) [13]. Regardless of the inherent properties of the drug candidates,

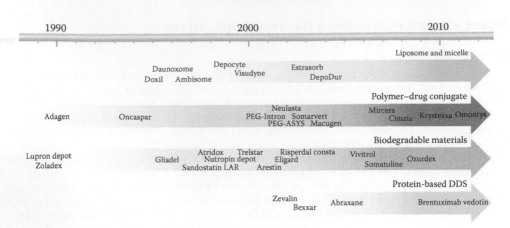

Figure 4.1 Timeline showing FDA-approved DDS in the market.

the pharmacokinetics and distribution pattern upon systemic administration will be dictated by the properties of the nanocarrier system. For instance, particle size and surface charge of tailor-made nanocarriers regulate the biodistribution and pharmacokinetic properties of the nanosystems in the body [14].

4.3 POLYMER-BASED NANOCARRIER SYSTEMS

A large number of polymers are available to form various nanocarrier systems and can be categorized into either natural or synthetic polymers. Natural materials used for the nanoparticle formulation include chitosan, dextran, gelatin, alginate agar agarose, carrageenan, chitosan, gum arabic, heparin, pullulan, and starch. Poly(lactide) (PLA), poly(glycolide) (PGA), poly(lactide-coglycolide) (PLGA), poly(cyanoacrylate) (PCA), polyethylenimine (PEI), and polycaprolactone (PCL) are the synthetic polymers that are used in the design of nanocarriers (Figure 4.6a,b) [15].

4.3.1 Novel Use of Natural Polymers in Drug Delivery

Use of natural polymers as drug carriers has a long history. The use of polysaccharides such as heparin, chondroitin sulfate, and chitosan as carriers, and coupled with the use of antibody and transferrin as targeting motif has all brought significant clinical benefits. Nonetheless, the tremendous potential of natural polymers as drug carriers is still under-represented and deserves more attention [16,17].

Natural polysaccharides, due to their nontoxicity, biocompatibility, and biodegradability, are widely being studied as biomaterial for drug delivery and tissue engineering applications.

Among them, carboxymethyl chitosan (CMCS), a water-soluble derivative of chitosan, has attracted booming interests in several fields such as in vitro diagnostics, theranostics bioimaging, biosensors, wound healing, gene therapy, and food technology, but its greatest impact has been in the area of drug delivery and tissue engineering. CMCS is a potential biologically compatible material, because of presence of chemically versatile ($-NH_2$ and $-COOH$) groups with various molecular weight (MW) [18]. The positive facets of increased water solubility, excellent biocompatibility, admirable biodegradability, high moisture retention ability, improved antioxidant property, enhanced antibacterial and antifungal activity, and nontoxicity as compared to chitosan has provided ample opportunities to the drug delivery and tissue engineering scientists to create a plethora of formulations and scaffolds. In addition, it is also known to be more bioactive, promotes osteogenesis, and its safety evaluation on compounds, in vitro models, blood systems, and tumor application has been well established. All these favorable physical, chemical, and biological properties of CMCS make it a promising biomedical material for drug delivery applications in several formulations [19–21].

CMCS has been shown to improve the dissolution rate of many otherwise poorly soluble drugs, and thus can be exploited for bioavailability improvement of drugs. Various therapeutic agents, such as anticancer, anti-inflammatory, antibiotics, antithrombotic, proteins, and amino acids have been effectively incorporated in CMCS-based systems to increase bioavailability and

Table 4.1: List of Commercially Used Biopolymers Based System in Drug Delivery

Product Name and Category	Year of Approval	Technology	Indication
Liposome and Micelle			
Doxil	1995	PEGylated liposomal doxorubicin	Various types of cancer
Daunoxome	1996	Liposomal daunorubicin	Advanced HIV-associated Kaposi's sarcoma
Ambisome	1997	Liposomal amphotericin B	Fungal infections
Depocyt	1999	Liposomal cytarabine	Lymphomatous meningitis
Visudyne	2000	Liposomal verteporfin	Age-related macular degeneration
Estrasorb	2003	Estradiol micellar nanoparticles	Moderate-to-severe vasomotor symptoms of menopause
DepoDur	2004	Liposomal morphine sulfate	Postoperative pain
Polymer–Drug Conjugate			
Adagen	1990	PEGylated adenosine deaminase	Adenosine deaminase deficiency causing severe combined immunodeficiency disease
Oncaspar	1994	PEGylated L-asparaginase	Acute lymphoblastic leukemia
PEG-intron	2001	PEGylated interferon alfa-2b	Chronic hepatitis C
PEG-ASYS	2002	PEGylated interferon alfa-2a	Chronic hepatitis C and B
Neulasta	2002	PEGylated granulocyte colony-stimulating factor analog	Neutropenia
Somavert	2003	PEGylated recombinant analogue of the human growth hormone	Acromegaly
Macugen	2004	Pegylated anti-VEGF aptamer	Age-related macular degeneration
Mircera	2007	PEGylatederythropoetin receptor activators	Anemia associated with chronic kidney disease
Cimzia	2008	PEGylated tumor necrosis factor alpha inhibitor	Crohn's disease
Krystexxa	2010	PEGylatedurate oxidase	Gout
Omontys	2012	PEGylatedpeginesatide	Anemia caused by chronic kidney disease

(Continued)

Table 4.1: (Continued) List of Commercially Used Biopolymers Based System in Drug Delivery

Product Name and Category	Year of Approval	Technology	Indication
Biodegradable Materials			
Zoladex	1989	PLGA/goserelin acetate	Prostate and breast cancer
Lupron depot	1989	PLGA/leuprolide acetate	Prostate cancer and endometriosis
Gliadel	1996	Polifeprosan 20/carmustine	High-grade and recurrent glioblastomamultiforme
Sandostatin LAR	1998	PLGA-glucose/octreotide acetate	Acromegaly
Atridox	1998	PLA/doxycycline hyclate	Periodontal disease
Nutropin depot	1999	PLGA/recombinant human growth hormone	Growth hormone deficiency
Trelstar	2000	PLGA/triptorelinpamoatea	Advanced prostate cancer
Arestin	2001	PLGA/minocycline	Adult periodontitis
Eligard	2002	PLGA/leuprolide acetate	Advanced prostate cancer
Risperdal Consta	2003	PLGA/risperidone	Schizophrenia and bipolar I disorder
Vivitrol	2006	PLGA/naltrexone	Alcohol dependence and opioid dependence
Somatuline	2007	PLGA/lanreotide	Acromegaly
Ozurdex	2009	PLGA/dexamethasone	Macular edema
Protein-Based DDS			
Zevalin	2002	Anti-CD20 monoclonal antibody/yttrium-90	Non-Hodgkin's lymphoma
Bexxar	2003	Anti-CD20 monoclonal antibody/iodine-131	Non-Hodgkin's lymphoma
Abraxane	2005	Albumin/paclitaxel	Breast cancer
Brentuximab vedotin	2011	Anti-CD30 monoclonal antibody/monomethyl auristatin E	Hodgkin's lymphoma and systemic anaplastic large cell lymphoma

Source: US Food and Drug Administration website (http://www.accessdata.fda.gov/scripts/cder/drugsatfda/). Websites of various pharmaceutical companies supplying the drugs.

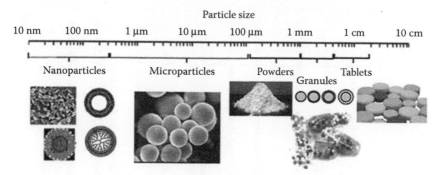

Figure 4.2 Relative sizes of various pharmaceutical particles ranging from nanoparticles to tablets.

to achieve targeted and/or controlled release. Figure 4.7a,b illustrates the route followed by different CMCS-based formulations during their delivery to the targeted site of action in human body [22–24].

4.3.2 Amphiphilically Modified Chitosan

One promising class of materials that has been developed is amphiphilically modified chitosan (AMC) for biomedical applications. With excellent colloidal stability for well-encapsulated therapeutic substances, AMC formulations are highly promising for practical drug delivery uses, especially for modified polymers that retain the biocompatibility of chitosan (Figure 4.8).

AMC can self-assemble into nanoparticles. Conceptual nanoparticle structures are presented, including a hydrophobic core–hydrophilic shell particle, a bilayer capsule, and a particle with hydrophobic and hydrophilic nanodomains. The nanoparticles can be loaded with drugs, which will distribute to minimize the chemical potential. The nanoparticles can carry surface modifications for targeting. The hydrophobic and hydrophilic modifications can also be groups that induce functionality, such as targeting or imaging capability. For visual clarity, the components in the figure are not depicted at scale [25]. An informative list of multiple AMC, colloidal structures, and biomedical applications is given in Table 4.4.

To summarize, an ideal polymeric nanoparticle matrix for drug delivery would exhibit the following characteristics:

1. Allow for the incorporation of the drug into the nanoparticles.

2. Provide protection of the drug from enzyme degradation.

3. Facilitate cellular uptake in target cells.

4. Release drug at the site of action (i.e., to increase the local drug concentration and prolong the duration of drug activity) [51,52].

5. Decrease drug toxicities.

6. Provide low manufacturing costs. To achieve these properties, chitosan has been modified to produce nanoparticles and widely investigated for use as a drug carrier [29,53].

Recently the significant difference in the redox environment has been explored for developing redox-responsive DDS. Redox-responsive crosslinking is introduced into DDS via disulfide-containing cross-linkers, oxidization of thiol group, and disulfide–thiol exchange reaction. The crosslinking can render good stability to the DDS such as polymeric micelles, which have compact structure, to provide secure encapsulation of drugs in the absence of thiol group.

Redox-responsive self-assembly of amphiphilic polymers in the form of micelles or polymersomes is explored for drug delivery [54]. One way is to combine hydrophobic segment and hydrophilic segment via disulfide bond. Hydrophobic poly(ε-caprolactone) was combined with poly(ethylene glycol) (PEG) or dextran via the disulfide bonds. Figure 4.9 shows that amphiphilic polymers were obtained by grafting different groups to polymer backbones via the disulfide bond. The polymer backbone can be water-soluble biopolymer like chitosan, hyaluronic acid (HA), and chondroitin sulfate [55].

Table 4.2: Drug Delivery Routes Explored by Nanocrystals

Drug	Manufacturing Technique	Mean Particle Size	Use/Benefits
Oral Delivery			
Danazol	Media milling	169 nm	Hypoestrogenic and hyperandrogenic activity/a 16-fold increase in bioavailability in comparison to danazol suspension
Ketoprofen	Media milling	265 nm	Rheumatoid arthritis/1.2-fold increase in C_{max} and 2-fold reduction in T_{max} in comparison with microcrystalline ketoprofen
Fenofibrate	HPH	356 nm	Lipid-lowering agent/12.5-fold increase in C_{max} and 17-fold increase in bioavailability
Cyclosporine	HPH	962 nm	Autoimmune disease
Itraconazole	Precipitation	267 nm	Antifungal/1.5- and 1.8-fold higher bioavailability from commercial product in the fed and fasted states
Icaritin	Antisolvent-crystallization method under ultrasonication	220 nm	Prevent osteoporosis/faster dissolution, improved absorption and grater in vivo bioactivity than raw suspension
Paraterphenyl derivative	Precipitation followed by HPH	200 nm	Promising anticancer agent/increased saturation solubility, accelerated dissolution and 5-fold higher AUC with significantly longer MRT in comparison to its solution
Cilostazol	Antisolvent and high-pressure homogenization method	326 nm	Vasodilator/enhanced AUC and C_{max} was observed in comparison to marketed formulation
Intravenous Delivery			
Oridonin	HPH	103.3 nm	Anticancer/improved bioavailability in comparison to its solution
Ascularine	HPH	133 nm	Anticancer/2.3-, 6.2-, 2.7-, and 2.7-fold increase in t1/2, Vd, CL, and MRT in comparison to ascularine solution
Curcumin	HPH	210.2 nm	Anticancer/3.1-fold increase in C_{max} 11.2-fold increase in MRT, and 4.8-fold increase in AUC
Flurbiprofen	HPH	–	Rheumatoid arthritis/improved bioavailability

(Continued)

Table 4.2: (*Continued*) Drug Delivery Routes Explored by Nanocrystals

Drug	Manufacturing Technique	Mean Particle Size	Use/Benefits
Atovaquone	HPH	279 nm	Improved activity against toxoplasma encephalitis due to enhanced bioavailability
Pulmonary Delivery			
Itraconazole	Precipitation	Less than 1 μm	Antifungal
Budesonide	–	Less than 1 μm	Anti-asthmatic
Buparvaquone	–	–	Antiprotozoal
Sildenafil	Precipitation	–	Erectile dysfunction and pulmonary hypertension
Carvedilol	Solvent precipitation ultrasonication method	190 nm	Antihypertensive
Ocular Delivery			
Hydrocortisone	Precipitation	300 nm	Steroid/1.8-fold increase in AUC
Forskolin	Wet milling	164 nm	Antiglaucoma agent/improved intraocular pressure lowering efficacy than its solution form
Cyclosporin A	In-situ precipitation	505 nm	Immunosuppressant/improved bioavailability
Mycophenolatemofetil	HPH	440 nm	Immunosuppressant/modified corneal drug disposition
Dermal Delivery			
L-Ascorbic acid	Emulsification + homogenization	148 nm	Antioxidant/long-term stable topical formulation without decomposition
Lutein	HPH	429 nm	Antioxidant
Hesperetin	HPH	300 nm	Antioxidant and antiallergic
Tretinoin	Precipitation	324 nm	Anti-acne agent
Ibuprofen	Wet milling	284 nm	Analgesic

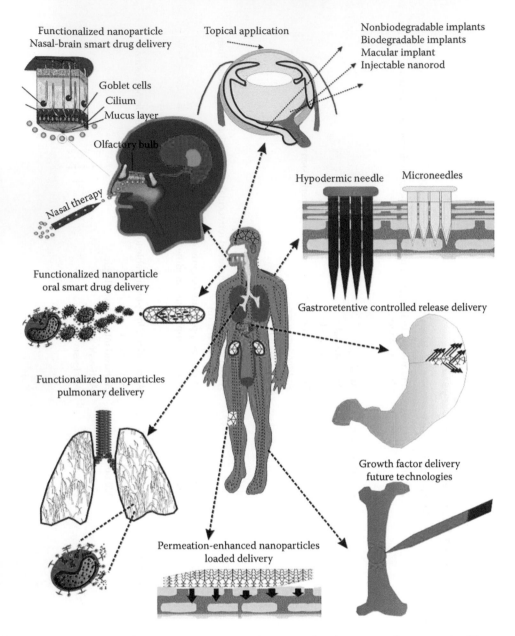

Figure 4.3 Schematic diagrams representing the recent developments of various significant routes of administration and targeting strategies.

4.3.3 Cyclodextrins (CDs)

Cyclodextrins (CDs) are water-soluble cyclic oligosaccharides with six, seven, or eight a-1,4-linked D-glucopyranose units, and named a-, b-, and g-cyclodextrin, respectively. These are also called cycloamyloses, cyclomaltoses, or Schardinger dextrins and are nonreducing in nature. The geometry of CDs gives a hydrophobic inner cavity having a depth of 7.8 Å, and an internal diameter of 5.7 Å. Due to their unique property to include hydrophobic guest molecules in their internal cavity, natural cyclodextrins have been widely used as carriers for drugs to enhance their solubilization, stabilization, and bioavailability [56,57]. β-CD is by far the most widely used host compound due to the optimal size of its internal cavity. However, because of its low aqueous solubility, chemical derivatives of β-CDs were prepared in order to extend its physicochemical properties as well as inclusion ability (Figure 4.10) [58].

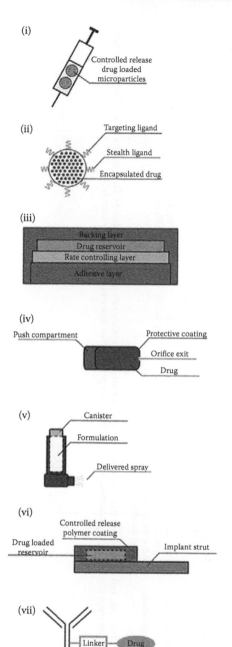

Microparticle-based depot systems comprise formulations of drugs, peptides, or proteins encapsulated in biodegradable polymeric particles. These systems allow for the sustained and controlled release of therapeutics over a long period of time, allowing for a reduced number of treatments.

Nanoparticles are drug carriers that are capable of encapsulating and protecting drugs from rapid degradation in vivo, improving both targeting and circulation profiles via surface modification with application-specific ligands, and controlling the rate of drug release from the particle.

Transdermal patches contain a backing layer that prevents drug leakage, a reservoir to store the drug, a rate controlling layer that controls drug release and an adhesive layer that attaches to the skin. Transdermal patches allow for a painless, patient–compliant interface to facilitate systemic administration of drugs.

OROS® technology is an osmotically driven system that controls the rate of drug release via the design of the osmotic pump and the osmotic properties of the drug. OROS® allows for the controlled release of therapeutics, via the oral route, which decreases dosing frequency and side effects.

Inhalers are compact devices that are used to store drug formulations which can be delivered as inhalable aerosolized sprays. Inhalers permit rapid absorption of drugs through the lungs, control over drug delivery via fixed doses, and the convenience of self-administration

Implants are devices that either passively, through material properties, or actively, through various actuation methods, control drug release rates. Implants allow for long-term delivery of therapeutics, often reducing the number of invasive procedures required to maintain similar therapeutic effect.

Antibody drug conjugates are chemical conjugates of monoclonal antibodies and cytotoxic agents. Antibodies allow targeted delivery of highly potent cytotoxic drugs, thereby reducing systemic toxicity.

Figure 4.4 Schematics and brief descriptions of the seven highlighted DDS: (i) microparticle-based depot formulations, (ii) nanoparticle-based cancer drugs, (iii) transdermal systems (patches highlighted here), (iv) oral DDS (OROS® highlighted here), (v) pulmonary DDS (inhalers highlighted here), (vi) implants, and (vii) antibody–drug conjugates.

As the knowledge in CDs progresses, novel applications are envisioned. For example, some CDs have been designed to provide by themselves certain controlled-release features when orally administered, delaying the release or providing site-specific delivery. Drug–CD conjugates may render colon-targeting prodrugs, while complexes of plasmids and cationic CDs have been shown as efficient carriers for gene therapy. Amphiphilic CDs can self-assemble creating supramolecular aggregates and nanospheres that can be loaded with high proportions of hydrophobic drugs forming complexes or interacting with other complexed drug molecules [59]. It is interesting to

Table 4.3: Routes of Administration

Route of Administration	Advantages	Disadvantages	Targets	Examples	Number of Top 100 Commercial Drugs
Injections: IV, IM, and SQ	Rapid onset (IV) up to 100% bioavailability Controlled depot release (IM, SQ) Suitable for most therapeutic molecules	Difficult for patient to self-administer (IV) Patients' fear of needles leads to noncompliance Higher instance of infection	Tissue with blood access (IV) Systemic	Vaccines (IM) Chemotherapy (IV) Insulin (SQ)	42
Oral	Patient compliant and most convenient	Poor bioavailability Generally nontargeted Not viable for larger therapeutics (peptides/proteins) Potentially inconsistent due to the presence of food	Systemic	Pills Liquid medications	54
Inhalation	Direct target to the lungs Fast absorption	Inconsistent delivery stemming from variation in patient-to-patient technique	Lungs Brain Systemic	Inhalers Anesthetics	7
Transdermal	Less side-effects due to direct delivery to the skin Bypasses first-pass degradation	Patients can potentially use incorrect dose (creams) Absorption dependent on skin condition and location	Skin Systemic	Patches Creams	4

Note: Advantages, disadvantages, potential targets, and examples of the most commonly used routes of administration for drug delivery. The number of top 100 commercial drugs and their routes of administration were determined by counting the best selling drugs in 2013 as determined by Drugs.com [11].

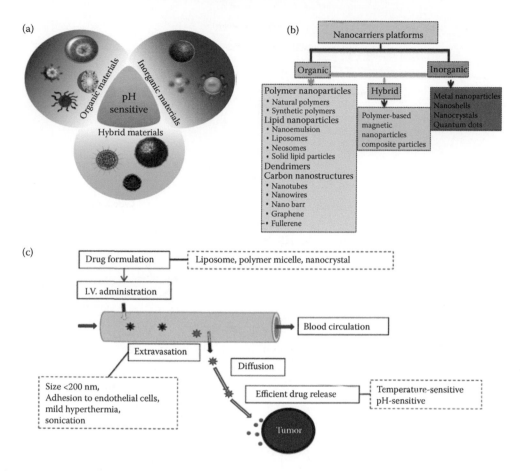

Figure 4.5 (a) and (b) Different types of nanocarrier platforms used in DDS. (c) Ideal sequence of targeted drug delivery to a tumor.

note that CDs can cooperatively work when they are close together, provoking a displacement in the complex formation equilibrium toward the complexed species. This latter finding makes CDs outstanding building blocks for the development of novel supramolecular DDS with a therapeutic potential still to be fully explored (Figure 4.11) [60].

4.3.4 Aerogel-Based Drug Delivery Systems

Aerogel-based systems constitute an emerging platform for drug delivery. The studies carried out so far show that aerogel-based materials are promising due to their high drug-loading capacities, their ability for controlled drug release, their capability to increase the bioavailability of low solubility drugs, and to improve both their stability and their release kinetics. Not only their unique properties, such as very high porosities and high surface areas, but also the flexibility of sol–gel chemistry play an important role [61]. Organic aerogels, mainly polysaccharide-based ones like starch aerogels, alginate aerogels, and cellulose aerogels, are promising for drug delivery applications. Drug delivery vehicles based on aerogels can be prepared by different methods such as the addition of the drug during the conventional sol–gel process or during the post-treatment of the synthesized aerogels as shown in Figure 4.12a,b [62]. A summary of the studies on aerogel-based DDS is given in Table 4.5 indicating the polymer type of the aerogel, the drug, and the loading method used in each study [63].

4.3.5 Hydrogel-, Microgel-, and Nanogel-Based Drug Delivery Systems

Hydrogels, microgels, and nanogels with excellent biocompatibility, a microporous structure with tunable porosities and pore sizes, and dimensions spanning from human organs, cells, to viruses

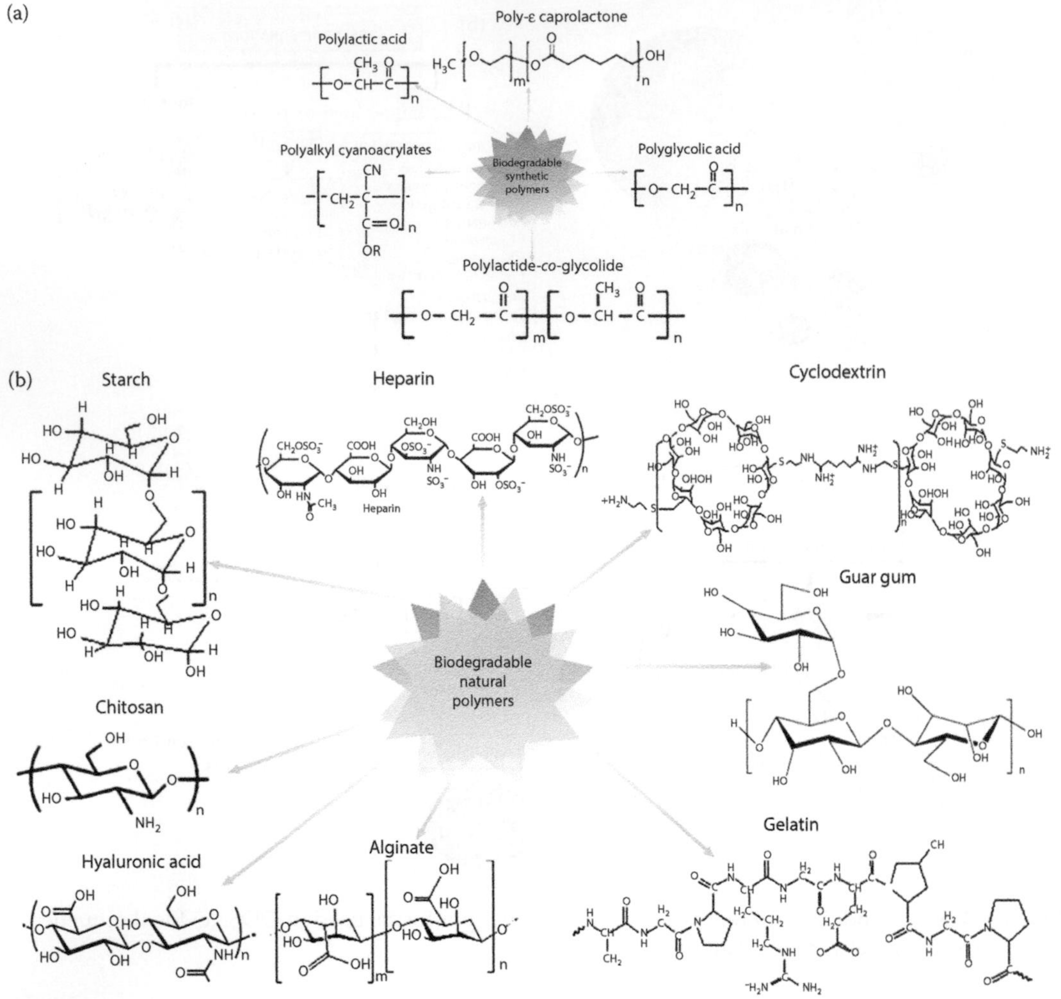

Figure 4.6 (a) and (b) Biodegradable natural and synthetic polymers in drug delivery.

have emerged as a most versatile and viable platform for sustained protein release, targeted drug delivery, and tissue engineering.

In recent years, click chemistry due to its high reactivity, superb selectivity, and mild reaction conditions has appeared as the most promising strategy to prepare hydrogels with varying dimensions and patterns (Figure 4.13). Hydrogels based on natural polymers (also called natural hydrogels), due to their excellent biocompatibility and biodegradability, have attracted great interest for drug delivery and tissue engineering. The unique bio-orthogonality of click reaction renders thus formed hydrogels highly compatible with encapsulated bioactive compounds including living cells, proteins, and drugs. For example, HA hydrogels developed via copper(I)-catalyzed azide-alkene cycloaddition (CuAAC) have been used as drug reservoir. Bisphosphonate-functionalized dextran nanogels crosslinked via CuAAC achieved significant localization in both femur and spine, and provided a possible antiosteoporotic effect toward bone disease [64]. The wide variety of work reported has demonstrated the beauty of click chemistry in creating novel hydrogel materials with dimensions spanning from human organs, cells, to viruses [65].

4.3.6 Polymer Micelles-Based Drug Delivery Systems

Polymeric micelles are nanoscopic (>100 nm) amphiphilic block copolymers with a core–shell structure. Recently, polymer micelles have gained considerable attention as a versatile nanomedicine platform with greatly improved drug pharmacokinetics and efficacious response in cancer

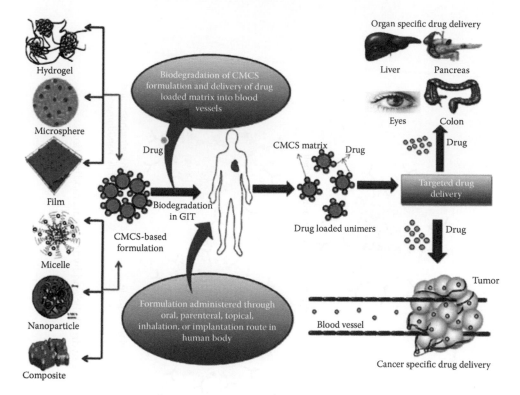

Figure 4.7 The route followed by different CMCS-based formulations during their delivery to the targeted site of action in human body.

treatment. Typical chemotherapeutic agents have low water solubility, short blood half-lives, narrow therapeutic indices, and high systemic toxicity, which lead to patient morbidity and mortality while compromising the desirable therapeutic outcome of the drugs. Polymer micelles have been shown to increase the aqueous solubility of chemotherapeutic agents and prolong their in vivo half-lives with lessened systemic toxicity. Polymer micelles are composed of amphiphilic macromolecules that have distinct hydrophobic and hydrophilic block domains, with the structure of the copolymers usually being a di-block, tri-block, or graft copolymer. Within each copolymer system, aqueous exposure induces the hydrophobic and hydrophilic segments to phase separate and form nanoscopic supramolecular core–shell structures (Figure 4.14).

The core–shell structure of polymer micelles affords several advantages for drug delivery applications. First, drug encapsulation within the micelle core allows for solubilization of water-insoluble drugs. For example, the water solubility of paclitaxel can be increased by several orders of magnitude from 0.0015 to 2 mg/mL through micelle incorporation [66]. Second, micelles have prolonged blood half-lives because PEG prevents opsonization, effectively reducing micelle uptake by the reticuloendothelial system (RES). Third, their small size (10–100 nm) makes them suitable for injection and enhanced tumor deposition due to the enhanced permeability and retention (EPR) effect stemming from the leakiness of tumor vasculature [67]. Finally, their chemistry allows for the development of multifunctional modalities that can enhance micelle accumulation in cancerous tissues and facilitate drug internalization inside cancer cells.

The unique characteristics of polymeric micelles, such as size in the nanometer range, relatively high stability due to low critical association concentrations (CMC), and core–shell arrangement, make them attractive for use in DDS in clinical applications, especially for hydrophobic drugs with very low solubility in water [68].

4.3.7 Dendrimer-Based Drug Delivery Systems

In the last two decades of the scientific research, the development of dendrimers as potential drug vehicles is one of the most active areas of biomedical and pharmaceutical sciences. Dendrimers are unimolecular, monodisperse, micellar nanostructures, around 20 nm in size, with a well-defined,

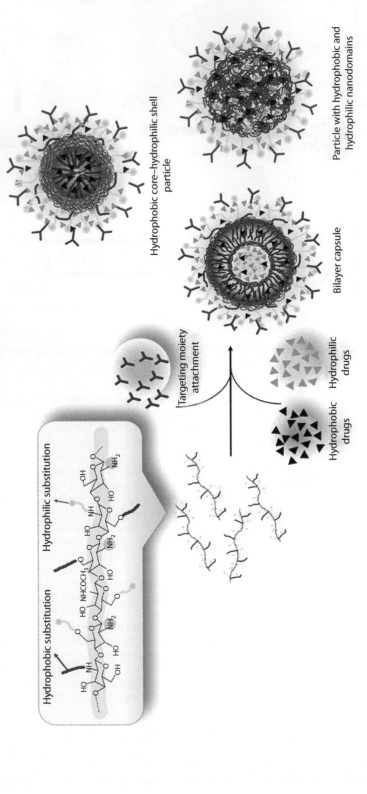

Figure 4.8 Schematic diagram illustrating the structure of AMC with possible sites for hydrophilic and hydrophobic modifications.

Table 4.4: List of Selected AMCs with Colloidal Properties and Biomedical Applications [26–50]

AMC	Colloidal Properties	Biomedical Applications
Acylated chitosan	Nanoparticles, spun nanofibers, microporous	Drug delivery
Acylated carboxymethyl chitosan	Nanoparticles	Drug delivery
Alkyl chain modified succinyl chitosan	Nanoparticles	Drug delivery
Carboxymethyl chitosan-6-mercaptopurine	pH-dependent nanoparticle formation	Drug delivery
Carboxymethylhexanoyl chitosan	Nanocapsules, nanoparticles, shell constituent in core–shell nanoparticles, nanomicrostructured macroscopic gels	Drug delivery, injectable depot gels, wound dressings, injectable cell scaffolds
Carboxymethyl-hexanoyl chitosan–silica	Multilayered nanoparticles	Drug delivery
Deoxycholic acid modified carboxymethylated chitosan	Nanoparticles	Drug delivery
Deoxycholic acid-N,O-hydroxyethyl chitosan	Nanoparticles	Drug delivery
DOX-conjugated stearic acid-g chitosan	Nanoparticles	Drug delivery
Glycidol chitosan deoxycholic acid	Nanoparticles	Drug delivery
Hydrophobically modified glycol chitosan	Nanoparticles	Drug delivery
Folate decorated succinyl chitosan	Nanoparticles	Drug delivery
Lauroyl sulfated chitosan	Nanoparticles	Drug delivery
Linoleic acid-carboxymethyl chitosan	Nanoparticles	Drug delivery
Linoleic acid grafted chitosan oligosaccharides	Nanoparticles	Drug delivery
Linoleic acid/poly(β-malic acid) double grafted chitosan	Nanoparticles	Drug delivery
N-alkyl-O-sulfate chitosan	Nanoparticles	Drug delivery
N-laurylcarboxymethyl chitosan	Nanoparticles	Drug delivery
N-octyl-O-sulfate chitosan	Nanoparticles	Drug delivery
Ocarboxymethyl chitosan methotrexate	Nanoparticles	Drug delivery
Octadecyl quaternized lysine modified chitosan	Nanoparticles together with cholesterol, multilamellar structure, could have folate-PEG coating	Drug delivery

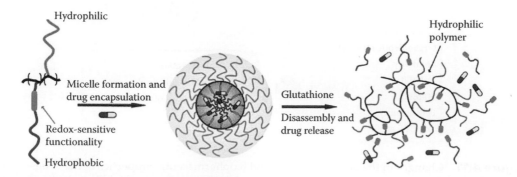

Figure 4.9 Amphiphilic block polymer with redox-responsive linkage.

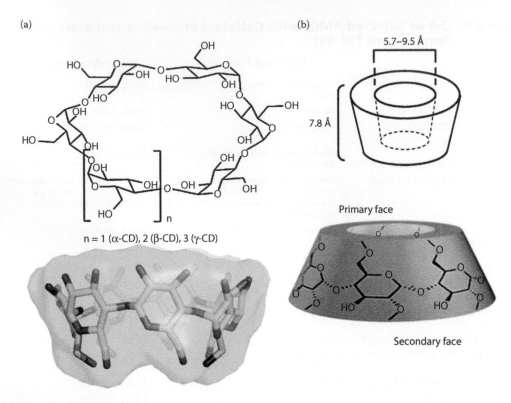

Figure 4.10 Structure of β-CD and schematic representation of CD molecules exhibiting the shape of a truncated cone or torus (a) chemical structure and (b) 3D structure.

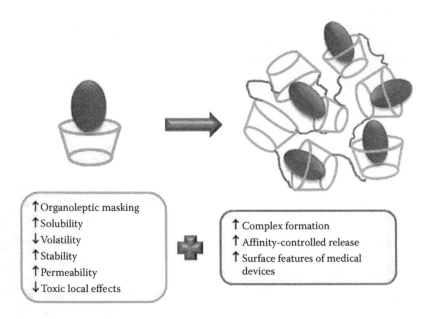

Figure 4.11 Changes in the physicochemical and biopharmaceutic properties of the drugs caused by inclusion complex formation with cyclodextrins in solution, and additional advantages provided by cross-linked cyclodextrin networks.

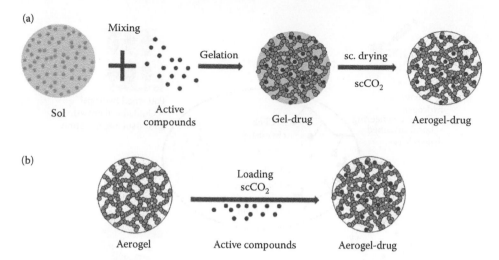

Figure 4.12 Drug loading of aerogels: (a) during the sol–gel process (cogelation) and (b) in the aerogel matrix by supercritical impregnation post-treatment method.

regularly branched symmetrical structure and a high density of functional end groups at their periphery. The structure of dendrimers consists of three distinct architectural regions as a focal moiety or a core, layers of branched repeat units emerging from the core, and functional end groups on the outer layer of repeat units. They are known to be robust, covalently fixed, 3D structures possessing both a solvent-filled interior core (nanoscale container) as well as a homogenous, mathematically defined, exterior surface functionality (Figure 4.15) [69].

Dendrimers offer several featured advantages as drug carrier candidates. These advantages include the following:

1. High density and reactivity of functional groups on the periphery of dendrimers that make multifarious bioactive molecules to be easily modified on to the surface.

2. Well-defined globular structure, predictable molecule weight, and monodispersity of dendrimers ensure reproductive pharmacokinetics.

3. Controllable size (generation-dependent) of dendrimers satisfies various biomedical applications.

4. High penetration abilities of dendritic structures through the cell membrane cause increased cellular uptake level of the drugs complexed or conjugated to them.

5. The lack of immunogenicity of dendrimers makes them much safer choices than synthesized peptide carriers and natural protein carriers.

6. EPR effect of dendrimers offers preferential uptake of the materials by cancer tissues.

Table 4.5: Studies about the Polymer-Based Aerogels as Drug Delivery Vehicles in the Literature

Aerogel Type Drug Loaded	Drug Loaded	Loading Method
Starch aerogel, alginate aerogel	Ibuprofen	Post-treatment
Starch aerogel	Paracetamol	Solvent exchange
Starch aerogel		Post-treatment
Alginate aerogel	Nicotinic acid	Gel preparation
Alginate aerogel	Ketoprofen, ketoprofenlysinate	Gel preparation
Multimembrane alginate aerogel	Nicotinic acid	Gel preparation
Bacterial cellulose aerogels	Dexpanthenol, L-ascorbic acid	Solvent exchange
Whey protein-based aerogel	Ketoprofen	Post-treatment
Amine-modified silica aerogel	Ketoprofen	Post-treatment

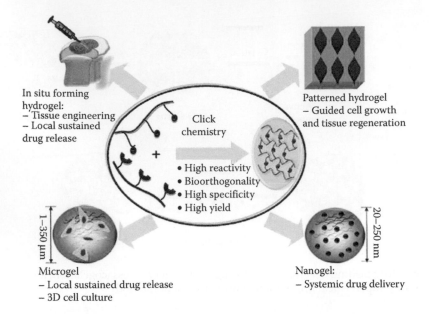

In situ forming
hydrogel:
– Tissue engineering
– Local sustained
drug release

Click
chemistry

• High reactivity
• Bioorthogonality
• High specificity
• High yield

Patterned hydrogel
– Guided cell growth
and tissue regeneration

1–350 μm

20–250 nm

Microgel
– Local sustained drug release
– 3D cell culture

Nanogel:
– Systemic drug delivery

Figure 4.13 Preparation and potential biomedical applications of click hydrogels, microgels, and nanogels.

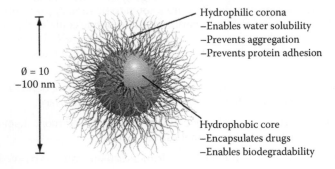

Hydrophilic corona
–Enables water solubility
–Prevents aggregation
–Prevents protein adhesion

Ø = 10
–100 nm

Hydrophobic core
–Encapsulates drugs
–Enables biodegradability

Figure 4.14 Schematic illustration of the core–shell structure of a polymer micelle with intended functions of each component.

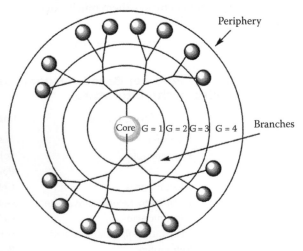

Periphery

Core G = 1 G = 2 G = 3 G = 4

Branches

Figure 4.15 Typical architecture of a fourth-generation dendrimer.

7. Well-established methodologies proposed to construct nanodevices with various functional moieties based on dendrimers provide miscellaneous biomedical applications of these promising materials, such as cancer-targeting therapy, magnetic response imaging, photodynamic therapy, and neutron capture therapy.

8. Perfectly programed release of drugs molecules or other bioactive agents from dendrimers leads to reduced toxicity, increased bioavailability, and a simplified dosing schedule. Prolonged residence time of the drug in the blood and protection of the bioactives from their environment with increased stability are other potential advantages of dendrimeric architecture. An ideal dendritic drug carrier must be nontoxic, nonimmunogenic, preferably biodegradable, present an adequate biodistribution, and allow tissue targeting. Dendrimers used in drug delivery studies typically incorporate one or more of the following polymers: polyamidoamine (PAMAM), melamine, poly L-glutamic acid (PG), polyethyleneimine (PEI), polypropyleneimine (PPI), and polyethylene glycol (PEG), chitin. Dendrimers may be used in two major modalities for targeting vectors for diagnostic imaging, drug delivery, gene transfection also detection, and therapeutic treatment of cancer and other diseases, namely by (1) passive targeting—nanodimension mediated via EPR effect involving primary tumor vascularization or organ-specific targeting and (2) active targeting—receptor-mediated cell-specific targeting involving receptor-specific targeting groups. There are several potential applications of dendrimers in the field of imaging, drug delivery, gene transfection, and nonviral gene transfer. Few applications are included in Table 4.6.

Table 4.6: Biomedical Application of Dendrimers

Dendrimers Composition	Drug	Application
PAMAM (polyamidoamine)	Chelated gadolinium	Diagnose certain disorders of the heart, brain, and blood vessels
Poly(L-glutamic acid), polyamidoamine and poly(ethyleneimine)	Folic acid	Breast cancer
PAMAM	Antibodies specific to CD14 and PSMA	Cell binding and internalization
PAMAM	Sulfamethoxazole	Strep throat (*Streptococcus*), staph infection (*Staphylococcus aureus*), and flu (*Haemophilus influenza*)
PAMAM (polyamidoamine)	Nadifloxacin, prulifloxacin	Various bacteria
PAMAM (polyamidoamine) PPI (polypropyleneimine generation)	Nystatin and terbinafine	Antifungal against *Candida albicans*, *Aspergillus niger*, and *Saccharomyces cereviseae*
PAMAM (polyamidoamine)	Propranolol	Hypertension
Polyamidoamine (PAMAM) dendrimers	Niclosmide	Tapeworm
Pegylated lysine-based copolymeric dendrimer	Artemether	*Plasmodium falciparum*
PAMAM dendrimers with carboxylic or hydroxyl surface groups	Pilocarpine	Glaucoma
PAMAM	Enoxaparin	Pulmonary embolism
PAMAM	Ketoprofen, diflunisal	Inflammation
PAMAM	Indomethacin	Inflammation
Polylysine dendrimer	VivaGel (SPL7013 Gel)	HIV, HSV, and sexually transmitted infections
Dendrimer	High-resolution x-ray image	Diagnostic tool for arteriosclerotic vasculature, tumors, infarcts, kidneys, or efferent urinary
Dendrimer	Gene transfer of cytokine genes (tumor necrosis factor, interleukin-2, granulocyte–macrophage colony-stimulating factor)	Induce a systemic antitumor immune response against residual tumor cells
PAMAM	5-Fluorouracil	Tumor
Dendrimer	Isotope of boron (10B)	Cancer

Source: Mudshinge SR, Deore AB, Patil S, Bhalgat CM. *Saudi Pharm J* 2011;19:129–141.

Table 4.7: Drug Formulations of Guar Gum in Drug Delivery

S. No.	Natural Gum	Model Drug	Dosage Form
1	Guar gum (97.3%)	Dexamethasone	Tablets
2	Guar gum (77.19%)	Indomethacin	Matrix tablets
3	Guar gum (125%)	Indomethacin	Tablets
4	Guar gum (20%)	Albendazole	Matrix tablets
5	Guar gum (75%)	Diltiazem	Matrix tablets
6	Guar gum (80%)	5 FU	Tablets
7	Guar gum	Tinidazole	Tablets
8	Guar gum	Calcium sennosides	Matrix tablets
9	Guar gum	Mesalazine	Tablets
10	Guar gum	Rofecoxib	Matrix tablets
11	Guar gum	Albendazole–cyclodextrin	Matrix tablets
12	Guar gum	Ondansetron	Matrix tablets
13	Guar gum (44%)	Indomethacin pellets	(coated with Eudragit FS 30D)
14	Guar gum	Itraconazole	Mucoadhesive tablet

4.3.8 Guar Gum-Based Drug Delivery Systems

Guar gum is a nonionic polysaccharide that is found abundantly in nature and has many properties derived from the seeds of *Cyamopsis tetragonolobus*, family *Leguminosae*. It consists of linear chains of (1→4)-β-D-mannopyranosyl units with α-D-galactopyranosyl units attached by (1→6) linkages. GG contains about 80% galactomannan, 12% water, 5% protein, 2% acidic insoluble ash, 0.7% ash, and 0.7% fat. In pharmaceutical formulations, GG is used as a binder, disintegrant, suspending agent, thickening agent, and stabilizing agent [70].

GG and its derivatives are stable, safe, and biodegradable. Due to these favorable properties, they are widely considered as potential target-specific drug delivery carriers. GG can be used as a colon-specific drug carrier in the form of matrix and compression-coated tablets as well as microspheres due to its viscous colloidal dispersions in aqueous solution. To reduce the enormous swelling properties of GG that limits its application as drug delivery carriers, various approaches of chemical medications have been taken. Among these, crosslinking GG polymer chains with crosslinking agents is quite promising. The viscosity of GG was found to be decreased even in the presence of enzymes by crosslinking with borax, glutaraldehyde, and trisodium trimetaphosphate. These cross-linked GG formulations can be useful for the controlled release of several antihypertensive drugs. In order to achieve pH and temperature-responsive GG hydrogels, GG has been grafted with pH-responsive polymers such as poly(acrylamide) and poly(acrylic acid) and a temperature-responsive polymer, poly(N-isopropyl acrylamide). These chemically modified stimuli responsive GG hydrogels can be used in the area of the site-specific drug delivery to specific regions of the gastrointestinal tract, especially in the colon-specific delivery of low-molecular-weight protein drugs. Since GG and its derivatives have good film forming and controlled drug release abilities, they have potential to be used as transdermal drug delivery devices [71].

Pharmaceutical applications of some guar gums that are used commercially as adjuvants in pharmaceutical formulations are summarized in Table 4.7.

4.3.9 Niosomes-Based Drug Delivery Systems

Niosomes are vesicles composed mainly of hydrated nonionic surfactants in addition to, in many cases, cholesterol (CHOL) or its derivatives. The unique structures of niosomes make it capable of encapsulating both hydrophilic and lipophilic substances. This can be achieved by entrapping hydrophilic in vesicular aqueous core or adsorbed on the bilayer surfaces while the lipophilic substances are encapsulated by their partitioning into the lipophilic domain of the bilayers. According to niosome size, they can be divided into three categories: small unilamellar vesicles (SUV) (10–100 nm), large unilamellar vesicles (LUV) (100–3000 nm), and multilamellar vesicles (MLV) where more than one bilayer is present (Figure 4.16) [72]. Niosomes have been one of the illustrious vesicles into all vesicular systems, being the focus of a great attention as potential DDS for different routes of administration, in recent years. This is due to the fact that niosomes do not have the many disadvantages that others have and are a very useful DDS with numerous applications. Niosomes have the ability of entrapping various types of drugs, genes, proteins, and vaccines.

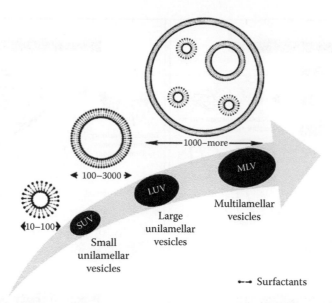

Figure 4.16 Schematic structure of SUVs, LUVs, and MLVs.

4.3.9.1 *Advantages of Niosomes*

Niosomes have attracted a great deal of attention in controlled DDS because of many advantages, such as biodegradability, nonimmunogenicity nature, bioavailability, and effective in the modulation of drug release properties. Niosomes offer numerous advantages as presented below:

1. Niosomes are osmotically active, chemically stable, and have long storage time compared to liposomes.

2. Their surface formation and modification are very easy because of the functional groups on their hydrophilic heads.

3. They have high compatibility with biological systems and low toxicity because of their nonionic nature.

4. Also, they are biodegradable and nonimmunogenic.

5. They can entrap lipophilic drugs into vesicular bilayer membranes and hydrophilic drugs in aqueous compartments.

6. They can improve the therapeutic performance of the drug molecules by protecting the drug from biological environment, resulting in better availability and controlled drug delivery by restricting the drug effects to target cells in targeted carriers and delaying clearance from the circulation in sustained drug delivery.

7. Access to raw materials is convenient.

8. They exhibit a high patient compliance because of the water-based suspension of niosomes.

9. Unlike phospholipids, the handling of surfactants requires no special precautions and conditions.

10. They increase the oral bioavailability and skin penetration of drugs.

11. The variable characteristics of the niosomes can be controlled. Characteristics, such as the type of the niosomes according to their size, entrapment efficiency, and stability, can be controlled by the type of preparation method, of surfactant, cholesterol content, size, surface charge, and suspension concentration.

12. Niosomes can enhance absorption of some drugs across cell membranes, to localize in targeted tissues and to elude the reticuloendothelial system.

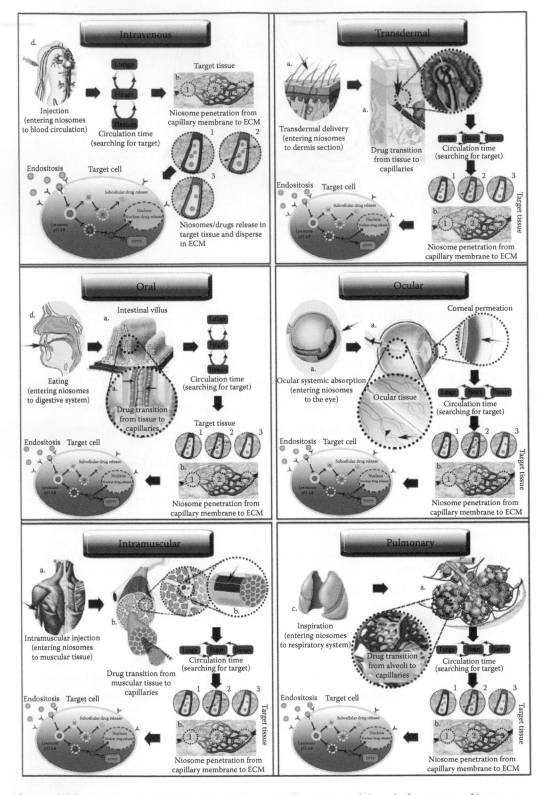

Figure 4.17 Routes of administration. Schematic illustration of the whole process of intravenous, ocular, and transversal, oral, pulmonary and intramuscular drug delivery in vivo, involving stages of systemic penetration, circulation time, tissue, and intracellular targeting.

13. Also, they can regulate the drug delivery rate in the external nonaqueous phase by emulsifying an aqueous phase in anon-aqueous phase.

Niosomes can encapsulate various drugs including doxorubicin, insulin, monoxide, ovalbumin, oligonucleotide, EGFP, hemagglutinin, DNA vaccine, α-interferon, bovine basic pancreatic inhibitor, and many others [73]. These can have various applications such as antioxidant, anticancer, anti-inflammatory, anti-asthma, antimicrobial, anti-amyloid, anti-Alzheimer, antibacterial, etc. [74]. Schematic illustration of the whole process of administrations has been shown in Figure 4.17 [75].

4.3.10 Liposome-Based Drug Delivery Systems

Liposomes are the commonest lipid-based formulation for drug delivery and the most successful DDS, known till date. Liposomes as carriers of therapeutic drugs have attracted attention for more than 40 years. As a DDS, liposomes have many advantages as follows: delivering both hydrophilic and lipophilic drugs (Figure 4.18), possessing targeting, controlled release properties, cell affinity, tissue compatibility, reducing drug toxicity, and improving drug stability. During the researches, the conventional structures of the liposomes have some changes, which have brought out a series of new type liposomes, such as long-circulating liposomes, stimuli-responsive liposomes, cationic liposomes, and ligand-targeted liposomes. There are more than 20 commercialized liposomal formulations and many more are under clinical and preclinical trials [76,77]. Their success can be attributed to the remarkable flexibility of lipid-based delivery systems, ability to efficiently encapsulate both small molecules and macromolecules, biodegradability and biocompatibility, possibility to be manufactured in components in a predictable manner [78].

Liposomes are small artificial vesicles of spherical shape with a membrane composed of phospholipid bilayers. They can be made of natural nontoxic phospholipids and cholesterol in the form of one or multiple concentric bilayers capable of encapsulating hydrophilic and hydrophobic drugs. The size of liposomes depends on their composition and preparation method with diameters ranging from around 50 nm to more than 100 nm (Figure 4.1). Among all the nanomedicine platforms, liposomes have demonstrated one of the most established nanoplatforms with several FDA-approved formulations for cancer treatment, and had the greatest impact on oncology to date because of their size, biocompatibility, biodegradability, hydrophobic and hydrophilic character, low toxicity, and immunogenicity [79].

Main classification of liposomes is based on structure. Multilamellar vesicles (MLV) range from 500 to 5000 nm and consist of several concentric bilayers. Large unilamellar vesicles (LUV) consist

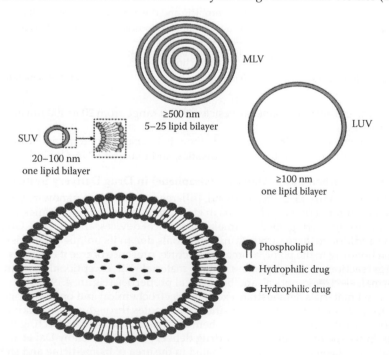

Figure 4.18 Schematic representation of liposome.

Table 4.8: Biomedical Application of Liposomes

Liposome Composition	Drug	Application
Hydrogenated soya, phosphatidylcholine, cholesterol, and distearoyl phosphatidylglycerol (DSPG)	Amphotericin B	*Aspergillus fumigatus*
1,2-Dipalmitoyl-*sn*-glycero-3-phosphocholine (DPPC) and cholesterol	Polymyxin B	*Pseudomonas aeruginosa*
Hydrogenated soya phosphatidylcholine (PC) and cholesterol	Ampillicin	*Micrococcus luteus* and *Salmonella typhimurium*
Dipalmitoyl-phosphatidylcholine, dipalmitoylphosphatidylglycerol and cholesterol	Ciprofloxacin	*Salmonella dublin*
Dipalmitoyl-phosphatidylcholine (DPPC), cholesterol and dimethylammonium ethane carbamoyl cholesterol (DC-chol)	Benzyl penicillin	*Staphylococcus aureus*
Phosphatidylcholine, cholesterol, and phosphatidylinositol	Netilmicin	*Bacillus subtilis* and *Escherichia coli*
Partially hydrogenated egg phosphatidylcholine (PHEPC), cholesterol, and 1,2-distearoyl-*sn*-glycero-3-phosphoethanolamine-*N*-(polyethylene glycol-2000) (PEGDSPE)	Gentamicin	*Klebsiella pneumoniae*
Phosphatidyl glycerol, phosphatidyl choline, and cholesterol	Streptomycin	*Mycobacterium avium*
Hydrogenated soy phosphatidylcholine, cholesterol and distearoylphos-phatidylglycerol (DSPG)	Amikacin	Gram-negative bacteria
Stearylamine (SA) and dicetyl phosphate	Zidovudine	Human immunodeficiency virus
Egg phosphatidylcholine, diacetylphosphate and cholesterol	Vancomycin or teicoplanin	Methicillin-resistant *Staphylococcus aureus* (MRSA)
DC-Chol liposome	Plasmid DNA	Gene transfer in subcutaneous tumor
Liposome	Daunorubicin and doxorubicin	Breast cancer
Liposome	Anti-GD2 immunoliposomes, liposomes entrapping fenretinide (HPR), gold-containing liposomes	Neuroblastoma
Hepatically targeted liposomes	Insulin	Diabetes mellitus

more than 100 nm, and small unilamellar vesicles (SUV) range from 20 to 100 nm and are formed by a single bilayer [80].

These versatile properties of liposomes made them to be used as potent carrier for various drugs like antibacterials, antivirals, insulin, antineoplastics, and plasmid DNA (Table 4.8).

4.3.11 Carbon-Based Materials (Graphene) in Drug Delivery Systems

Carbon-based materials like graphite, diamond, fullerenes, nanotubes, nanowires, and nanoribbons have been used for various applications in electronic, optics, optoelectronics, biomedical engineering, tissue engineering, medical implants, medical devices, and sensors. Graphene is an important new addition to these carbon family materials due to its unique properties. The strong carbon–carbon bonding in the plane, aromatic structure, presence of free π electrons, and reactive sites for surface reactions make graphene a unique material with exceptional mechanical, physicochemical, thermal, electronic, optical, and biomedical properties (Figure 4.19) [81].

Graphene-based materials demonstrate excellent electrochemical and optical properties, as well as the capability to adsorb a variety of aromatic biomolecules through a p–p stacking interaction and/or electrostatic interaction, which make them ideal materials for constructing biosensors and loading drugs. Since the first application for drug delivery was reported by Dai et al., graphene-based materials have been intensively investigated in the area of biomedicine and show promising potential in this field [82].

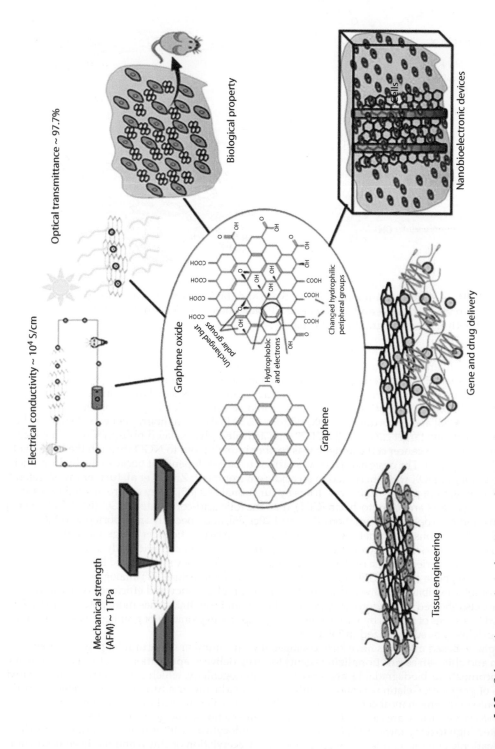

Figure 4.19 Schematic overview of various applications of graphene.

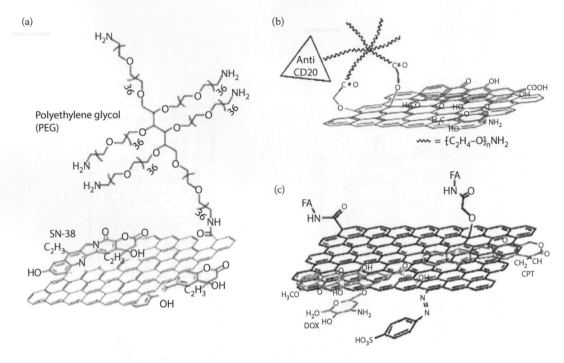

Figure 4.20 A schematic illustration of (a) SN38 and (b) doxorubicin (DOX) loading onto NGO–PEG–Rituxan via p-stacking and (c) DOX and CPT load onto FA-NGO (note that drugs can be loaded on both sides of the graphene sheets).

The major advantage of graphene over other nanomaterials is their ultrahigh surface area ($2630\ m^2/g$) and sp^2 hybridized carbon area, which make it an efficient drug carrier to load large amount of drug molecules on both sides of the single atom layer sheet. For example, Dai's group found that simple physisorption via p-stacking could be used for loading anticancer drugs SN38 (Figure 4.20a) [83] and doxorubicin (DOX) (Figure 4.20b) [84] onto nanographene oxide (NGO). In order to selectively target cancer cells, CD20+ (an activated-glycosylated phosphor protein which is overexpressed in cancer cells) antigen was further immobilized to NGO through the linkage of polyethylene glycol. The designed DDS was proved to be pH dependent because the hydrophilicity and solubility of DOX were increased in an acidic environment. Zhang et al. further investigated targeted delivery of mixed anticancer drugs by functional GO [85]. They control loaded two anticancer drugs, DOX and camptothecin (CPT), onto the folic acid-conjugated NGO (FA-NGO) via p–p stacking and hydrophobic interactions (Figure 4.20c) [86], and specially transported it to MCF-7 cells. Results demonstrated that FA-NGO loaded with the two anticancer drugs showed remarkably higher cytotoxicity against target cells compared to NGO loaded with only a single drug.

Liu et al. [87] carried out one of the earliest work in this field. They synthesized PEG-functionalized nanoscale graphene oxide (NGO) sheets loaded with a camptothecin (CPT) analog, SN38. NGO–PEG–SN38 complex exhibited good water solubility retaining high potency and efficiency of SN38. The complex also showed high cytotoxicity in HCT-116 cells and was 1000 times more potent than CPT. This led to a series of studies by various research groups for exploration of graphene-based materials in drug delivery as summarized in Table 4.9.

Graphene-based materials have been conjugated with a number of natural biopolymers like gelatin and chitosan as functionalizing agents for drug delivery applications. Natural biopolymers are biocompatible, biodegradable, and have low immunogenicity, which can greatly reduce the toxic effects of graphene. Gelatin was successfully used as a reducing and functionalizing agent to load DOX onto grapheme nanosheets (gelatin–GS) [88]. Gelatin–GS showed higher drug-loading capacity due to large surface area and relatively higher π interactions. The gelatin–GS–DOX complex also exhibited high toxicity toward MCF-7 cells through endocytosis. Chitosan is a naturally occurring linear cationic polysaccharide obtained by alkaline deacetylation of chitin and has been used with graphene for loading various drugs like ibuprofen, 5-fluorouracil [89], and CPT [90]. Rana et al.

Table 4.9: Drug and Applications of Graphene-Based Composites [81–87]

Graphene Composites	Drug	Graphene Composites Drug/Gene Cargo Highlights of the Study
NGO–PEG–RB–DOX	DOX	pH-dependent targeted drug release achieved using rituxan (CD20+ antibody)
PEG–BPEI–rGO–DOX	DOX	Photothermally induced cytosolic DOX delivery via endosome disruption
PEG–GO–DOX	DOX	Real time monitoring of in vitro and in vivo intracellular glutathione triggered controlled DOX release via label-free fluorescence live-cell imaging technique
DOX–GO–CHI–FA	DOX	pH-sensitive drug release with faster DOX release in acidic environment
NGO–SS–PEG–DOX	DOX	Demonstrate rapid intracellular release of DOX from GO composite at tumor relevant glutathione concentrations in HeLa cells
GO–FA–βCD–DOX	DOX	In vivo study of DOX-loaded GO–folic acid β cyclodextrin complex Demonstrates good cytocompatibility in vitro and tumor growth inhibition in vivo
Gelatin–GS–DOX	DOX	Gelatin-functionalized graphene for cellular imaging and delivery of DOX
GO–Fe_3O_4	DOX	Inorganic functionalization-based drug delivery
FeCo–GC–DOX	DOX	Photothermally enhanced drug delivery via FeCo–GC nanocomposite with enhanced delivery at elevated temperatures achieved by NIR laser irradiation
Chitosan–GO	Ibuprofen, 5FU, CPT, and pDNA delivery	Controlled release of chemically diverse drugs from chitosan–GO complexes, condensation of pDNA with chitosan–GO complex demonstrating satisfactory transfection efficiency in vitro
ADR–GO	DOX	Drug-resistance reversal in MCF-7/ADR cells using GO as DOX carrier. High drug loading capacity with pH-sensitive drug release
PEI–GO siRNA	DOX	Sequential delivery. Sequential gene and drug codelivery with high transfection efficiency and enhanced anticancer activity

Abbreviations: NGO, nanographene oxide; PEG, polyethylene glycol; RB, rituxan (CD20+antibody); DOX, doxorubicin; BPEI, branched polyethylenimine; rGO, reduced graphene oxide; CHI, chitosan; FA, folic acid; SS, disulfide linkages; βCD, β cyclodextrin; GS, graphene sheet; CPT, camptothecin; PNIPAM, poly(N-isopropylacrylamide); 5FU, 5-fluorouracil; ADR, adriamycin/doxorubicin (DOX); CNT, carbon nanotubes; Ce6, chlorin e6; PEI, polyethylenimine; Ti, titanium; BMP2, bone morphogenetic protein-2.

[89] used chitosan-functionalized GO for ibuprofen (IBU) and 5-fluorouracil (5-FU) delivery. 5-FU showed a lower drug-loading capacity due to relatively hydrophilic character, lower π–π interaction, and presence of diamide group. In another study, Bao and coauthors [90] synthesized chitosan–GO–CPT complex, which showed remarkably higher toxicity in HepG2 and HeLa cell lines compared to the pure CPT. Use of graphene-based materials has also been explored for codelivery of multiple drugs for chemotherapeutic efficacy. Zang et al. [91] functionalized GO with sulfonic acid groups followed by covalent bonding of folic acid molecules for targeted drug delivery. Controlled loading of DOX and CPT inside the same drug delivery vehicle resulted in remarkably higher toxicity in MCF-7 cells compared with GO-loaded only with DOX or CPT. Thus, graphene and GO-modified magnetic nanoparticles find wide biomedical applications in drug delivery, MRI, and bioimaging.

GO possesses unique features, such as easy synthesis, high dispersibility in water as well as in physiological environments, excellent biocompatibility and easily tunable surface functionalization, which are highly propitious to biological applications [92]. Importantly, both sides of a GO sheet can be available for drug loading, which contributes to the high drug-loading amount. Moreover, the dynamic bonding interactions (e.g., p–p stacking, hydrophobic, hydrogen bonding, and electrostatic interactions) between GO and the drugs show controlled response to external stimuli (such as pH, temperature, chemical substances, and electric fields) [93,94]. Therefore, the controlled drug release from GO can be achieved by various routes. All these positive attributes make GO much more efficacious than other carbonaceous nanomaterials as drug carriers for in vitro and in vivo biological applications [95]. Polymer-coated GO nanosheets have also been used as therapeutic carriers as the coating can improve the biocompatibility of GO. Chitosan-coated GO was used to load and deliver hydrophobic and aromatic drugs, proving to be both biocompatible and highly effective in cancer cell reduction [96]. Remarkable progress in synthesis and functionalization of graphene materials has opened new avenues exploring their use in drug delivery.

4.3.12 Core–Shell Nanoparticles-Based Drug Delivery Systems

Core–shell nanoparticles have a core made of a material coated with another material on top of it. In biological applications, core–shell nanoparticles have major advantages over simple nanoparticles leading to the improvement of properties such as (i) less cytotoxicity [97], (ii) increase in dispersibility, bio- and cyto-compatibility, (iii) better conjugation with other bioactive molecules, (iv) increased thermal and chemical stability, and so on [98]. More elaborately

1. When the desired nanoparticles are toxic which may cause plenty of trouble to the host tissues and organs. The coating of a benign material on top of the core makes the nanoparticles much less toxic and biocompatible. Sometimes shell layer not only acts as nontoxic layer but also improves the core material property.

2. Hydrophilicity of nanoparticles is very important to disperse them in biological systems (aqueous). The increase in biodispersivity, bio-, and cytocompatibility makes it a useful alternative to conventional drug delivery vehicle. The ease of synthesis also plays an important role in attracting the attention of researchers to this class of materials. The core–shell nanoparticles are mainly designed for biomedical applications based on the surface chemistry, which increases its affinity to bind with drugs, receptors, ligands, etc. [99,100]. The biocompatibility and cytocompatibility increase its therapeutic value opening a whole new avenue for the synthesis of novel drug carrier with enhanced properties such as increased residence time, increased bioavailability, and reduction of dosing quantity as well as frequency along with increased specificity. As a specific example, the bio-inspired polymeric coat on hydrophobic drug can facilitate the proper release of the drug at its targeted site because of ion-, temperature-, and pH-specific degradation of the polymer [101,102]. A schematic presentation of a core–shell nanoparticle for multipurpose biomedical applications is shown in Figure 4.21 [103].

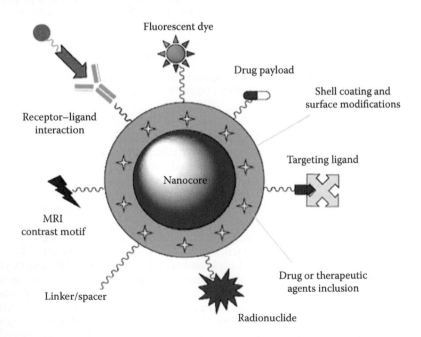

Figure 4.21 Scheme of multifunctional nanoparticle for molecular imaging, drug delivery, and therapy. Optionally functionalized and devised nanoparticles could be achieved for individualized diagnosis and treatments.

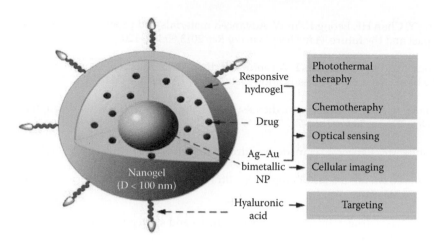

Figure 4.22 Schematic illustration of multifunctional core–shell hybrid nanogels.

4.3.12.1 Core–Shell Nanogels

Core–shell nanogels are composed of a metal core and a hydrophilic shell such as PEG, poly(*N*-isopropyl acrylamide-*co*-acrylic acid), etc. Wu et al. [104] constructed hybrid nanogels by coating the Ag–Au bimetallic NP core with a thermo-responsive nonlinear poly(ethylene glycol) (PEG)-based hydrogel as shell. They then loaded the nanogel with anticancer drug temozolomide and used it for drug delivery as well as fluorescence imaging of mouse melanoma cells (B16F10 cell-line). The drug release can be induced by both the heat generated by external NIR irradiation and the temperature increase of local environmental media. In one of their works, Wu and his fellow workers [105] developed core–shell structured hybrid nanogels (40–80 nm) composed of Ag nanoparticles as core and smart gel of poly(*N*-isopropylacrylamide-*co*-acrylicacid) as shell, which can overcome cellular barriers to enter the intracellular region and light up the mouse melanoma cells, including the nuclear regions. The pH-responsive hybrid nanogels exhibit not only a high drug-loading capacity but also a pH-controllable drug releasing behavior, clearly visualized in Figure 4.22 [106].

4.4 CONCLUSIONS AND FUTURE PROSPECTS

This chapter has attempted the compilation of the most recent advances performed in the field of smart polymers and their application in the biomaterials area as drug delivery carriers. With the advancement of novel DDS, smart biomaterial-based DDS provide a link between therapeutic need and drug delivery. This chapter highlights the current literature and describes the principles and applications of smart materials. While there are many exciting challenges faced by this field, there are a number of opportunities for the development of smart polymeric DDS. Smart biomaterials DDS have a very wide range of applications and are likely to have an exciting future. There is a wide range of nanoparticulate materials and structures being developed for the delivery of therapeutic compounds. Each has its own particular advantages, but as these nanoparticles become optimized for their specific application, the outcome will be better controlled therapy as a result of targeted delivery of smaller amounts of effective drugs to the required sites in the body. This is being made possible through the use of advanced material, improved control of particle size, increased half-life, high biocompatibility, minimum immunogenicity, site targeting, overcome the membrane barriers, better understanding of interface between the biological and material surfaces, and their effects in vivo. Some nanoparticle-based products are already approved by the US FDA, while several others are currently under development and clinical assessment.

REFERENCES

1. Felice B, Prabhakaran MP, Rodríguez AP, Ramakrishna S. Drug delivery vehicles on a nano-engineering perspective. *Mater Sci Eng C* 2014;41:178–195.

2. Zhang Y, Chan HF, Leong Kam W. Advanced materials and processing for drug delivery: The past and the future. *Adv Drug Delivery Rev* 2013;65:104–120.

3. Dokoumetzidis A, Macheras P. A century of dissolution research: From Noyes and Whitney to the biopharmaceutics classification system. *Int J Pharm* 2006;321:1–11.

4. Patton JS, Byron PR. Inhaling medicines: Delivering drugs to the body through the lungs. *Nat Rev Drug Discov* 2007;6(1):67–74.

5. Prausnitz MR, Langer R. Transdermal drug delivery. *Nat Biotechnol* 2008;26(11):1261–1268.

6. Gaudana R, Ananthula HK, Parenky A, Mitra AK. Ocular drug delivery. *AAPS J* 2010;12(3):348–360.

7. Illum L. Nasal drug delivery: New developments and strategies. *Drug Discov Today* 2002;7(23):1184–1189.

8. Pawar VK, Singh Y, Meher JG, Gupta S, Chourasia MK. Engineered nanocrystal technology: In-vivo fate, targeting and applications in drug delivery. *J Controll Release* 2014;183:51–66.

9. Tuan-Mahmood TM, McCrudden MT, Torrisi BM, McAlister E, Garland MJ, Singh TR, Donneyll RF. Microneedles for intradermal and transdermal drug delivery. *Eur J Pharm Sci* 2013;50(5):623–637.

10. Anselmo AC, Mitragotri S. An overview of clinical and commercial impact of drug delivery systems. *J Control Release* 2014;190:15–28.

11. U.S. Pharmaceutical Sales—2013. January 17, 2014. Available from: http://www.drugs.com/stats/top100/2013/sales.

12. Juan L, Huang Y, Kumar A, Tan A, Jin S, Mozhi A, Liang XJ. pH-sensitive nano-systems for drug delivery in cancer therapy. *Biotechnol Adv* 2014;32:693–710.

13. Lee BK, Yun YH, Park K, Sturek M. Introduction to biomaterials for cancer therapeutics. In: Park K, editor. *Biomaterials for Cancer Therapeutics*. Oxford, UK: Woodhead Publishing Ltd.; 2013.

14. Jabr Milane Lara S, Van Vlerken Lilian E, Yadav S, Amiji Mansoor M. Multi-functional nanocarriers to overcome tumor drug resistance. *Cancer Treat Rev* 2008;34:592–602.

15. Jong WHD, Borm PJ. Drug delivery and nanoparticles: Applications and hazards. *Int J Nanomed* 2008;3:133–149.

16. Liu Z, Jiao Y, Wang Y, Zhou C, Zhang Z. Polysaccharides-based nanoparticles as drug delivery systems. *Adv Drug Deliv Rev* 2008;60:1650–1662.

17. Agrawal U, Sharma R, Gupta M, Vyas SP. Is nanotechnology a boon for oral drug delivery?. *Drug Discov Today* 2014;19(10):1530–1546.

18. Khanjari A, Karabagias IK, Kontominas MG. Combined effect of N,O-carboxymethyl chitosan and oregano essential oil to extend shelf life and control Listeria monocytogenes in raw chicken meat fillets. LWT-*Food Sci Technol* 2013;53:94–99.

19. Luo Y, Teng Z, Wang X, Wang Q. Development of carboxymethyl chitosan hydrogel beads in alcohol-aqueous binary solvent for nutrient delivery applications. *Food Hydrocollloid* 2013;31:332–339.

20. Zhao D, Huang J, Hu S, Mao J, Mei L. Biochemical activities of N,O-carboxymethyl chitosan from squid cartilage. *Carbohydr Polym* 2011;85:832–837.

21. Li P, Liu DH, Miao L, Liu CX, Sun XL, Liu Y, Zheng N. A pH-sensitive multifunctional gene carrier assembled via layer-by-layer technique for efficient gene delivery. *Int J Nanomed* 2012;7:925–939.

22. Wang F, Chen Y, Zhang D, Zhang Q, Zheng D, Hao L. Folate-mediated targeted and intracellular delivery of paclitaxel using a novel deoxycholic acid-O-carboxymethylated chitosan-folic acid micelles. *Int J Nanomed* 2012;7:325–337.

23. Maya S, Kumar LG, Sarmento B, Rejinold NS, Menon D, Nair SV. Cetuximab conjugated O-carboxymethyl chitosan nanoparticles for targeting EGFR overexpressing cancer cells. *Carbohydr Polym* 2013;93:661–669.

24. Upadhyaya L, Singh J, Agarwal V, Tewari RP. The implications of recent advances in carboxymethyl chitosan based targeted drug delivery and tissue engineering applications. *J Control Release* 2014;186:54–87.

25. Larsson M, Huang WC, Hsiao MH, Wang YJ, Nydén M, Chiou SH, Liu DM. Biomedical applications and colloidal properties of amphiphilically modified chitosan hybrids. *Prog Polym Sci* 2013;38:1307–1328.

26. Shelma R, Sharma CP. Acyl modified chitosan derivatives for oral delivery of insulin and curcumin. *J Mater Sci Mater Med* 2010;21:2133–2140.

27. Zhang Y, Huo M, Zhou J, Yu D, Wu Y. Potential of amphiphilically modified low molecular weight chitosan as a novel carrier for hydrophobic anticancer drug: Synthesis, characterization, micellization and cytotoxicity evaluation. *Carbohydr Polym* 2009;77:231–238.

28. Xiangyang X, Ling L, Jianping Z, Shiyue L, Jie Y, Xiaojin YR., Jinsheng R. Preparation and characterization of N-succinyl-N'-octyl chitosan micelles as doxorubicin carriers for effective anti-tumor activity. *Colloids Surf B Biointerfaces* 2007;55:222–228.

29. Zheng H, Rao Y, Yin Y, Xiong X, Xu P, Lu B. Preparation, characterization, and in vitro drug release behavior of 6-mercaptopurine-carboxymethyl chitosan. *Carbohydr Polym* 2011;83:1952–1958.

30. Tan YL, Liu CG. Self-aggregated nanoparticles from linoleic acid modified carboxymethyl chitosan: Synthesis, characterization and application in vitro. *Colloids Surf B Biointerface* 2009;69:178–182.

31. Hsiao MH, Tung TH, Hsiao CS, Liu DM. Nano-hybrid carboxymethyl-hexanoyl chitosan modified with (3-aminopropyl)triethoxysilane for camptothecin delivery. *Carbohydr Polym* 2012;89:632–639.

32. Jin YH, Hu HY, Qiao MX, Zhu J, Qi JW, Hu CJ, Zhang Q,Chen DW. pH-sensitive chitosan-derived nanoparticles as doxorubicin carriers for effective anti-tumor activity: Preparation and in vitro evaluation. *Colloids Surf B* 2012;94:184–191.

33. Li H, Huo M, Zhou J, Dai Y, Deng Y, Shi X, Masoud J. Enhanced oral absorption of paclitaxel in N-deoxycholic acid-N, O-hydroxyethyl chitosan micellar system. *J Pharm Sci* 2010;99:4543–4553.

34. Hu FQ, Liu LN, Du YZ, Yuan H. Synthesis and antitumor activity of doxorubicin conjugated stearic acid-g-chitosan oligosaccharide polymeric micelles. *Biomaterials* 2009;30:6955–6963.

35. Sahu SK, Maiti S, Maiti TK, Ghosh SK, Pramanik P. Folate-decorated succinylchitosan nanoparticles conjugated with doxorubicin for targeted drug delivery. *Macromol Biosci* 2011;11:285–295.

36. Zhou H, Yu W, Guo X, Liu X, Li N, Zhang Y, Ma X. Synthesis and characterization of amphiphilic glycidol–chitosan–deoxycholic acid nanoparticles as a drug carrier for doxorubicin. *Biomacromolecules* 2010;11:3480–3486.

37. Kim K, Kwon S, Park JH, Chung H, Jeong SY, Kwon IC, Kim IS. Physicochemical Characterizations of self-assembled nanoparticles of glycol chitosan–deoxycholic acid conjugates. *Biomacromolecules* 2005;6:1154–1158.

38. Shelma R, Sharma CP. Development of lauroyl sulfated chitosan for enhancing hemocompatibility of chitosan. *Colloids Surf B Biointerfaces* 2011;84:561–570.

39. Liu C, Fan W, Chen X, Liu C, Meng X, Park HJ. Self-assembled nanoparticles based on linoleic-acid modified carboxymethyl-chitosan as carrier of adriamycin (ADR). *Curr Appl Phys* 2007;7(S1):e125–e129.

40. Du YZ, Wang L, Yuan H, Wei XH, Hu FQ. Preparation and characteristics of linoleic acid-grafted chitosan oligosaccharide micelles as a carrier for doxorubicin. *Colloids Surf B Biointerfaces* 2009;69:257–263.

41. Zhao Z, He M, Yin L, Bao J, Shi L, Wang B, Tang C, Yin C. Biodegradable nanoparticles based on linoleic acid and poly(beta-malic acid) double grafted chitosan derivatives as carriers of anticancer drugs. *Biomacromolecules* 2009;10:565–72.

42. Zhang C, Ding Y, Yu L, Ping Q. Polymeric micelle systems of hydroxycamptothecin based on amphiphilic N-alkyl-N-trimethyl chitosan derivatives. *Colloids Surf B Biointerfaces* 2007;55:192–9.

43. Zhang C, Ping Q, Zhang H, Shen J. Preparation of N-alkyl-O-sulfate chitosan derivatives and micellar solubilization of taxol. *Carbohydr Polym* 2003;54:137–141.

44. Miwa A, Ishibe A, Nakano M, Yamahira T, Itai S, Jinno S, Kawahara H. Development of novel chitosan derivatives as micellar carriers of taxol. *Pharm Res* 1998;15:1844–1850.

45. Zhang C, Qu G, Sun Y, Yang T, Yao Z, Shen W, Shen Z, Ding Q, Zhou H, Ping Q. Biological evaluation of N-octyl-O-sulfate chitosan as a new nano-carrier of intravenous drugs. *Eur J Pharm Sci* 2008;33:415–423.

46. Zhang C, Qu G, Sun Y, Wu X, Yao Z, Guo Q, Ding Q, Yuan S, Shen Z, Ping Q, Zhou H. Pharmacokinetics, biodistribution, efficacy and safety of N-octyl-O-sulfate chitosan micelles loaded with paclitaxel. *Biomaterials* 2008;29:1233–1241.

47. Mo R, Jin X, Li N, Ju C, Sun M, Zhang C, Ping Q. The mechanism of enhancement on oral absorption of paclitaxel by N-octyl-O-sulfate chitosan micelles. *Biomaterials* 2011;32:4609–4620.

48. Zhang C, Qineng P, Zhang H. Self-assembly and characterization of paclitaxel-loaded N-octyl-O-sulfate chitosan micellar system. *Colloids Surf B Biointerfaces* 2004;39:69–75.

49. Wang Y, Yang X, Yang J, Wang Y, Chen R, Wu J, Liu Y, Zhang N. Self-assembled nanoparticles of methotrexate conjugated O-carboxymethyl chitosan: Preparation, characterization and drug release behavior in vitro. *Carbohydr Polym* 2011;86:1665–1670.

50. Wang H, Zhao P, Liang X, Gong X, Song T, Niu R, Chang J. Folate-PEG coated cationic modified chitosan—cholesterol liposomes for tumor-targeted drug delivery. *Biomaterials* 2010;31:4129–4138.

51. Peniche H, Peniche C. Chitosan nanoparticles: A contribution to nanomedicine. *Polym Int* 2011;60:883–889.

52. Sashiwa H, Aiba Si. Chemically modified chitin and chitosan as biomaterials. *Prog Polym Sci* 2004;29:887–908.

53. Aranaz I, Harris R, Heras A. Chitosan amphiphilic derivatives: Chemistry and applications. *Curr Org Chem* 2010;14:308–330.

54. Ryu JH, Roy R, Ventura J, Thayumanavan S. Redox-sensitive disassembly of amphiphilic copolymer based micelles. *Langmuir* 2010;26:7086–7092.

55. Wei H, Zhuo R-X, Zhang X-Z. Design and development of polymeric micelles with cleavable links for intracellular drug delivery. *Prog Polym Sci* 2013;38:503–535.

56. Brewster ME, Loftsson T. Cyclodextrins as pharmaceutical solubilizers. *Adv Drug Deliv Rev* 2007;59:645–666.

57. Vyas A, Saraf S, Saraf S. Cyclodextrin based novel drug delivery systems. *J Inclusion Phenom Macrocyclic Chem* 2008;62(1–2):23–42.

58. Nadish Z, Hatem F, Abdelhamid E. Cyclodextrin containing biodegradable particles: From preparation to drug delivery applications. *Int J Pharm* 2014;461:351–366.

59. Sawada SI, Sasaki Y, Nomura Y, Akiyoshi K. Cyclodextrin-responsive nanogelas an artificial chaperone for horseradish peroxidase. *Colloid Polym Sci* 2011;289:685–691.

60. Concheiro A, Alvarez-Lorenzo C. Chemically cross-linked and grafted cyclodextrin hydrogels: From nanostructures to drug-eluting medical devices. *Adv Drug Deliv Rev* 2013;65:1188–1203.

61. Aegerter MA, Leventis N, Koebel MM. Advances in sol–gel derived materials and technologies. In: Aegerter MA, Prassas M, editors. *Aerogel Handbook*. New York: Springer; 2011.

62. García-González CA, Alnaief M, Smirnova I. Polysaccharide-based aerogels—Promising biodegradable carriers for drug delivery systems. *Carbohydr Polym* 2011;86:1425–1438.

63. Ulker Z, Erkey C. An emerging platform for drug delivery: Aerogel based systems. *J Control Release* 2014;177:51–63.

64. Heller DA, Levi Y, Pelet JM, Doloff JC, Wallas J, Pratt GW, Jiang S et al. Modular 'click-in-emulsion' bone-targeted nanogels. *Adv Mater* 2012;25:1449–1454.

65. Jiang Y, Chen J, Deng C, Suuronen Erik J, Zhong Z. Click hydrogels, microgels and nanogels: Emerging platforms for drug delivery and tissue engineering. *Biomaterials* 2014;35:4969–4985.

66. Soga O, Van Nostrum CF, Fens M, Rijcken CJ, Schiffelers RM, Storm G, Hennink WE. Thermosensitive and biodegradable polymeric micelles for paclitaxel delivery. *J Control Release* 2005;103:341Y353.

67. Maeda H, Greish K, Fang J. Polymer therapeutics: Polymers as drugs, conjugates and gene delivery systems. *Adv Polym Sci* 2006;192:1–8.

68. Safari J, Zarnegar Z. Advanced drug delivery systems: Nanotechnology of health design A review. *J Saudi Chem Soc* 2014;18:85–99.

69. Mudshinge SR, Deore AB, Patil S, Bhalgat CM. Nanoparticles: Emerging carriers for drug delivery. *Saudi Pharm J* 2011;19:129–141.

70. Prabaharan M. Prospective of guar gum and its derivatives as controlled drug delivery systems. *Int J Biol Macromol* 2011;49:117–124.

71. Prajapati VD, Jani GK, Moradiya NG, Randeria NP. Pharmaceutical applications of various natural gums, mucilages and their modified forms. *Carbohydr Polym* 2013;92:1685–1699.

72. Kaur IP, Garg A, Singla AK, Aggarwal D. Vesicular systems in ocular drug delivery: An overview. *Int J Pharm* 2004;269:1–14.

73. Srinivasan BP, Shilpa S, Chauhan M. Niosomes as vesicular carriers for delivery of proteins and biologicals. *Int J Drug Deliv* 2011;3:14–24.

74. Ammar HO, El-Nahhas SA, Higazy IM. Proniosomes as a carrier system for transdermal delivery of tenoxicam. *Int J Pharm* 2011;405:142–152.

75. Moghassemi S, Hadjizadeh A. Nano-niosomes as nanoscale drug delivery systems: An illustrated review. *J Control Release* 2014;185:22–36.

76. Food and Drug Administration. Available from: www.accessdata.fda.gov.

77. Buse J, El-Aneed A. Properties, engineering and applications of lipid-based nanoparticle drug-delivery systems: Current research and advances. *Nanomedicine* 2010;5(8):1237–1260.

78. Allen TM, Cullis PR. Liposomal drug delivery systems: From concept to clinical applications. *Adv Drug Deliv Rev* 2013;65(1):36–48.

79. Muthu MS, Singh S. Targeted nanomedicines: Effective treatment modalities for cancer, AIDS and brain disorders. *Nanomedicine-UK* 2009;4:105–118.

80. Li J, Wang X, Zhang T, Wang C, Huang Z, Luo X, Deng Y. A review on phospholipids and their main applications in drug delivery systems. *Asian J Pharm Sci* 2015;10(2):81–98.

81. Goenka S, Sant V, Sant S. Graphene-based nanomaterials for drug delivery and tissue engineering. *J Control Release* 2014;173:75–88.

82. Shen H, Zhang L, Liu M, Zhang Z. Biomedical applications of graphene. *Theranostics* 2012;2(3):283–294.

83. Liu Z, Robinson JT, Sun X, Dai H. PEGylated nano-graphene oxide for delivery of water insoluble cancer drugs. *J Am Chem Soc* 2008;130(33):10876–10877.

84. Sun X, Liu Z, Welsher K, Robinson JT, Goodwin A, Zaric S, Dai H. Nano-graphene oxide for cellular imaging and drug delivery. *Nano Res* 2008;1(3):203–212.

85. Zhang L, Xia J, Zhao Q, Liu L, Zhang Z. Functional graphene oxide as a nanocarrier for controlled loading and targeted delivery of mixed anticancer drugs. *Small* 2010;6(4):537–544.

86. Zhang L, Lu Z, Zhao Q, Huang J, Shen H, Zhang Z. Enhanced chemotherapy efficacy by sequential delivery of siRNA and anticancer drugs using PEI-grafted graphene oxide. *Small* 2011;7(4):460–464.

87. Liu Z, Robinson JT, Sun X, Dai H. PEGylated nano-graphene oxide for delivery of water insoluble cancer drugs. *J Am Chem Soc* 2008;130:10876–10877.

88. Liu KP, Zhang J-J, Cheng F-F, Zheng T-T, Wang C, Zhu J-J. Green and facile synthesis of highly biocompatible graphene nanosheets and its application for cellular imaging and drug delivery. *J Mater Chem* 2011;21:12034–12040.

89. Rana VK, Choi M-C, Kong J-Y, Kim GY, Kim MJ, Kim S-H, Mishra S, Singh RP, Ha CS. Synthesis and drug-delivery behavior of chitosan-functionalized graphene oxide hybrid nanosheets. *Macromol Mater Eng* 2011;296:131–140.

90. Bao H, Pan Y, Ping Y, Sahoo NG, Wu T, Li L, Li J, Gan LH. Chitosan-functionalized graphene oxide as a nanocarrier for drug and gene delivery. *Small* 2011;7:1569–1578.

91. Zhang L, Xia J, Zhao Q, Liu L, Zhang Z. Functional graphene oxide as a nanocarrier for controlled loading and targeted delivery of mixed anticancer drugs. *Small* 2010;6:537–544.

92. Georgakilas V, Otyepka M, Bourlinos AB, Chandra V, Kim N, Kemp KC, Hobza P, Zboril R, Kim KS. Functionalization of graphene: Covalent and non-covalent approaches, derivatives and applications. *Chem Rev.* 2012;112(11):6156–6214.

93. Huang X, Qi X, Boey F, Zhang H. Graphene-based composites. *Chem Soc Rev* 2012;41(2):666–686.

94. Ostrikov K, Neyts EC, Mayyappan M. Plasma nanoscience: From nano-solids in plasmas to nano-plasmas in solids. *Adv Phys* 2013;62(2):113–224.

95. Yang Y, Asiri AM, Tang Z, Du D, Lin Y. Graphene based materials for biomedical applications. *Mater Today* 2013;16(10):365–373.

96. Justin R, Chen B. Characterisation and drug release performance of biodegradable chitosan-graphene oxide nanocomposites. *Carbohydr Polym* 2014;103:70–80.

97. Law W-C, Yong K-T, Roy I, Xu G, Ding H, Bergey EJ, Zeng H, Prasad PN. Optically and magnetically doped organically modified silica nanoparticles as efficient magnetically guided biomarkers for two-photon imaging of live cancer cells. *J Phys Chem C* 2008;112:7972–7977.

98. Sounderya N, Zhang Y. Use of core/shell structured nanoparticles for biomedical applications. *Recent Pat Biomed Eng* 2008;1:34–42.

99. Sahoo SK, Labhasetwar V. Nanotech approaches to drug delivery and imaging. *Drug Discov Today* 2003;8:1112–1120.

100. Gilmore JL, Yi X, Quan L, Kabanov AV. Novel nanomaterials for clinical neuroscience. *J Neuroimmune Pharmacol* 2008;3:83–94.

101. Mahmud A, Xiong X-B, Aliabadi HM, Lavasanifar A. Polymeric micelles for drug targeting. *J Drug Target* 2007;15:553–584.

102. Van Tomme SR, Storm G, Hennink WE. In situ gelling hydrogels for pharmaceutical and biomedical applications. *Int J Pharm* 2008;355:1–18.

103. Liu G, Swierczewska M, Lee S, Chen X. Functional nanoparticles for molecular imaging guided gene delivery. *Nano Today* 2010;5:524–539.

104. Wu W, Shen J, Banerjee P, Zhou S. Core–shell hybrid nanogels for integration of optical temperature-sensing, targeted tumor cell imaging, and combined chemo-photothermal treatment. *Biomaterials* 2010;31:7555–7566.

105. Wu W, Zhou T, Berliner A, Banerjee P, Zhou S. Smart core-shell hybrid nanogels with Ag nanoparticle core for cancer cell imaging and gel shell for pH-regulated drug delivery. *Chem Mater* 2010;22:1966–1976.

106. Chatterjee K, Sarkar S, Rao JK, Paria S. Core/shell nanoparticles in biomedical applications. *Adv Colloid Interface Sci* 2014;209:8–39.

5 Wound-Dressing Implants

5.1 WOUNDS

A wound can be described as a defect or a break in the skin, resulting from physical or thermal damage or as a result of the presence of an underlying medical or physiological condition. According to the Wound Healing Society, a wound is the result of "disruption of normal anatomic structure and function" [1]. Based on the nature of the repair process, wounds can be classified as acute or chronic wounds. Acute wounds are usually tissue injuries that heal completely, with minimal scarring, within the expected time frame, usually 8–12 weeks [2]. The primary causes of acute wounds include mechanical injuries due to external factors such as abrasions and tears which are caused by frictional contact between the skin and hard surfaces. Mechanical injuries also include penetrating wounds caused by knives and gun shots and surgical wounds caused by surgical incisions to, for example, remove tumors. Another category of acute wounds includes burns and chemical injuries that arise from a variety of sources such as radiation, electricity, corrosive chemicals, and thermal sources. Wounds are also classified on basis of the number of skin layers and area of skin affected [3,4]. A pictorial representation of wound has been shown in Figure 5.1.

Injury that affects the epidermal skin surface alone is referred to as a superficial wound, whilst injury involving both the epidermis and the deeper dermal layers, including the blood vessels, sweat glands, and hair follicles is referred to as partial thickness wound. Full thickness wounds occur when the underlying subcutaneous fat or deeper tissues are damaged in addition to the epidermis and dermal layers.

5.2 TYPES OF WOUND

Wounds can be divided into four categories based on their appearance and stage of healing. Each wound type has slightly different characteristics and a wound healing by secondary infection will progress through these different stages over time. There is no "one size fits all" dressing; hence, wounds must be re-evaluated regularly in order to identify and respond to any changes.

5.2.1 Necrotic Wounds

Necrotic wounds (Figure 5.2a) are usually black or dark green and contain devitalized tissue. Infected necrotic wounds require sharp surgical debridement back to viable tissue in order to prevent systemic sepsis. In the absence of infection, necrotic tissues will eventually separate from the wound bed by autolysis. Necrotic wounds are particularly susceptible to dehydration, and autolysis is inhibited if the wound is allowed to dry out; the main priority of a dressing is to maintain sufficient moisture in the local environment of the wound [5].

5.2.2 Sloughing Wounds

Sloughing wounds (Figure 5.2b) contain a mixture of leukocytes, wound exudates, dead bacteria and fibrin, typically forming a glutinous yellow layer of tissue over the wound. The presence of slough predisposes to wound infection because it provides a nutrient-rich environment for bacterial proliferation. The formation of granulation tissue is delayed in a sloughing wound compared with a clean wound, and, hence, the optimal dressing will contribute toward wound debridement and the maintenance of a clean wound bed [6].

5.2.3 Granulating Wounds

Granulating wounds (Figure 5.2c) are highly vascularized and are a rich pink or red color. The amount of exudate produced is often substantial, and a dressing with the capacity to absorb excess exudate is desirable. Significant heat loss may occur with wounds covering large areas, requiring a dressing with insulating properties.

Overgranulating wounds have the following properties:

■ Contain excessive friable granulation tissue

■ Are prone to recurrent episodes of bleeding

■ Suffer from delayed epithelialization

In this situation, caustic pencils containing silver nitrate or topical corticosteroid can be applied directly to the affected areas in order to control the excess tissue [7].

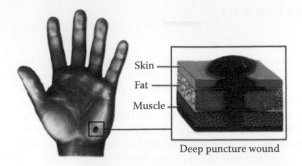

Figure 5.1 Pictorial presentation of anatomy of wound.

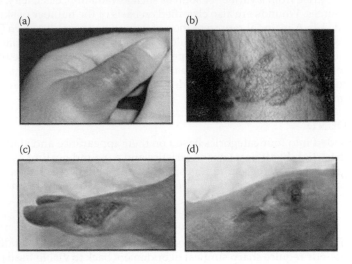

Figure 5.2 Different types of wounds. (a) Necrotic wound, (b) sloughing wounds, (c) granulating wounds, and (d) epithelializing wounds

5.2.4 Epithelializing Wounds

Epithelializing wounds (Figure 5.2d) contain new epithelial tissue (formed by the migration of keratinocytes from the wound margins) or contain islands of tissue (formed from skin appendages in the wound bed). The main priorities for dressing are the maintenance of a warm, moist environment around the wound, and the use of low-adherence dressings (see below) to minimize the trauma of dressing changes. In addition to the type of wound, the location, size, and depth of the wound may vary considerably. Along with the condition of the surrounding skin, these should also be considered when deciding the most suitable dressing [8].

5.3 WOUND HEALING

Wound healing (Figure 5.3) is a complex biological sequence of events in a closely orchestrated cascade to repair damage [9]. This process is divided into five overlapping but well-choreographed phases including hemostasis, inflammatory, maturation proliferative, and remodeling and scar formation [10]. For the normal healing process, it is essential to progress thorough sequential events which results in the immediate healing of the gap. Acute wound healing follows a predictable chain of events in a well-organized fashion, whereas chronic wounds will have prolonged inflammatory or proliferative phases, resulting in tissue fibrosis and nonhealing ulcers [11].

5.4 PHASES OF WOUND HEALING

The entire wound-healing process is a complex series of events that begins at the moment of injury and can continue for months to years. This overview will help in identifying the various phases of wound healing (Figure 5.4).

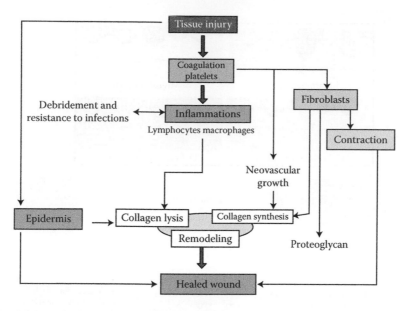

Figure 5.3 Outline diagram of healing process.

5.4.1 Hemostasis

Bleeding usually occurs when the skin is injured and serves to flush out bacteria and/or antigens from the wound. In addition, bleeding activates hemostasis that is initiated by exudate components such as clotting factors. Fibrinogen in the exudate elicits the clotting mechanism resulting in the coagulation of the exudates (blood without cells and platelets) and, together with the formation of a fibrin network, produces a clot in the wound causing bleeding to stop. The clot dries to form a scab and provides strength and support to the injured tissue. Hemostasis, therefore, plays a protective role as well as contributes to successful wound healing [12].

5.4.2 Inflammation

The inflammatory phase occurs almost simultaneously with hemostasis, sometimes from within a few minutes of injury to 24 h and lasts for about 3 days. It involves both cellular and vascular responses. The release of protein-rich exudates into the wound causes vasodilation through the release of histamine and serotonin, and allows phagocytes to enter the wound and engulf dead cells (necrotic tissue). Necrotic tissue is hard and is liquefied by enzymatic action to produce a yellow-colored mass described as sloughy. Platelets liberated from damaged blood vessels become activated as they come into contact with mature collagen and form aggregates as part of the clotting mechanism [13].

5.4.3 Migration

The migration phase [14] involves the movement of epithelial cells and fibroblasts to the injured area to replace damaged and lost tissue. These cells regenerate from the margins, rapidly growing over the wound under the dried scab (clot) accompanied by epithelial thickening.

5.4.4 Proliferation

The proliferative phase occurs almost simultaneously or just after the migration phase (day 3 onward) and basal cell proliferation, which lasts for between 2 and 3 days. Granulation tissue is formed by the in-growth of capillaries and lymphatic vessels into the wound and collagen is synthesized by fibroblasts giving the skin strength and form. By the fifth day, maximum formation of blood vessels and granulation tissue has occurred. Further epithelial thickening takes place until collagen bridges the wound. The fibroblast proliferation and collagen synthesis continue for up to 2 weeks by that time blood vessels decrease and edema recedes [15].

5.4.5 Maturation

This phase (also called the "remodeling phase") involves the formation of cellular connective tissue and strengthening of the new epithelium which determines the nature of the

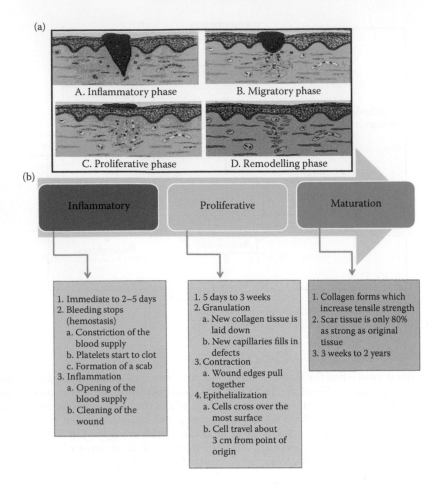

Figure 5.4 (a) Schematic representation of the phases of wound-healing: (A) infiltration of neutrophils into the wound area, (B) invasion of wound area by epithelial cells, (C) epithelium completely covers the wound, and (D) many of the capillaries and fibroblasts, formed at early stages have all disappeared (Adapted from Gandour—unpublished.) and (b) flow chart of various phase of wound healing.

final scar. Cellular granular tissue is changed to a cellular mass from several months up to about 2 years [16,17].

5.5 ROLE OF OXYGEN IN WOUND HEALING

Oxygen's key role (Figure 5.5) in the healing of wounds is well understood [18]. Wound healing is an energy demanding process and oxygen is needed to support the respiration essential to release the required energy [19,20]

Its role in healing is multifaceted and it is needed for

1. *Energy metabolism*: Important for the cellular processes of repair.

2. *Collagen synthesis*: Important for tissue regeneration.

3. *Neovascularization*: Important for tissue regeneration.

4. *Polymorphonuclear cell function*: Important for the first-line defence against microorganisms.

5. *Antimicrobial action*: Many of the pathogenic and malodorous bacteria found in wounds are obligate anaerobes which will be killed in an oxygenated environment. Some antibiotics need the presence of oxygen to exert their antimicrobial effects.

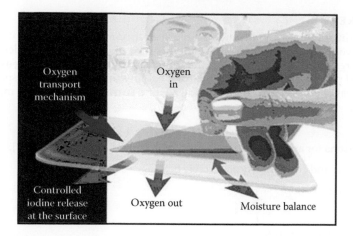

Figure 5.5   Schematic presentation of oxygen transport in case of wound healing.

5.6 REQUIREMENT FOR WOUND HEALING

The successful wound dressing (Figure 5.6) must perform the following functions:

- Seal the wound and prevent the introduction of external stresses and loss of energy
- Remove excess exudates and toxic components
- Maintain a high humidity at the wound-dressing interface
- Provide thermal insulation
- Act as a barrier to microorganism
- Be free from particulates and toxic wound contamination
- Be removable without causing trauma at dressing change

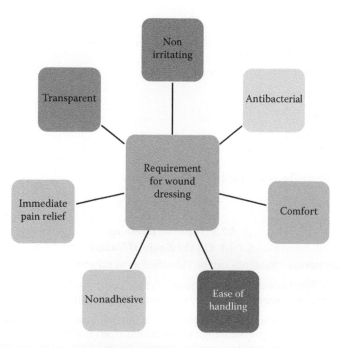

Figure 5.6   Diagrammatic presentation of requirements of wound healing.

5.7 WOUND DRESSING

The perfect dressing provides and maintains a moist environment and an adequate gaseous exchange at the wound surface that favors the proliferative phase of repair, particularly epithelialization. The dressing should also protect the wound from infection by acting as a bacterial shield and should provide thermal insulation. An ideal dressing occludes dead space, permits the atraumatic removal of excessive exudate from the wound surface, and is easy to manipulate and nonantigenic [21].

5.7.1 Reasons for Applying a Dressing

The principal reasons for applying a dressing can be summarized as follows [22]:

- To produce rapid and cosmetically acceptable healing
- To remove or control odor
- To reduce pain
- To prevent or combat infection
- To contain exudates
- To cause minimum stress or disturbance to the patient
- To hide or cover a wound for cosmetic reasons
- A combination of two or more of the above

5.7.2 Properties of the "Ideal" Wound Dressing

A dressing is an adjunct used by a person for application to a wound to promote healing and/or prevent further harm. A dressing is designed to be in direct contact with the wound, which makes it different from a bandage, which is primarily used to hold a dressing in place. The ideal dressing can be summarized as follows [23]:

- Removes excess exudate, but prevents the saturation of the dressing to its outer surface (strike through)
- Permits diffusion of gases
- Protects wound from microorganisms
- Provides mechanical protection
- Controls local temperature and pH
- Is easy and comfortable to remove/change
- Minimizes pain from the wound
- Controls wound odor
- Is cosmetically acceptable
- Is nonallergenic
- Does not contaminate the wound with foreign particles
- Is cost-effective

5.7.3 Types of Dressing

5.7.3.1 On the Basis of Nature

On the basis of their nature, dressings can be classified as synthetic, semisynthetic, and biologic.

1. *Synthetic dressings*: Synthetic dressings (Figure 5.7a) are composed of man-made fabric or plastic materials in the form of gauze, films, sprays, foams, and gels [24].

2. *Semisynthetic dressings*: Semisynthetic dressings (Figure 5.7b) are a combination of synthetic and biologic products. Biologic dressings are obtained from natural sources and include amnion, allografts, and xenografts as well as bioengineered tissues composed of various

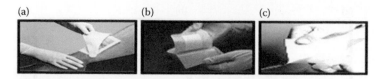

Figure 5.7 Picture of various types of dressing on the basis of nature (a) synthetic dressing, (b) semisynthetic dressing, and (c) bilogic dressing.

proteins (particularly collagen) or cultured wound-healing cells (primarily fibroblasts and keratinocytes) [25].

3. *Biologic dressing*: Biologic dressings (Figure 5.7c) often exert a beneficial effect on the wound in addition to providing protective covering [26].

5.7.3.2 *According to Their Ability to Adhere to a Wound*

According to their ability to adhere to a wound, dressings are also classified as adherent, low-adherent, and nonadherent.

1. *Adherent dressings*: Adherent dressings (Figure 5.8a) should be restricted to the initial inflammatory and debridement phases because they facilitate the removal of debris and excess exudates but may damage fragile tissues formed in subsequent phases [27].

2. *Low-adherent dressings*: Low-adherent (Figure 5.8b) products with a wound-contact surface that is designed specifically to reduce adherence, for example, some absorbent wound dressings [28].

3. *Nonadherent dressings*: A dressing (Figure 5.8c) that maintains a moist-gel layer over the wound that is not expected to adhere, provided that it is not allowed to dry out. In other words, those dressings that maintain a moist-gel layer over the wound, for example, hydrocolloids, hydrogels, and alginates. These would not be expected to adhere provided that they are not allowed to dry out. The performance of some of these materials will be largely determined by the choice of a secondary dressing where this is required [29].

5.7.3.3 *According to Their Ability to Permit the Passage of Exudates and Vapor*

According to their ability to permit the passage of exudates and vapors, dressings are further classified as occlusive and nonocclusive (permeable).

1. *Occlusive dressings*: Occlusive dressings (Figure 5.9a) are impermeable to water vapors, fluid, and oxygen, thus providing an environment that favors the proliferation of anaerobic bacteria. Because occlusive dressings encourage the formation of exuberant granulation tissue in equine wounds [30], it is recommended to restrict their use to the first 6–48 h after dressings.

2. *Nonocclusive dressings*: Nonocclusive dressings (Figure 5.9b) were developed to manage the moisture level at the wound surface. These dressings are designed to absorb excess exudates and to allow the evaporation of water vapors from the outside surface. They are, therefore, designed to handle a lot of fluid without feeling at all wet on their outside surface.

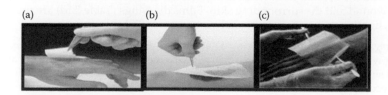

Figure 5.8 Various types of dressings on the basis of ability to adhere: (a) adherent dressing, (b) low-adherent dressing, and (c) nonadherent dressing.

(a)　　　　　　　　　　　　　(b)

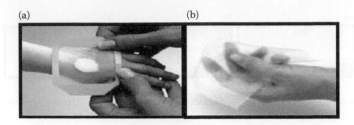

Figure 5.9 Pictures of various types of dressings on the basis of ability to permit passage of exudates and vapor: (a) occlusive dressing and (b) nonocclusive dressing.

The combined benefits of absorption and water vapor transmission allow large quantities of exudates to be "managed" without maceration, while maintaining the moist wound-healing environment that is conducive to repair [31].

5.7.3.4 Modern Dressings

Modern dressings are discussed under the type of material (hydrocolloid, alginate, and hydrogel) employed to produce the dressing and the physical form (film and foam) of the dressing.

1. *Tulle dressings*: Tulle dressings are cotton or viscose gauze dressings impregnated with paraffin (antiseptic or antibiotic may also be incorporated). Paraffin lowers the dressing adherence, but this property is lost if the dressing dries out. The hydrophobic nature of paraffin prevents the absorption of moisture from the wound, and frequent dressing changes are usually needed. Skin sensitization is also common in medicated types. Tulle dressings (Table 5.1a) are mainly indicated for superficial clean wounds, and a secondary dressing is usually needed [32].

2. *Hydrocolloids dressings*: Hydrocolloids contain a hydrocolloid matrix of gelatin, pectin, and cellulose mixed together to form a waterproof adhesive dressing that interacts with the wound bed and patients experience less pain, require less analgesia, and are able to carry out their normal daily activities. Exudates produced by the wound absorb into the dressing, which dissolve and form a gel. The moisture from this gel enhances the autolytic debridement of necrotic and sloughing tissues and promotes the formation of granulation tissue. Hydrocolloid dressings (Table 5.1b) absorb light-to-moderate levels of exudate, do not require a secondary dressing, and are shower proof, but on the absorption of wound exudate, a change in the physical state occurs with the formation of a gel covering the wound. Therefore, they are used to pressure sores, minor burns, and traumatic injuries [33].

3. *Hydrofibres dressings*: Hydrofibers (Table 5.1c) are produced from similar materials to hydrocolloids and also form a gel on contact with the wound, but are softer and more fibrous in appearance, with a greater capacity to absorb exudate. Moisture from the gel assists in debridement and facilitates nontraumatic removal [34].

4. *Films dressings*: Films are made from a thin polyurethane film coated with adhesive. Film dressings are highly comfortable, shower proof, and their transparency allows for wound monitoring without dressing removal. Vapor-permeable films allow the diffusion of gases and water vapor, but are minimally absorbed. Problems can arise if these dressings are applied to heavily exuding wounds because fluid tends to accumulate underneath the film, leading to maceration of the wound and the surrounding skin. Films dressings (Table 5.1d) are thus suited to superficial, lightly exudating, or epithelializing wounds [35].

5. *Foam dressings*: A foam dressing is constructed from polyurethane and absorbs exudate without interacting with the wound bed. They absorb low-to-moderate amounts of fluid and usually have a semipermeable backing to allow the escape of moisture. Foams (Table 5.1e) do not require a secondary dressing and are often used as an outer dressing with other products [36].

6. *Alginates dressings*: Alginates are derived from a calcium salt of alginic acid, producing highly absorbent dressings (occur either in the form of freeze-dried porous sheets (foams) or as flexible fibers due to their ability to form gels upon contact with wound exudates (high absorbency

Table 5.1: Types of Modern Dressings

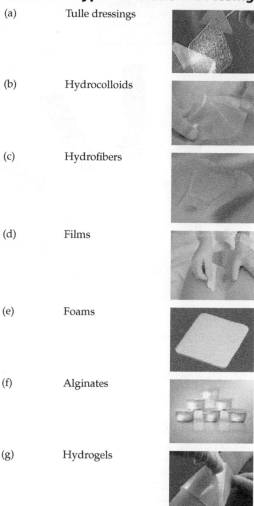

(a)	Tulle dressings	
(b)	Hydrocolloids	
(c)	Hydrofibers	
(d)	Films	
(e)	Foams	
(f)	Alginates	
(g)	Hydrogels	

via strong hydrophilic gel formation, which limits wound secretions and minimizes bacterial contamination)) suitable for heavily exudating wounds; some alginates also possess hemostatic properties. As they absorb exudate, alginates change from a soft fibrous texture into a gel, facilitating easy removal and preventing dressing fibers from contaminating the wound. Alginates (Table 5.1f) are manufactured as flat sheets or as rope, and are suitable for packing cavities [37].

7. *Hydrogel dressings*: Hydrogels are excellent materials and have all the properties required for wound dressings. These are capable of absorbing contaminated exudates and safely retaining them within the gel structure, which provides microclimate that stimulates and regulates all cellular activities and nutritional processes during the individual phases of wound healing. Hydrogels are removed from the wound without pain, thus avoiding the risk of wound irritation [38–41].

The removal of hydrogel dressing (Table 5.1g) is almost painless because hydrogel does not adhere to the wound surface. Hydrogel stays permanently moist and can be easily removed after prolonged application without pain and risk of wound irritation. Due to the above reasons, the hydrogel dressings are highly accepted by the patient [42].

Hydrogels are prepared from synthetic and natural polymers. But blends of both represent a new class of materials with better mechanical properties, biocompatibility and flexibility than

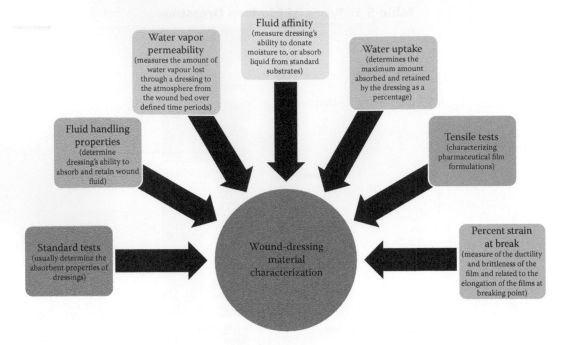

Figure 5.10 Physical tests applied for characterization of wound-dressing materials.

those of the single components [43]. Recently, blends of the synthetic polymers with natural polymers such as starch [44], cellulose [45], chitin [46], chitosan [47,48], cotton [49], gelatin [50,51], alginate [52], and dextran [53] have been reported for the development of wound dressings.

5.8 PHYSICAL CHARACTERIZATION OF WOUND DRESSINGS

The physical properties of wound-dressing materials depend on the nature of materials, and surface to which apply, that play a significant role for its desired properties and applications. Therefore, wound-dressing materials are characterized by various tests before approval as wound-dressing materials. These tests include fluid-handling properties, moisture vapor permeability, fluid affinity, water uptake, compressive tests, rheological tests, bioadhesive strength, and gelling properties (Figure 5.10).

5.9 NATURAL POLYMERS IN WOUND DRESSINGS

Natural polymers used in wound dressing provide a waterproof covering and prevents: (1) invasion of exogenous bacteria; (2) loss of water by evaporation; (3) protein loss by exudation; (4) pain from exposed nerve endings; (5) loss of heat, thereby reducing metabolic requirements; and (6) immobility that would be produced by heavy protective dressing. Natural polymers (such as alginate, chitosan, gelatin and collagen, as well as some of their derivatives) are the most commonly used materials to prepare wound dressing [54].

5.9.1 Chitosan

Chitosan (Figure 5.11) [poly-(b-1/4)-2-amino-2-deoxy-D-glucopyranose] is a collective name for a group of partially and fully deacetylated chitin compounds [55]. Due to its unique biological characteristics, including biodegradability and nontoxicity, many applications have been found either alone or blended with other natural polymers (starch, gelatin, and alginates) in the food, pharmaceutical, textile, agriculture, water treatment, and cosmetic industries [56–61]. Antimicrobial activity of chitosan has been demonstrated against many bacteria, filamentous fungi, and yeasts [62–65]. Chitosan has a wide spectrum of activity and high killing rate against Gram-positive and Gram-negative bacteria, but lower toxicity toward mammalian cells [66,67]. Ever since the broad-spectrum antibacterial activity of chitosan was first proposed by Allen [68], along with great commercial potential, the antimicrobial property of chitosan and its derivatives have been attracting great attention from researchers.

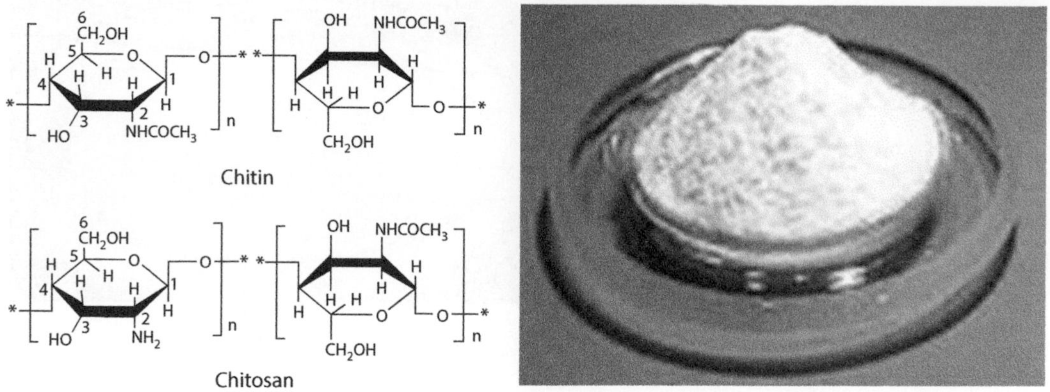

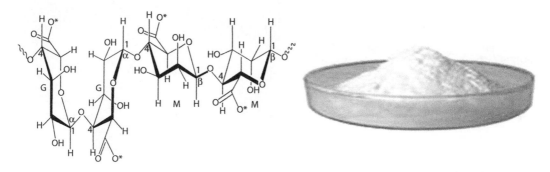

Figure 5.11   Chemical structure of chitin and chitosan.

Figure 5.12   Structure of alginate.

5.9.2 Alginates

Alginates (Figure 5.12) are produced from the naturally occurring calcium and sodium salts of alginic acid found in a family of brown seaweed (Phaeophyceae). They generally fall into one of two kinds: those containing 100% calcium alginate or those that contain a combination of calcium with sodium alginate, usually in a ratio of 80:20. Alginates are rich in either mannuronic acid or guluronic acid, the relative amounts of each influencing the amount of exudate absorbed and the shape the dressing will retain. Alginates partly dissolve on contact with wound fluid to form a hydrophilic gel as a result of the exchange of sodium ions in wound fluid for calcium ions in the dressing. Those high in mannuronic acid (such as Kaltostat) can be washed off the wound easily with saline, but those high in guluronic acid (such as Sorbsan) tend to retain their basic structure and should be removed from the wound bed in one piece. Alginates can absorb 15–20 times their weight of fluid, making them suitable for highly exuding wounds. They should not be used, however, on wounds with little or no exudate as they will adhere to the healing wound surface, causing pain and damaging healthy tissue on removal [69].

5.9.3 Gelatin

Gelatin (Figure 5.13) is a natural polymer that is derived from collagen, and is commonly used for pharmaceutical and medical applications because of its biodegradability and biocompatibility in physiological environments as reviewed by Tabata and Mikos [70,71]. These characteristics have contributed to gelatin's safety as a component in drug formulations or as a sealant for vascular prostheses [72]. Moreover, gelatin has relatively low antigenicity because of being denatured in contrast to collagen which is known to have antigenicity due to its animal origin. Gelatin contains a large number of glycine, proline, and 4-hydroxyproline residues.

5.9.4 Carboxymethylcellulose

Carboxymethylcellulose (Figure 5.14) is a major commercial derivative of cellulose. It is a highly water-soluble anionic polysaccharide which is widely used in pharmaceutical, cosmetics, and food

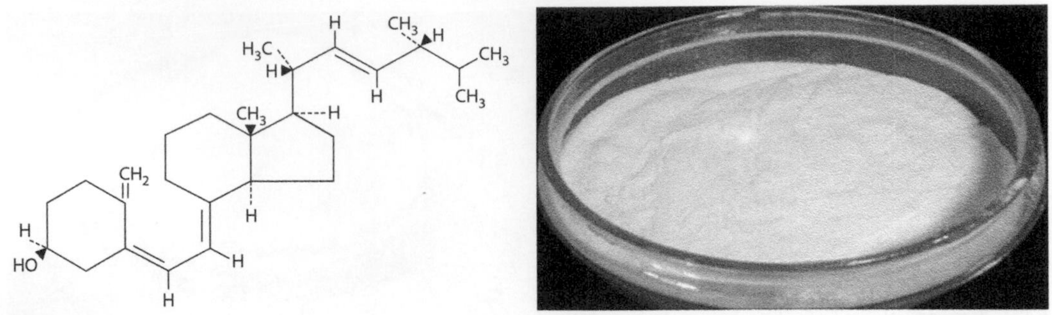

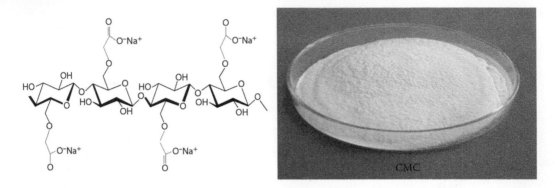

Figure 5.13 Structure of gelatin.

Figure 5.14 Structure of carboxymethylcellulose.

applications [73]. In biomedical fields, it is used to prevent the postoperative adhesion [74] and epidermal scarring. Moreover, its nontoxic, biocompatible, hydrophilic, chiral, and semirigid nature makes it a functional material of first choice [75].

5.9.5 Sterculia Gum

Sterculia gum (Figure 5.15), a medicinally important naturally occurring polysaccharide, has unique features such as high swelling and water retention capacity, high viscosity, and inherent nature of antimicrobial activity [76]. These features can be exploited for developing the wounds dressing. It has been used to prepare the controlled release matrix and has shown superior muco-adhesion than guar gum [77]. Sterculia gum composed of galacturonic acid, b-D-galactose, glucuronic acid, L-rhamnose, and other residues [78]. It is obtained from the tree *Sterculia urens* and is commonly known as karaya gum or sterculia gum [79].

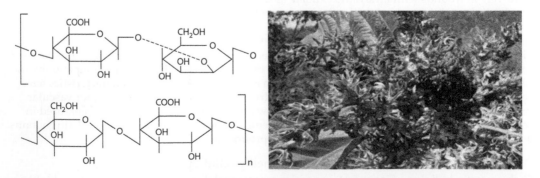

Figure 5.15 Structure of sterculia gum.

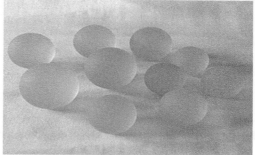

Figure 5.16 Structure of polyurethane.

5.10 SYNTHETIC POLYMERS AS WOUND DRESSINGS

Synthetic polymer-based dressings have a long shelf-life, inducing minimal inflammatory reaction and carry almost no risk of pathogen transmission [80]. In recent years, researchers have focused on biological synthetic dressings, which are bi-layered and consist of high polymer and biological materials [81–83]. These three categories of wound dressings are all used frequently in the clinical settings, but none is without disadvantages. Synthetic polymers such as poly(urethanes), poly(ethylenes), poly(β-caprolactone), poly(lactic acid), poly(glycolic acid), poly(glycolic-lactic acid), poly(acrylonitrile), poly(amino acids), silicone rubbers are used as dressing materials.

5.10.1 Polyurethane

Polyurethane (Figure 5.16) dressings are highly conformable, nonadherent, and semiocclusive. The foam can be used to absorb exudate from the wound, thereby decreasing tissue maceration; simultaneously, they maintain a moist environment while, with the sheet form, exudating pools beneath the dressing. These dressings can be used in the early inflammatory phase as well as in the proliferative phase of repair because they do not adhere to the regenerating tissue and leave it undisturbed at bandage changes. In heavily exuding wounds, these dressings should be replaced frequently to increase comfort, whereas the frequency of dressing change decreases as healing progresses and less fluid is produced by the wound [84].

5.10.2 Silicones

Silicone (Figure 5.17) dressings are used as an effective alternative to intralesional corticosteroids, surgical excision, laser surgery, and cryosurgery for the management of excessive scarring in man. It appears that this type of synthetic, nonadherent, and fully occlusive dressing surpasses other modalities in decreasing the amount of scar tissue while exerting no negative side effects. In a recent study performed in wounds of the distal limbs of horses, the silicone dressing surpassed a conventional permeable, nonadherent dressing in preventing the formation of exuberant granulation tissue and improving tissue quality [85].

5.10.3 Polyvinyl Pyrrolidone

Polyvinyl pyrrolidone (PVP) (Figure 5.18) is a synthetic polymer that has been shown to be biocompatible; UV-cured films of N-vinyl pyrrolidone copolymers have been proposed as a potential

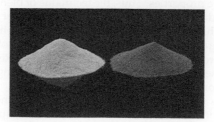

Figure 5.17 Structure of silicone.

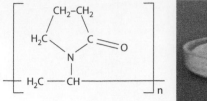
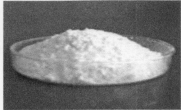

Figure 5.18 Structure of polyvinyl pyrrolidone.

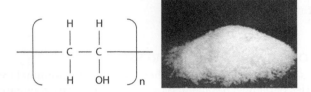

Figure 5.19 Structure of PVA.

bioadhesive wound-dressing matrix [86]. Due to its lubricity and viscous properties, PVP has been used to coat tissue contacting surfaces [87] and as a vitreous humor substitute [88].

5.10.4 Polyvinyl Alcohol

Polyvinyl alcohol (PVA) (Figure 5.19) has several useful properties including nontoxicity, biocompatibility, high hydrophilicity, fiber/film forming ability, and the chemical and mechanical resistance. It has been widely commercialized and studied in the chemical and medical industries for the productions of fibers, films, coatings, cosmetics, pharmaceuticals, and so on [89]. PVA hydrogels are produced by using the freezing–thawing technique to form a matrix of physically crosslinked polymeric chains containing uncrosslinked polymer and water. The use of freeze–thawed PVA hydrogels has been explored for biomedical and pharmaceutical applications. These gels are nontoxic, noncarcinogenic, have good biocompatibility, and have desirable physical properties such as rubbery nature and high degree of swelling in water [90]. PVA must be crosslinked if it is to be used in biodegradable materials. PVA hydrogels have excellent transparency and is smooth as membrane, and it is also biologically inactive and biocompatible. It has attracted much attention to be widely used as a good material for temporary skin covers or burn dressings [91].

5.11 POLYMER BLENDS AS WOUND-DRESSING MATERIALS

Blending of polymers has emerged as an important route to design new, high-performance polymeric materials over the last 50 years. Blends are, in fact, attractive materials because their properties can be easily adjusted by varying the ratio and nature of constituent components [92]. This class of materials also has a considerable potential owing in part to the large number of polymers that can be mixed.

Blending is a simple method to combine the advantages of different polymers, depending on the proportion of components and condition of mixing [93]. The resulting polymer blends show synergistic properties. Thus, the technique of blending polymers offers means to obtain tailor-made products with a good range of properties at low cost for specific applications. The blending of hydrophilic/hydrophobic polymer produces phase-separated composite hydrogels. Polymer blend hydrogels are mostly composed of water-soluble polymers such as alginate, starch-(EVOH), hydroxypropyl lignin, PVA, alkyl cellulose, etc. Recently, there has been an increasing interest in starch-based biodegradable blends [94,95], offering a method to modify both the properties and degradation rates.

There is a growing interest in developing engineered actuation systems that have properties more in common with soft biological materials, such as muscles and tendons, than with traditional engineering materials. In an aqueous environment, blend hydrogels may undergo a reversible phase transformation that results in dramatic volumetric swelling and shrinking upon the exposure and removal of a stimulus. Thus, these materials, normally composed of ionic polymers, can be used as muscle-like actuators, fluid pumps, and valves. Interest in blend hydrogels has gained momentum recently because these materials can be actuated by a variety of stimuli such as pH, salinity, electrical current, temperature, and antigens [96].

Zeng and coworkers [97] prepared microporous chitosan membrane by selective dissolution of its blend. Two synthetic polymers, for example, PVP and polyethylene glycol (PEG), were chosen to be the counterpart polymers. Results of Fourier transform infrared (FTIR) characterization, differential scanning calorimeter (DSC) analysis, and wide angle x-ray diffraction (WAXD) measurements showed that there are special interactions between chitosan and the counterpart polymers. Singh and Pal [98] studied the modification of sterculia gum by PVA–PVP through radiation crosslinking, to develop the hydrogels meant for the delivery of antimicrobial agent to the wounds. The hydrogels were characterized by scanning electron microscopy (SEM), FTIR, TGA, and swelling studies. Witthayaprapakorn and coworkers [99] designed the synthetic hydrogels for biomedical use as wound dressings. Crosslinked polymers of 2-acrylamido-2-methylpropane sulfonic acid (AMPS) and its sodium salt (Na-AMPS) were prepared via free radical polymerization in aqueous solution using photo initiation.

Ezequiel and coworkers [100] studied the development and characterization of novel polymer blends based on chitosan and PVA and chemically crosslinked by glutaraldehyde for possible use in a variety of biomedical applications. Mansur and coworkers [101] reported the preparation, characterization, and cytocompatibility of novel polymeric systems based on blends of chitosan and PVA and chemically crosslinked by glutaraldehyde. The structure of the hydrogels was characterized through FTIR spectroscopy and their swelling behavior was investigated. Sikareepaisana and coworkers [102] successfully prepared the wound-dressing materials from alginate, a natural polymer capable of forming hydrogels, and asiaticoside (PAC), a substance from the plant *Centella asiatica* which is commonly used in traditional medicine to heal wounds. Liua and coworkers [103] prepared the PVA/gelatin hydrogels as potential vascular cell culture biomaterials, tissue models, and vascular implants. The PVA/gelatin hydrogels were physically crosslinked by the freeze–thaw technique, which is followed by a coagulation bath treatment. In this study, the thermal behavior of the gels was examined by DSC and dynamic mechanical thermal analysis (DMTA). Fathia and coworkers [104] designed the physically crosslinked hydrogels composed of different amounts of dextran in the PVA matrix by applying freeze–thaw cycles to their aqueous solutions. Morphology, thermal properties, and FTIR spectra of the resulting blend xerogels were examined by SEM, DSC, TGA, and FTIR spectroscopy.

Wu and coworkers [105] prepared the porous gelatin scaffolds with a microtubule orientation structure by unidirectional freeze-drying technology, and their porous structure was characterized by SEM. Sung and coworkers [106] developed a minocycline-loaded wound dressing with an enhanced healing effect. The crosslinked hydrogel films were prepared with PVA and chitosan using the freeze–thawing method. Their gel properties, in vitro protein adsorption, release, in vivo wound-healing effect, and histopathology were then evaluated. Saha et al. [107] focused on the significant properties of hydrogels prepared with polymeric biomaterials: solely biopolymers (gelatin [G] and sodium alginate [SA] as base polymer) or in combination with synthetic and bio polymers PVP and carboxymethylcellulose (CMC) for biomedical application. Singh et al. [108] studied the modification of sterculia gum to develop novel wound dressings for the delivery of antimicrobial agent (tetracycline hydrochloride). The sterculia crosslinked PVA (sterculia-cl-PVA) hydrogels were characterized by FTIR and swelling studies. Yang and coworkers [109] prepared the PVA/water-soluble chitosan (ws-chitosan)/glycerol hydrogels by γ-irradiation followed by the freeze–thawing method. The effects of irradiation dose and the contents of PVA and agar on the swelling, rheological, and thermal properties of these hydrogels were investigated. Mc Gann and coworkers [110] prepared the physically crosslinked hydrogels composed of 75% PVA and 25% poly(acrylic acid) by a freeze–thaw treatment of aqueous solutions. Between 0.5 and 1 wt% of aspirin was incorporated into the systems. The purpose of the research was the development of a novel pH-sensitive hydrogel composite for the delivery of aspirin to wounds. Jayakumar and coworkers [111] studied the wound dressing of chitin and chitosan. The adhesive nature of chitin and chitosan, together with their antifungal and bactericidal character, and their permeability to oxygen, is a very important property associated with the treatment of wounds and burns. Kofuji and coworkers [112] obtained a transparent wound-dressing sheet by forming a complex between b-glucan and chitosan (CS). These materials were chosen for their biocompatible, bioabsorbable, and biodegradable properties, expected to promote the therapeutic efficacy of the dressing by increasing the wound-healing response.

Table 5.2: Tissue-Engineered Skin Substitutes Available Commercially

Dressing	Type	Major Components	Manufacturers
Integra™	Artificial skin	Collagen/chondroitin-6 sulfate matrix overlaid with a thin silicone sheet	Integra LifeScience (Plainsborough, NJ)
Biobrane™	Biosynthetic skin substitute	Silicone, nylon mesh, collagen	Dow Hickham/Bertek Pharmaceuticals (Sugar Land, TX)
Alloderm™	Acellular dermal graft	Normal human dermis with all the cellular material removed	Lifecell Corporation (Branchberg, NJ)
Dermagraft™	Dermal skin substitute	Cultured human fibroblasts on a biodegradable polyglycolic acid or polyglactin mesh	Advanced Tissue Sciences (LaJolla, CA)
Epicel™	Epidermal skin substitute	Cultured autologous human keratinocytes	Genzyme Biosurgery (Cambridge, MA)
Myskin™	Epidermal skin substitute	Cultured autologous human keratinocytes on medical grade silicone polymer substrate	Celltran Limited (University of Sheffield, Sheffield, UK)
TranCyte™	Human fibroblast-derived skin substitute (synthetic epidermis)	Polyglycolic acid/polylactic acid, extracellular matrix proteins derived from allogenic human fibroblasts and collagen	Advanced Tissue Sciences
Apligraf™	Epidermal and dermal skin substitutes	Bovine type I collagen mixed with a suspension of dermal fibroblasts	Organogenesis (Canton, MA)
Hyalograft 3-D™	Epidermal skin substitute	Human fibroblasts on a laser-microperforated membrance of benzyl hyaluronate	Fidia Advanced Biopolymers (Padua, Italy)
Laserskin™	Epidermal skin substitute	Human keratinocytes on a laser-microperforated membrane of benzyl hyaluronate	Fidia Advanced Biopolymers
Bioseed™	Epidermal skin substitute	Fibrin sealant and cultured autologous human keratinocytes	BioTissue Technologies (Freiburg, Germany)

Source: Boateng JS, Matthews KH, Stevens HNE, Eccleston GM. *J Pharm Sci* 2008;97(8):2892–2923.

Tsaob and coworkers [113] present a novel design for an easily stripped polyelectrolyte complex (PEC), which consists of chitosan as a cationic polyelectrolyte and poly (glutamic acid) (PGA) as an anionic polyelectrolyte, as a wound-dressing material. Sirousazara and coworkers [114] prepared the hydrogel wound dressings based on PVA by the cyclic freezing–thawing method and their dehydration process was investigated by experimental and mathematical methods. Mishra and coworkers [115] prepared the hydrogels of carboxymethyl cellulose (CMC)/(PVA)/gelatin and crosslinked polyacrylamide (PAM). The prepared hydrogels were loaded with povidone-iodine for using as wound dressing. Release and swelling characteristics were also studied for loaded hydrogels and found to be dependent on chemical architecture. Blood compatibility was also studied by clot formation and hemolysis assay.

5.12 TISSUE-ENGINEERED SKIN SUBSTITUTES

Traditional and modern dressings are applied in many burn but they have some limitations such as they cannot be applied at severe burn (chronic wounds) cases where large tissue have lost. Therefore, to cure such types of burns, wound-dressing materials based on "smart" polymers can be applied which act as biomaterials or as skin substitutes because these can replace lost tissue rather than just facilitate wound healing as well as able to mimic normal physiologic responses during wound healing by providing help for natural cell and tissue regeneration [116–119]. Presently, there are two types of acellular and cell-containing matrices produced either from synthetic collagen and extracellular matrix combinations such as hyaluronic acid, gradually degrade, leaving behind a matrix of connective tissue with the appropriate structural and mechanical properties, for example, Integra™, Alloderm™, Apligraf™, are employed in tissue-engineered skin substitutes as well as useful for the delivery of additional bioactive materials such as growth factors and genetic materials [120,121]. Some of the developed tissue-engineered products and skin substitutes available are summarized in Table 5.2.

REFERENCES

1. Lazarus GS, Cooper DM, Knighton DR, Margolis DJ, Percoraro ER, Rodeheaver G, Robson MC. Definitions and guidelines for assessment of wounds and evaluation of healing. *Arch Dermatol* 1994;130:489–493.

2. Percival JN. Classification of wounds and their management. *Surgery* 2002;20:114–117.

3. Bolton L, van Rijswijk L. Wound dressings: Meeting clinical and biological needs. *Dermatol Nurs* 1991;3:146–161.

4. Krasner D, Kennedy KL, Rolstad BS, Roma AW. The ABCs of wound care dressings. *Wound Manag* 1993;66:68–69.

5. Zhao-fan XIA, Dao-feng BEN, Bing MA, Heng-yu LI, Liu LIU. Low-grade thermal injury. *Chinese Med J* 2009;122(3):359–360.

6. Zahedia P, Rezaeiana I, Ranaei-Siadat SO, Jafaria SH Supaphol P. A review on wound dressings with an emphasis on electrospun nanofibrous polymeric bandage. *Polym Adv Technol* 2010;21:77–95.

7. Stein HD, Keiser HR. Collagen metabolism in granulating wounds. *J Surg Res* 1971;11:277–283.

8. Garg VK, Paliwal SK. Wound-healing activity of ethanolic and aqueous extracts of Ficus benghalensis. *J Adv Pharm Technol Res* 2011;2:110–114.

9. Falabella A, Kirsner R. *Basic and Clinical Dermatology*. Boca Raton, FL: Taylor & Francis; 2005.

10. Enoch S, Leaper DJ. Basic science of wound healing. *Surgery* (Oxford) 2005;23:37–42.

11. Lineen E, Namias N. Biologic dressing in burns. *J Craniofac Surg* 2008;19:923–928.

12. Chandrasinghe PC, Ariyaratne MHJ. Current concepts in management of chronic wounds. *Sri Lanka J Surg* 2010;28:2–5.

13. Atiyeh BS, Amm CA, El Musa KA. Improved scar quality following primary and secondary healing of cutaneous wounds. *Aesthetic Plast Surg* 2003;27:411–417.

14. Monaco JL, Lawrence WT. Acute wound healing an overview. *Clin Plastic Surg* 2003;30:1–12.

15. Midwood KS, Williams LV, Schwarzbauer JE. Tissue repair and the dynamics of the extracellular matrix. *Int J Biochem Cell Biol* 2004;36:1031–1037.

16. Musset JH, Winfield AJ. Wound management, stoma and incontinence products. In: Winfield AJ, Richards RME, editors. *Pharmacy Practice*. 2nd edition. UK: Churchill Livingstone; 1998, pp. 176–187.

17. Eccleston GM. Wound dressing. In: Aulton ME, editor. *Pharmaceutics: The Science of Dosage Form Design*. 3rd edition. UK: Churchill Livingstone; 2007, pp. 264–271.

18. Ueno C, Hunt TK, Hopf HW. Using physiology to improve surgical wound outcomes. *Plast Reconstr Surg* 2006;117:59S–71S.

19. Trabold O, Wagner S, Wicke C, Scheuenstuhl H, Hussain MZ, Rosen N, Seremetiev A, Becker HD, Hunt TK. Lactate and oxygen constitute a fundamental regulatory mechanism in wound healing. *Wound Repair Regen* 2003;11:504–509.

20. Hunt TK, Ellison EC, Sen CK. Oxygen: At the foundation of wound healing—Introduction. *World J Surg* 2004;28:291–293.

21. Purna SK, Babu M. Collagen based dressings—A review. *Burns* 2000;26:54–62.

22. Kent DJ. Wound and Skin Care: Basic ostomy management, part 2. Nursing 2010;40:62–63.

23. Ehrenreich M, Ruszczak Z. Tissue-engineered wound coverings. Important options for the clinics. *Acta Dermatoven, APA* 2006;15:5–13.

24. Queen D, Evans JH, Gaylor JDS, Courtney JM, Reid WH. Burn wound dressings—A review. *Burns* 1987;13:218–228.

25. Jorge H, Gomez MVZ, Reid Hanson R. Use of dressings and bandages in equine wound management. *Vet Clin Equine* 2005;21:91–104.

26. Edward L, Nicholas N. Honey in the Management of Infections. *J Craniofac Surg* 2008;19:923–928.

27. Thomas S. *Wound Management and Dressings*. London: Pharmaceutical Press; 1994.

28. Letouze A, Voinchet V, Hoecht B, Muenter KC, Vives F, Bohbot S. Using a new lipidocolloid dressing in paediatric wounds: Results of French and German clinical studies. *J Wound Care* 2004;13:221–225.

29. Walsh N, Blanck AW, Smith L. Use of a sacral silicone border foam dressing as one component of a pressure ulcer prevention programme in an intensive care setting. *J Ostomy Wound Continence Nurs* 2012;9(2):146–149.

30. Hutchinson JJ, Maryanne McGuckin MT. Occlusive dressings: A microbiologic and clinical review. *Am J Infect Control* 1990;18:257–268.

31. Kelsey MC, Gosling, M. A comparison of the morbidity associated with occlusive and nonocclusive dressings applied to peripheral intravenous devices. *J Hosp Infect* 1984;5:313–321.

32. Hoekstra MJ, Hermans MH, Richters CD, Dutrieux RP. A histological comparison of acute inflammatory responses with a hydrofibre or tulle gauze dressing. *J Wound Care* 2002;11:113–117.

33. Packard S, Douma C. Skin care. In: Cloherty JP, Eichenwald EC, Stark AR, editors. *Manual of Neonatal Care*, 5th edition. Philadelphia, PA: Lippincott Williams & Wilkins; 2004.

34. Meaume S, Vallet D, Morere MN, Teot L. Evaluation of a silver-releasing hydroalginate dressing in chronic wounds with signs of local infection. *J Wound Care* 2005;14:411–419.

35. Thomas S, Fear M, Humphreys J. The effect of dressings on the production of exudate from venous leg ulcers. *Wounds* 1996;8(5):145–149.

36. Watson NFS, Hodgkin W. Wound dressings. *Surgery* 2005;23:52–55.

37. Thomas S. Alginate dressings in surgery and wound management—Part 1. *J Wound Care* 2000;9:56–60.

38. Jones A, Vaughan D. Hydrogel dressings in the management of a variety of wound types: A review. *J Orthop Nurs* 2005;9:S1–S11.

39. Lugao AB, Machado LDB, Miranda LF, Alvarez MR, Rosiak JM. Study of wound dressing structure and hydration/dehydration properties. *Radiat Phys Chem*, 1998;52:319–322.

40. Falanga V. Classifications for wound bed preparation and stimulation of chronic wounds. *Wound Repair Regen* 2000;8:347–352.

41. Gruen RL, Chang S, MacLellan DG. Optimizing the hospital management of leg ulcers. *Aust NZJ Surg* 1996;66:171–174.

42. Singh B, Pal L. Radiation crosslinking polymerization of sterculia polysaccharide-PVA-PVP for making hydrogel wound dressings. *Int J Biol Macromol* 2011;48:501–510.

43. Areekul SW, Prahsarn C. Development and in vitro evaluation of chitosan polysaccharides composite wound dressings. *Int J Pharm* 2006;313:123–128.

44. Zhai M, Yoshii F, Kume T, Hashim K. Synthesis of PVP/starch grafted hydrogels by irradiation. *Carbohydr Polym* 2002;50:295–303.

45. Jinghua Y, Xue C, Alfonso GC, Turturro A, Pedemonte E. Study of the miscibility and thermodynamics of cellulose diacetate-poly(vinyl pyrrolidone) blends. *Polymer* 1997;38:2127–2133.

46. Muzzarelli RA, Guerrieri M, Goteri G, Muzzarelli C, Armeni T, Ghiselli R, Corenlissen M. The biocompatibility of dibutyryl chitin in the context of wound dressings. *Biomaterials* 2005;26:5844–5854.

47. Mi FL, Shyu SS, Wu YB, Lee ST, Shyong JY, Huang RN. Fabrication and characterization of a sponge-like asymmetric chitosan membrane as a wound dressing. *Biomaterials* 2001;22:165–173.

48. Kim IY, Yoo MK, Seo JH, Park SS, Na HS, Lee HC, Kim SK, Cho CS. Evaluation of semi-interpenetrating polymer networks composed of chitosan and poloxamer for wound dressing application. *Int J Pharm* 2007;341:35–43.

49. Edwards JV, Howley P, Cohen IK. In vitro inhibition of human neutrophil elastase by oleic acid albumin formulations from derivatized cotton wound dressings. *Int J Pharm* 2004;284:1–12.

50. Lin FH, Tsai JC, Chen TM, Chen KS, Yang JM, Kang PL, Wu TH. Fabrication and evaluation of auto-stripped tri-layer wound dressing for extensive burn injury. *Mater Chem Phys* 2007;102:152–158.

51. Deng CM, He LZ, Zhao M, Yang D, Liu Y. Biological properties of the chitosangelatin sponge wound dressing. *Carbohydr Polym* 2007;69:583–589.

52. Hashimoto T, Suzuki Y, Tanihara M, Kakimaru Y, Suzuki K. Development of alginate wound dressings linked with hybrid peptides derived from laminin and elastin. *Biomaterials* 2004;25:1407–1414.

53. Varshney L. Role of natural polysaccharides in radiation formation of PVA-hydrogel wound dressing. *Nucl Instrum Meth Phys Res B* 2007;255:343–349.

54. Hoffman AS. Hydrogels for biomedical applications. *Adv Drug Deliv Rev* 2002;54:3–12.

55. Tikhonov VE, Stepnova EA, Babak VG, Yamskov IA, Palma-Guerrero J, Jansson HB, Lopez-Llorca LV, Salinas J, Gerasimenko DV, Avdienko ID, Varlamov VP. Bactericidal and antifungal activities of a low molecular weight chitosan and its N-/2(3)-(dodec-2-enyl)succinoyl/-derivatives. *Carbohydr Polym* 2006;64:66–72.

56. Arvanitoyannis IS. Totally and Partially Biodegradable Polymer Blends Based on Natural and Synthetic Macromolecules: Preparation, Physical Properties, and Potential as Food Packaging Materials. *J Macromol Sci Rev Macromol Chem Phys C* 1999;39:205–271.

57. Arvanitoyannis IS, Nakayama A, Aiba S. Chitosan and gelatin based edible films: State diagrams, mechanical and permeation properties. *Carbohyd Polym* 1998;37:371–382.

58. Haque T, Chen H, Ouyang W, Martoni C, Lawuyi B, Urbanska AM, Prakash S. Superior cell delivery features of poly(ethylene glycol) incorporated alginate, chitosan, and poly-l-lysine microcapsules. *Mol Pharmaceut* 2005;2:29–36.

59. Kim HJ, Chen F, Wang X, Rajapakse NC. Effect of chitosan on the biological properties of sweet basil (Ocimum basilicum L.). *J Agri Food Chem* 2005;53:3696–3701.

60. Roberts GAF. *Chitin Chemistry*. London: MacMillan Press; 1992, p. 350.

61. Yamada K, Akiba Y, Shibuya T, Kashiwada A, Matsuda K, Hirata M. Water purification through bioconversion of phenol compounds by tyrosinase and chemical adsorption by chitosan beads. *Biotech Prog* 2005;21:823–829.

62. Hirano S, Nagao N. Effects of chitosan, pectic acid, lysozyme, and chitinase on the growth of several phytopathogens. *Agric Biol Chem* 1989;53:3065–3066.

63. Kendra DF, Hadwiser LA. Characterization of the smallest chitosan oligomer that is maximally antifungal to Fusarium solani and elicits pisatin formation inPisum sativum. *Exp Mycol* 1984;8:276–281.

64. Uchida Y, Izume M, Ohtakara A. In: Skjak-Braek G, Anthonsen T, Sandford P, editors. *Chitin and Chitosan*. London, UK: Elsevier; 1989. p. 373.

65. Ueno K, Yamaguchi T, Sakairi N, Nishi N, Tokura S. In: Domard A, Roberts GAF, Varum KM, editors. *Advanced Chitin and Science*. Lyon, France: Jacques Andre; 1997. p. 156.

66. Franklin TJ, Snow GA. *Biochemistry of Antimicrobial Action*, 3rd edition. London: Chapman & Hall; 1981. p. 175.

67. Takemono K, Sunamoto J, Askasi M. *Polymers and Medical Care*. Mita: Tokyo; 1989; Chapter IV.

68. Allan CR, Hardwiger LA. The fungicidal effect of chitosan on fungi of various cell composition. *Exp Mycol* 1979;3:285–287.

69. Jones V, Grey JE, Harding KG. Wound Dressings. *BMJ* 2006;332:777–780.

70. Tabata Y, Ikada Y. Protein release from gelatin matrices. *Adv Drug Deliv Rev* 1998;31:287–301.

71. Young S, Wong M, Tabata Y, Mikos AG. Gelatin as a delivery vehicle for the controlled release of bioactive molecules. *J Control Release* 2005;109:256–274.

72. Djagny KB, Wang Z, Xu S. Gelatin: A valuable protein for food and pharmaceutical industries: Review. Gelatin: A valuable protein for food and pharmaceutical industries: Review. *Food Sci Nutr* 2001;41:481–492.

73. Wade A, Weller PJ. *Handbook of Pharmaceutical Experiments*. 2nd edition, The Pharmaceutical Press, Oxon, UK: Wallingford; 1994.

74. Heidrick GW, Pippit CH, Morgam MA. Efficacy of intraperitoneal sodium carboxymethylcellulose in preventing postoperative adhesion formation. *J Reprod Med* 1994;39:575–578.

75. Bajpai AK, Mishra A. Preparation and characterization of tetracycline-loaded interpenetrating polymer networks of carboxymethyl cellulose and poly(acrylic acid): Water sorption and drug release study. *Polym Inter* 2004;54:1347–1356.

76. Gauthami S, Bhat VR. A monograph on Gum Karaya. National Institute of Nutrition, Indian Council of Medical Research, Hyderabad; 1992.

77. Park CR, Munday DL. Evaluation of selected polysaccharide excipients in buccoadhesive tablets for sustained release of nicotine. *Drug Dev Ind Pharm* 2004;30:609–17.

78. Weiping W. Tragacanth and karaya. In: Philips GO, Williams PA, editors. *Handbook of Hydrocolloids*. Cambridge: Woodhead; 2000. p. 155–168.

79. Singh B, Pal L. Development of sterculia gum based wound dressings for use in drug delivery. *Eur Polym J* 2008;44:3222–3230.

80. Lu S, Gao W, Gu HY. Construction, application and biosafety of silver nanocrystalline chitosan wound dressing. *Burns* 2008;34:623–628.

81. Bruin P, Jonkman MF, Meijer HJ, Pennings AJ. A new porous polyetherurethane wound covering. *J Biomed Mater Res* 1990;24:217–226.

82. Suzuki S, Matsuda K, Isshiki N, Tamada Y, Ikada Y. Experimental study of a newly developed bilayer artificial skin. *Biomaterials* 1990;11:356–360.

83. Matsuda K, Suzuki S, Isshiki N, Yoshioka K, Okada T, Ikada Y. Influence of glycosaminoglycans on the collagen sponge component of a bilayer artificial skin. *Biomaterials* 1990;11:351–355.

84. Jorge H, Gomez MVZ, Reid Hanson R. Use of dressings and bandages in equine wound management. *Vet Clin Equine* 2005;21:91–104.

85. Ducharme-Desjarlais M, Celeste CJ, Lepault E, Theoret CL. Effect of a silicone-containing dressing on exuberant granulation tissue formation and wound repair in horses. *Am J Vet Res* 2005;66:1133–1139.

86. Risbud M, Hardikar A, Bhonde R. Growth modulation of fibroblasts by chitosan-polyvinyl pyrrolidone hydrogel: Implications for wound management?. *J Biosci* 2000;25(1):25–31.

87. Hong Y, Chirila TV, Vijayasekaran S, Shen W, Lou X, Dalton P.Biodegradation in vitro and retention in the rabbit eye of crosslinked poly(1-vinyl-2-pyrrolidinone) hydrogel as a vitreous substitute. *J Biomed Mater Res* 1998;39:650–659.

88. Kao FJ, Manivannan G, Sawan SP. UV curable bioadhesives: copolymers of N-vinyl pyrrolidone. *J. Biomed Mater Res (Appl Biomater)* 1997;38:191–196.

89. Yeo JH, Lee KG, Kim HC, Oh YL, Kim AJ, Kim SY. The effects of Pva/chitosan/fibroin (PCF)-blended spongy sheets on wound healing in rats. *Biol Pharm Bull* 2000;23:1220–1223.

90. Peppas NA, Stauffer SR. Reinforced uncross-linked poly(vinyl alcohol) gels produced by cyclic freezing-thawing processes: A short review. *J Control Release* 1991;16:305–310.

91. Peppas NA, Scott JE. Controlled release from poly(vinyl alcohol) gels prepared by freezing-thawing processes. *J Control Release* 1992;18:95–100.

92. Utracki LA. *Polymer Blends Hand Book*. Dordrecht: Kluwer Academic Publishers; Netherlands 2002.

93. Avella M, Errico ME. Preparation of PHBV/starch blends by reactive blending and their characterization. *J Appl Polym Sci* 2000;77:232–236.

94. Wong XL, Yang KK, Wang YZ. Properties of Starch Blends with Biodegradable Polymers. *J Macromol Sci Polym Rev* 2003;43:385–409.

95. Pedroso AG, Rosa DS. Mechanical, thermal and morphological characterization of recycled LDPE/corn starch blends. *Carbohdr Polym* 2005;59:1–9.

96. Johnson B, Niedermaier DJ, Crone WC, Moorthy J, Beebe DJ. Mechanical properties of a pH sensitive hydrogel. In Proceedings of the 2002 Society for Experimental Mechanics (SEM) Annual Conference, Milwaukee, WI, USA, 10–12 June 2002; pp. 1–2.

97. Zeng M, Fang Z, Xu C. Effect of compatibility on the structure of the microporous membrane prepared by selective dissolution of chitosan/synthetic polymer blend membrane. *J Membr Sci* 2004;230:175–181.

98. Singh B, Pal L. Radiation crosslinking polymerization of sterculia polysaccharide-PVA-PVP for making hydrogel wound dressings. *Int J Biol Macromol* 2011;48:501–510.

99. Witthayaprapakorn C. Design and preparation of synthetic hydrogels via photopolymerisation for biomedical use as wound dressings. *Phys Procedia* 2011;8:286–291.

100. Costa-Júnior ES, Barbosa-Stancioli EF, Mansur AAP, Vasconcelos WL, Mansur HS. Preparation and characterization of chitosan/poly(vinyl alcohol) chemically crosslinked blends for biomedical applications. *Carbohydr Polym* 2009;76:472–481.

101. Sailaja GS, Sreenivasan K, Yokogawa Y, Kumary TV, Varma HK. Bioinspired mineralization and cell adhesion on surface functionalized poly(vinyl alcohol) films. *Acta Biomater* 2009;5(5):1647–1655.

102. Sikareepaisana P, Ruktanonchaic U, Supaphola P. Preparation and characterization of asiaticoside-loaded alginate films and their potential for use as effectual wound dressings *Carbohydr Polym* 2011;83:1457–1469.

103. Liu Y, Geever LM, Kennedy JE, Higginbotham CL, Cahill PA, McGuinnessa GB. Thermal behavior and mechanical properties of physically crosslinked PVA/Gelatin hydrogels. *J Mech Behav Biomed Mater* 2010;3:203–209.

104. Fathia E, Atyabia N, Imani M, Alinejad Z. Physically crosslinked polyvinyl alcohol–dextran blend xerogels: Morphology and thermal behavior. *Carbohydr Polym* 2011;84:145–152.

105. Wu X, Liu Y, Li X, Wen P, Zhang Y, Long Y, Wang X, Guo Y, Xing F, Gao J. Preparation of aligned porous gelatin scaffolds by unidirectional freeze-drying method. *Acta Biomater* 2010;6:1167–1177.

106. Sung JH, Hwang MR, Kim JO, Lee JH, Kim YI, Kim JH, Chang SW, Jin SG, Kim JA, Lyoo WS, Han SS, Ku SK, Yong CS, Choi HG. Gel characterisation and in vivo evaluation of minocycline-loaded wound dressing with enhanced wound healing using polyvinyl alcohol and chitosan. *Int J Pharm* 2010;392:232–240.

107. Saha N, Saarai A, Roy N, Kitano T, Saha P. Polymeric biomaterial based hydrogels for biomedical applications. *J Biomater Nanobiotechnol* 2011;2:85–90.

108. Singh B, Pal L. Development of sterculia gum based wound dressings for use in drug delivery. *Eur Polym J* 2008;44:3222–3230.

109. Yang X, Zhu Z, Liu Q, Chen X, Maa M. Preparation and characterization of chitosan/poly(vinyl alcohol) blended films: Mechanical, thermal and surface investigations. *Rad Phys Chem* 2008;77:954–960.

110. Mc Gann MJ, Higginbotham CL, Geever LM, Nugent MJD. The synthesis of novel pH-sensitive poly(vinyl alcohol) composite hydrogels using a freeze/thaw process for biomedical applications. *Int J Pharm* 2009;372:154–161.

111. Jayakumar R, Prabaharan M, Sudheesh Kumar PT, Nair SV, Tamura H. Biomaterials based on chitin and chitosan in wound dressing applications. *Biotechnol Adv* 2011;29:322–337.

112. Kofuji K, Huang Y, Tsubaki K, Kokido F, Nishikawa K, Isob T, Murata Y. Preparation and evaluation of a novel wound dressing sheet comprised of β-glucan–chitosan complex. *React Funct Polym* 2010;70:784–789.

113. Tsao CT, Chang CH, Lin YY, Wu MF, Han JL, Hsieh KH. Kinetic study of acid depolymerization of chitosan and effects of low molecular weight chitosan on erythrocyte rouleaux formation. *Carbohydr Res* 2010;346(1):94–102.

114. Sirousazara M, Kokabia M, Yaric M. Mass transfer during the preusage dehydration of polyvinyl alcohol hydrogel wound dressings. *Iranian J Pharm Sci* 2008;4:51–56.

115. Mishra A, Chaudhary N. Study of povidone iodine loaded hydrogels as wound dressing material. *Trends Biomater Artif Organs* 2009;23:122–128.

116. Andreadis ST, Geer DJ. Biomimetic approaches to protein and gene delivery for tissue regeneration. *Trends Biotechnol* 2006;24:331–337.

117. Horch RE, Kopp J, Kneser U, Beier J, Bach AD. Tissue engineering of cultured skin substitutes. *J Cell Mol Med* 2005;9:592–608.

118. Whitaker MJ, Quirk RA, Howdle RA, Shakesheff KM. Growth factor release from tissue engineering scaffolds. *J Pharm Pharmacol* 2001;53:1427–1437.

119. Supp DM, Boyce ST. Engineered skin substitutes: practices and potentials. *Clin Dermatol* 2005;23:403–412.

120. Burke JF, Yannas IV, Quinby WC, Bondoc CC, Jung WK. Successful use of a physiologically acceptable artificial skin in the treatment of extensive burn injury. *Ann Surg* 1981;194:413–428.

121. Sefton MV, Woodhouse KA. Tissue engineering. *J Cutan Med Surg* 1998;3:18–23.

122. Boateng JS, Matthews KH, Stevens HNE, Eccleston GM. Wound healing dressings and drug delivery systems: A review. *J Pharm Sci* 2008;97(8):2892–2923.

6 Smart Biomaterials in Tissue-Engineering Applications

6.1 BASIC PRINCIPLES

Tissue engineering is an interdisciplinary field that applies the principles of engineering and life science toward the development of biological substitutes used to restore, maintain, or improve tissue functions [1,2]. Scaffolding materials (temporary synthetic extracellular matrices) are designed as a 3D mirror image, on which cells grow and regenerate the needed tissues. Because the scaffolding materials are biodegradable, they will resorb after fulfilling the template function and leave nothing foreign in the patient (Figure 6.1).

Tissue engineering, according to its recent definition suggested by Prof. Williams in 2006 [3], is the creation of new tissue for the therapeutic reconstruction of the human body by the deliberate and controlled stimulation of selected target cells through a systematic combination of molecular and mechanical signals. If regenerative medical paradigms based on this refined tissue-engineering concept are realized in routine clinical practice, a new therapeutic approach for disease therapy could be developed based on the regeneration of defective or lost tissues and on the biological substitution of organ functions. Although tissue engineering is not yet delivering significant progress in terms of clinical outcomes and commercialization, this fascinating field of research is bound to dramatically change clinical practice and the therapeutic choices made by clinicians, resulting in significant therapeutic benefits for patients for whom there are not currently any clinically effective therapies [4].

The main purpose of tissue engineering is to overcome the lack of tissue donors and the immune repulsion between receptors and donors. The basic principle of tissue engineering involves a "triad" wherein a combination of cells in a suitably engineered material scaffold with appropriate biochemical signals is used to provide viable therapeutic options for clinical applications. Advances in research have shown that the engineering and design of the scaffold matrices, and the mechanical signals that regulate engineered tissues, have an important role. A scaffold is "permanently placed, or temporary 3D porous and permeable natural or synthetic biomaterial that is biocompatible." It is of pivotal importance as it allows the attachment, migration, and differentiation of progenitor cells. Readers should be aware that the physical characteristics of scaffolds (such as biodegradability, porosity, stiffness, and strength) can greatly influence cell adhesion, migration, and proliferation (such as osteoconduction), which signals the delivery of molecules and therefore the subsequent overall clinical success of the graft [5].

In essence, tissue engineering is a technique of imitating nature. Natural tissues consist of three components: cells, extracellular matrix (ECM), and signaling systems. The ECM is made up of a complex of cell secretions immobilized in spaces and thus forming a scaffold for its cells. Hence, it is natural that the engineered tissue construct is a triad [6], the three constitutes of which correspond to the above-mentioned three basic components of natural tissues. Figure 6.2 illustrates the triad, that is, a scaffold, living cells, and signal molecules (such as growth factors and cytokines).

There are three approaches in tissue engineering (Figure 6.3):

■ The use of isolated cells or cell substitutes to replace those cells that supply the needed function.

■ The delivery of tissue-inducing substances, such as growth and differentiation factors, to targeted locations.

■ Growing cells in 3D scaffolds.

6.2 FOUNDATIONS OF TISSUE ENGINEERING

The three fundamental elements of tissue engineering are stem cells, scaffold, and cell signaling.

6.2.1 Stem Cells

Stem cells have added a new drive to tissue engineering. They have the ability to self-renew and commit to specific cell lineages in response to appropriate stimuli, providing excellent regenerative potential that will most likely lead to functionality of the engineered tissue [7]. Present biology and pathology reveal that many diseases originate from malfunctioned cells [8]. Differentiation of stem cells into different types of tissues or organs is still a major limiting factor in the area of tissue engineering mainly due to the complexity and multicellular structure of the tissues and organs [7,8]. Stem cells are clonogenic cells capable of self-renewal and generating

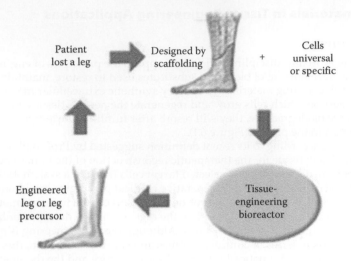

Figure 6.1 Schematic diagram showing the tissue-engineering concept using a hypothetical example of leg regeneration.

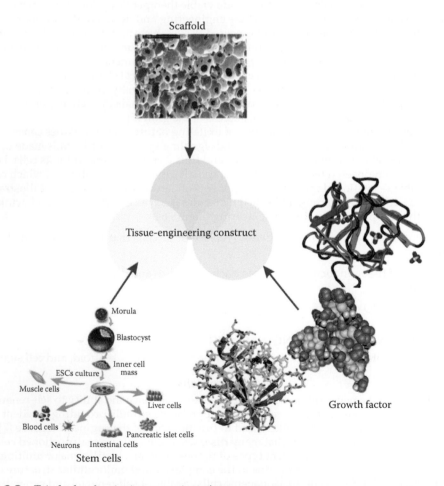

Figure 6.2 Triad of a classic tissue-engineering construct.

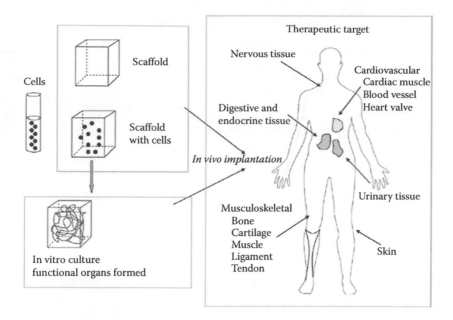

Figure 6.3 In the process of tissue engineering, cells are cultured on a scaffold to form a natural tissue, and then the formed tissue is implanted in the defect part in the patients. In some cases, a scaffold or a scaffold with cells is implanted *in vivo* directly, and the host's body works as a bioreactor to construct new tissues [2].

differentiated progenies. These cells are responsible for normal tissue renewal as well as for healing and regeneration after injuries. As a classical definition, a stem cell is an undifferentiated cell that can produce daughter cells that can either remain a stem cell in a process called self-renewal, or commit to a specific cell type via the initiation of a differentiation pathway leading to the production of mature progeny cells. Despite this acknowledged definition, the classification of stem cells has been a perplexing notion that may often raise misconception even among stem cell biologists.

6.2.1.1 Classification and Nomenclature of Stem Cells

The terminology used to classify the stem cells is somewhat perplexing. If someone uses the term embryonic stem cell (ESC), there is no doubt that he means a group of cells that are derived from the embryo. Thus, one of the most commonly used classifications is based upon their origin or location (Table 6.1). Depending on their residency, stem cells are classified in two categories:

Table 6.1: Stem Cell Types according to Their Origin, Differentiation Potency, and Progeny

Name	Cell Type (Location)	Differentiation Potency	Progeny
ESC	Cells at morula stage Cell of inner cell mass at blastocyte stage	Totipotent Pluripotent	Embryonic and extraembryonic tissues Embryo proper (all somatic and germ cells)
ESC	Cell of epiblast layer at gastrula stage	Pluripotent	Endoderm, mesoderm, and ectoderm
ESC	Cell of ectoderm, endoderm, or mesoderm	Pluripotent	All somatic cells
TSSC	Cell of specific tissues	Multipotent	One to several cell types depending on the residing tissue (e.g., hematopoietic stem cell)
TSSC	Resident cells in a given tissue	Unipotent	Single cell type (e.g., myosatellite cells of muscle

Abbreviations: ESC, embryonic stem cells and TSSc, tissue-specific stem cells.

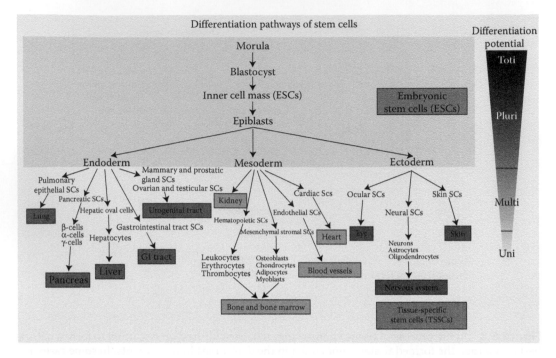

Figure 6.4 Differentiation pathways of stem cells.

ESCs and adult stem cells, which are also called TSSCs, derived either from a fetus or a postnatal individual (Figure 6.4). The second and more functional classification of stem cells is based according to their developmental potential as totipotent, pluripotent, multipotent, and unipotent [9]. Figure 6.5 depicts the tissue-engineering applications of stem cells-based scaffolds.

6.2.2 Scaffolds

Scaffolds are temporary frameworks used to provide a 3D microenvironment in which cells can proliferate, differentiate, and generate the desired tissue. Scaffolds might be defined as an artificial structure capable of supporting 3D tissue formation that allows cell attachment and migration, deliver and retain cells and biochemical factors enable diffusion of vital cell nutrients and expressed products. To achieve the goal of tissue reconstruction, scaffolds must meet some specific requirements. The design of the ideal scaffold for each tissue to be formed is a challenging task. Scaffolds are usually made from ceramics, natural or synthetic polymers, or composites of these materials. The choice of scaffold material depends on the desired outcome; thus physical as well as chemical characteristics must be considered [10]. Several fabrication technologies have been applied to process biodegradable and bioresorbable materials into 3D polymeric scaffolds of high porosity and surface area. The scaffold degradation is fundamental to achieve success in tissue-engineering therapies. It should ideally reabsorb once it has served its purpose of providing a template for tissue regeneration. The degradation must occur at a rate compatible with the new tissue formation [10]. A tissue-engineering approach is to use a scaffold, in combination with cells and other extrinsic factors to simulate the environment at the site of the injury. There are two approaches for tissue engineering to regenerate or repair the tissue or organ. The first approach is to regenerate tissue/organ using biomolecules with biomaterial scaffold. The second approach is to regenerate tissue/organ using donor cell or own cell with biomaterial scaffold (Figure 6.6). Whatever the approach being used in tissue engineering, the critical issues to optimize any tissue-engineering strategy toward producing a functional equivalent tissue are the source of the cells and substrate biomaterial to deliver the cells in particular anatomical sites where a regenerative process is required [11,12]. Both approaches require 3D scaffold or biomaterial to stitch the repaired tissue. The design of the scaffold depends on polymers, method of preparation, molecule size, etc.; hereby nanomedicine comes into the role of scaffold for tissue engineering (Figure 6.7) [13].

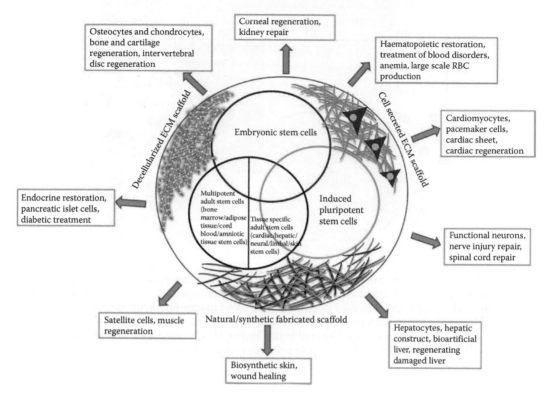

Figure 6.5 Applications of stem cells-based scaffolds in tissue engineering.

Scaffolds usually serve at least one of the following purposes:

1. Allow cell attachment and migration

2. Deliver and retain cells and biochemical factors

3. Enable diffusion of vital cell nutrients and expressed products

4. Exert certain mechanical and biological influences to modify the behavior of the cell phase [14]

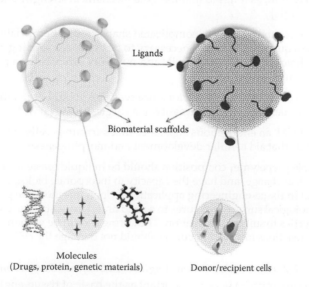

Figure 6.6 Approaches of tissue engineering.

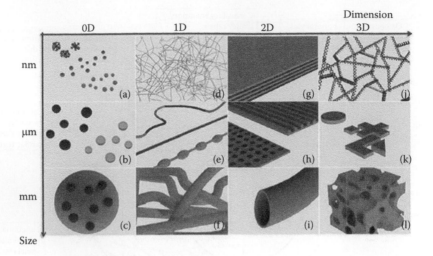

Figure 6.7 Development of biomaterials according to the dimension and size. (a–c) Spherical objects may be processed as nano- (a) or micro- (b) particles or capsules, or fabricated with higher sizes (c). (d–f) 1D structures fabricated as nano-, micro-, and macro-fibers. (g) 2D thin or nano-structured films. (h) Micro-patterned or micro-textured substrates. (i) 2D films may be arranged in thicker or higher scale objects. (j) 3D nanofibrilar hydrogels obtained by self-assembly. (k) Micro scale tissues used as building blocks to produce complex structures. (l) Traditional porous scaffolds.

6.2.2.1 Prerequisites of Scaffolds

1. Acceptable biocompatibility and toxicity profiles and having ability to support cell growth and proliferation [15].

2. Should have mechanical properties matching those of the tissue at the implantation site or mechanical properties that are sufficient to shield cells from damaging compressive or tensile forces without inhibiting appropriate biomechanical cues [14].

3. The absorption kinetics of scaffold should depend on tissue to be regenerated. For example, if scaffold is used for tissue engineering of skeletal system, degradation of scaffold biomaterial should be relatively slow, as it has to maintain the mechanical strength until tissue regeneration is almost completed [16].

4. It should have process ability to form complicated shapes with appropriate porosity. A high porosity and an adequate pore size are necessary to facilitate cell seeding and diffusion throughout the whole structure of both cells and nutrients. An optimum pore size is in the range between 100 and 500 µm [16].

5. Biodegradability is often an essential factor since scaffolds should preferably be absorbed by the surrounding tissues without the necessity of a surgical removal [17].

6. Mimic the native ECM, an endogenous substance that surrounds cells, bind them into tissues, and provide signals that aid cellular development and morphogenesis.

7. Ideally an injectable prepolymer composition should be in liquid/paste form, sterilizable without causing any chemical change, and have the capacity to incorporate biological matrix requirements to be useful in tissue-engineering applications. Upon injection, the prepolymer mixture should bond to biological surface and cures to a solid and porous structure with appropriate mechanical properties to suit the application. The curing should be with minimal heat generation and the chemical reactions involved in curing should not damage the cells or adjacent tissues [15].

6.2.2.2 Heart Valve Tissue-Engineered Scaffold Requirements

The scaffold architecture (matrix) is very important as the basic of tissue-engineering concept. The original heart valve cusps consist of an ECM. The following characteristics ensure the success of the scaffold: (i) the structure should provide extensive network of interconnecting pore; a channel should be designed throughout the scaffold matrix to provide the oxygen and nutrients to those cells which are far away from the surface (usually more than 1 mm); (ii) the materials should be biocompatible and biodegradable; and (iii) the shape and the size of the scaffold should associate the native tissue with appropriate mechanical properties [18].

6.2.2.3 Bone Tissue-Engineered Scaffold Requirements

Major advances in bone tissue engineering with scaffolds are achieved through growth factors and cells. The biomechanical system of bone is complex so that the following requirements of an ideal scaffold are diverse (Table 6.2).

6.2.2.4 Scaffolds Essential Properties

The following properties have been defined being essential [20–24].

6.2.2.4.1 Biocompatibility

Scaffolds should be well integrated in the host's tissue without eliciting an immune response.

6.2.2.4.2 Porosity

Scaffolds must possess an open pore, fully interconnected geometry in a highly porous structure with large surface-to-area-volume ratios that will allow cell ingrowth and an accurate cell distribution throughout the porous structure, and will facilitate the neovascularization of the construct from the surrounding tissue. Furthermore, the scaffolds should also exhibit adequate microporosity in order to allow capillary ingrowth. Porosity and interconnectivity are also important for an accurate diffusion of nutrients and gases and for the removal of metabolic waste resulting from the activity of the cells that had meanwhile grown into the scaffold. This is of particular importance regarding bone tissue engineering because, due to bone metabolic characteristics, high rates of mass transfer are expected to occur, even under in vitro culture conditions [25]. However, the degree of porosity always influences other properties of the scaffolds such as its mechanical stability, so, its value, should always be balanced with the mechanical needs of the particular tissue that is going to be replaced.

6.2.2.4.3 Pore Size

Pore size is also a very important issue because if the pores employed are too small, pore occlusion by the cells will happen, which will prevent cellular penetration, ECM production, and neovascularization of the inner areas of the scaffold.

It is well accepted that for bone tissue-engineering purposes, pore size should be in the 200–900 µm range. However, Holly et al. [26] reported a different concept. In the referred case the authors believe that bone reconstruction will only be achieved by having a 3D temporary matrix with a large macroporous interconnected structure with pore size ranging from 1.2 to 2.0 mm.

Table 6.2: Criteria of an Ideal Scaffold for Bone Tissue Engineering

1.	Ability to deliver and foster cells	The material should not only be biocompatible (i.e., nontoxic), but also foster cell attachment, differentiation, and proliferation
2.	Biodegradability	The composition of the material should lead biodegradation *in vivo* at rates appropriate to tissue regeneration
3.	Mechanical properties	The substrate should provide mechanical support to cells until sufficient new ECM is synthesized by cells
4.	Porous structure	The scaffold should have an interconnected porous structure for cell penetration, tissue ingrowth and vascularization, and nutrient delivery
5.	Fabrication	The material should possess desired fabrication capability, for example, being readily produced into irregular shapes of scaffolds that match the defects in bone of individual patients
6.	Commercialization	The synthesis of the material and fabrication of the scaffold should be suitable for commercialization

Source: Bruder SP, Caplan AI. Bone regeneration through cellular engineering. In: Lanza RP, Lannger R, Vacanti JP, editors. *Principles of Tissue Engineering* (2nd ed.). California: Academic Press; 2000. p. 683–696.

This approach has evident advantages due to its high surface-to-volume ratios that will facilitate cell, tissue, and blood vessels ingrowth. However, this affects the mechanical properties avoiding its use in areas that are very demanding from the mechanical point of view.

6.2.2.4.4 Surface Properties

Surface properties, both chemical and topographical, can control and affect cellular adhesion and proliferation [23]. Chemical properties are related with the ability of cells to adhere to the material as well as with the protein interactions with the latter. Topographical properties are of particular interest when the topic is osteoconduction. As defined by Davies et al., osteoconduction is the process by which osteogenic cells migrate to the surface of the scaffold through a fibrin clot, which is established right after the material implantation. This migration of osteogenic cells through the clot will cause retraction of the temporary fibrin matrix. Hence, it is of the utmost importance that the fibrin matrix is well secured to the scaffold or, otherwise, when osteogenic cells start to migrate the fibrin will detach from the scaffolds due to wound contraction. It has been previously shown [25] that a more rough surface will be able to imprison the fibrin matrix, better than a smooth surface, and hence facilitate the migration of osteogenic cells to the materials surface.

6.2.2.4.5 Osteoinductivity

Osteoinduction is the process by which mesenchymal stem and osteoprogenitor cells are recruited to a bone healing site, and stimulated to undergo the osteogenic differentiation pathway. However, when the portion of bone to regenerate is large, natural osteoinduction combined with a biodegradable scaffold may not be enough. Because of this the scaffold should be osteoinductive by itself.

6.2.2.4.6 Mechanical Properties and Biodegradability

In vitro, the scaffolds should have sufficient mechanical strength to withstand the hydrostatic pressures and to maintain the spaces required for cell ingrowth and matrix production. In vivo, and because bone is always under continuous stress, the mechanical properties of the implanted construct should ideally match those of living bone, so an early mobilization of the injured site can be made possible. Furthermore, the scaffolds degradation rate must be tuned appropriately with the growth rate of the neotissue in such a way that by the time the injury site is totally regenerated the scaffold is totally degraded [24].

6.2.3 Cell Signaling

Cell signaling is part of a complex system of communication that governs cell activities and organizes their interactions. The surface of scaffolding materials is important in tissue engineering because the surface can directly affect cellular response and ultimately the tissue regeneration. An ideal tissue-engineering scaffold should mimic ECM and positively interact with cells, including enhanced cell adhesion, growth, migration, and differentiated function. Although a variety of synthetic biodegradable polymers have been used as tissue-engineering scaffolding materials, they often lack biological recognition [27].

6.2.3.1 Strategies for Biomaterial Presentation of Growth Factors

Two distinct strategies for biomaterial presentation of growth factors in tissue engineering have been pursued: (i) chemical immobilization of the growth factor into or onto the matrix and (ii) physical encapsulation of growth factors in the delivery system (Figure 6.8). The former approach typically involves chemical binding or affinity interaction between the growth-factor-containing polymer substrate and a cell or a tissue. The latter approach is achieved by the encapsulation, diffusion, and preprogrammed release of growth factor from substrate into the surrounding tissue (Table 6.3). The efficacy of factor delivery can be significantly enhanced by 3D patterning of the growth factors on scaffolds [26–31].

The use of various forms of ECM scaffolds, with recent implementations including whole organs, derived from decellularized allogenic tissues/organs that retain structurally organized entities such as collagen, GAGs, and fibronectin, is increasingly routine, enabling natural templates that accommodating tissue-engineering and regenerative approaches [28,32–34] (Figure 6.9).

6.3 NATURAL MATERIALS IN TISSUE ENGINEERING

Biomaterials are materials designed to interact with cells, tissues, or body fluids intra- or extra corporeally and are applied in different settings such as for cell culture, dialysis, life-support systems, catheters, implants for permanent mechanical support, or regenerative therapies [35]. Biomaterials

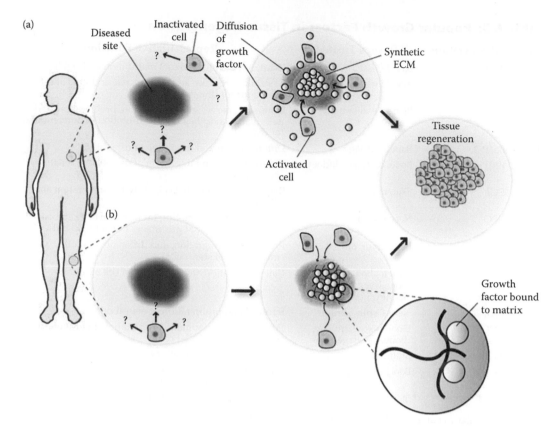

Figure 6.8 Schematic of two tissue-engineering approaches using synthetic ECMs to present growth factors to tissues. (a) Physically encapsulated bioactive factors can be released from synthetic ECMs to target specific cell populations to migrate and direct tissue regeneration. (b) Alternatively, growth factors can be chemically bound to the material system, making them available to cells that infiltrate the material.

are central components of many tissue-engineering strategies because they provide an architectural context in which ECM, cell–cell and growth–factor interactions combine to generate regenerative niches [36]. The use of naturally derived materials has been considered vital in technologies or methodologies for tissue engineering (Figure 6.10) [37]. One of the fundamental applications is the preparation of an artificial scaffold of cells for cell proliferation and differentiation. Why do we need tissue-engineered biomaterial? Natural materials owing to the bioactive properties have better interactions with the cells which allow them to enhance the cells' performance in biological system. Natural polymers can be classified as proteins (silk, collagen, gelatin, fibrinogen, elastin, keratin, actin, and myosin), polysaccharides (cellulose, amylose, dextran, chitin, and glycosaminoglycans), or polynucleotides (DNA, RNA) [38]. Cells residing around the scaffold infiltrate the scaffold and proliferate and differentiate there if the artificial ECM is biologically compatible. Natural polymers can mimic many features of ECM and thus can direct the migration, growth, and organization of cells during tissue regeneration and wound healing [39,40]. Here, the natural scaffold is a physical support for the cells and also provides a natural environment for cell proliferation and differentiation or morphogenesis, which contributes to tissue regeneration and organogenesis.

This chapter focuses on several natural protein-based polymers, including collagen, gelatin, and fibrin (fibrinogen), used for tissue engineering. These polymers can provide not only physical support for tissue regeneration but also biomimetic matrices with biological functions to actively induce tissue regeneration [40,41].

6.3.1 Polymeric and Natural Biomaterial

Tissue engineering can generally be classified into two parts: the polymer-based scaffold (which is constructed from synthetic polymeric materials) and the natural-based scaffold (which is

Table 6.3: Popular Growth Factors in Tissue Regeneration

No.	Abbreviation	Tissues Treated	Representative Function
1	Ang-1	Blood vessel	Heart, muscle blood vessel maturation and stability
2	Ang-2	Blood vessel	Destabilize, regress, and disassociate endothelial cells from surrounding tissues
3	FGF-2	Blood vessel muscle	Bone, skin, nerve, spine, migration, proliferation, and survival of endothelial cells, inhibition of differentiation of ESC
4	BMP-2	Bone, cartilage	Differentiation and migration of osteoblasts
5	BMP-7	Bone, cartilage, kidney	Differentiation and migration of osteoblasts, renal development
6	EGF	Skin, nerve	Regulation of epithelial cell growth, proliferation and differentiation
7	EPO	Nerve, spine	Wound healing promoting the survival of red blood cells and development of precursors to red blood cells
8	HGF	Bone, liver, muscle	Proliferation, migration, and differentiation of mesenchymal stem cells
9	IGF-1	Muscle, bone, cartilage, bone liver, lung, kidney, nerve, skin	Cell proliferation and inhibition of cell apoptosis
10	NGF	Nerve, spine, brain	Survival and proliferation of neural cells
11	PDGF-AB (or — BB)	Blood vessel, muscle, bone, cartilage, skin	Embryonic development, proliferation, migration, growth of endothelial cells
12	TGF-a	Brain, skin	Proliferation of basal cells or neural cells
13	TGF-b	Bone, cartilage	Proliferation and differentiation of bone-forming cells, antiproliferative factor for epithelial cells
14	VEGF	Blood vessel	Migration, proliferation, and survival of endothelial cells

Source: Hoshiba T et al. *Expert Opin Biol Ther* 2010;10:1717–1728.

constructed from the natural substances). It is not surprising that much research effort has been focused on naturally occurring polymers such as collagen [42] and chitosan [43] for tissue-engineering applications. Theoretically, naturally occurring polymers should not cause foreign materials response when implanted in humans. They provide a natural substrate for cellular attachment, proliferation, and differentiation in its native state. For the above-mentioned reasons, natural occurring polymers could be a favorite substrate for tissue engineering [44]. Table 6.4 presents major naturally occurring polymers, their sources, and applications.

Many advantages and disadvantages characterize these two different classes of biomaterials. Synthetic polymers have relatively good mechanical strength and their shape and degradation rate can be easily modified, but their surfaces are hydrophobic and lack cell-recognition signals. Naturally derived polymers have the potential advantage of biological recognition that may positively support cell adhesion and function, but they have poor mechanical properties. Many of them are also limited in supply and can, therefore, be costly. To design a tissue-engineering substrate, it is necessary to weight up the "pros and cons" of the potential precursor materials, which are summarized in Table 6.5 [49].

6.3.1.1 Collagen

Collagen is considered by many scientists as an ideal biocompatible scaffold or matrix for tissue engineering as it is the major protein component of the ECM, and multiple scaffolds based on collagen are currently available for clinical use, particularly for application in soft tissue such as skin [50,51]. For example, bilayered collagen gels seeded with human fibroblasts in the lower part and human keratinocytes in the upper layer have been used as the "dermal" matrix of an artificial skin product and are commercialized by Organogenesis in United States under the name of Apligraf®. Collagen sponges have been used also for the treatment of long bone fractures, for example, Collagraft®. Biomend® is a collagen membrane conventionally used in the regeneration of periodontal tissue [52]. Collagen is defined by high mechanical strength, good biocompatibility, low antigenicity and the ability of being cross-linked, and tailored for its mechanical degradation and water uptake properties; 27 types of collagens have been identified so far, but collagen type I is the most

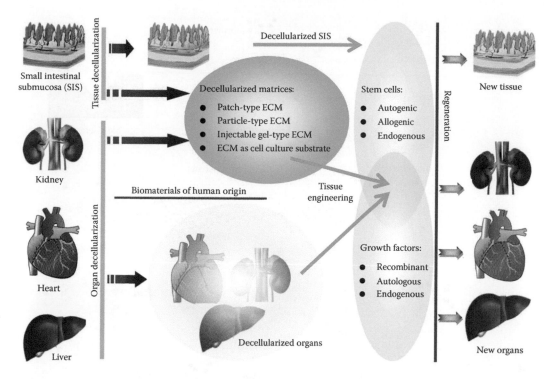

Figure 6.9 Decellularized matrices from tissues (e.g., small intestinal submucosa [SIS]) or organs (e.g., kidney, heart, and liver) that have native-like ECM microstructures, compositions, and biomechanical properties (schematic is not to scale). These decellularized ECMs may maintain the shapes of the original tissues and organs when used as scaffolding materials in tissue-engineering approaches for new tissue/organ regeneration. Alternatively, decellularized matrices derived from tissues and organs can be made into different types, such as a patch or particle, for tissue-engineering scaffolding biomaterials or can be designed as an injectable gel for cell culture substrates [28].

abundant and the most investigated for biomedical applications. Any desired physical and structural form (e.g., porous matrices, films, gels, or monofilaments) that can be fabricated from tissue-derived collagens can also be produced using recombinant collagens. Additionally, collagen has been combined with other materials for application. For example, collagen microsponges can be easily impregnated into previously prepared synthetic polymer scaffolds to enhance mechanical performance [53]. Also, growth factors may be incorporated into or added after the construction of the final forms. Growth factors and other active agents can be combined with collagen-based systems, including scaffolds and gels, to prolong the release rate of factors and increase their therapeutic effect [54].

Collagen has potential uses as follows [55]:

- Collagen gel matrix maintains its shape following cell seeding and culture

- Highly permeable bioscaffold design

- Production of tissue implants for reconstructive/cosmetic surgery applications

- Generation of spinal cord repair implants

More recently, collagen has found use as a hemostatic sealant [56]. Collagen is highly thrombogenic and plays a role in the body's natural clotting process by activating fibrogen conversion into fibrin, heavily cross-linked mesh networks of fibrogen. Fibrin captures activated platelets to make a clot. By creating a collagen-based sealant, wounds can be coated and blood flow halted much more quickly. The Food and Drug Administration (FDA) has approved a couple of collagen-containing solutions, including HelistatVR (Integra Life Sciences, NJ) and FloSealVR (Baxter, IL), for the treatment of bleeding during surgery.

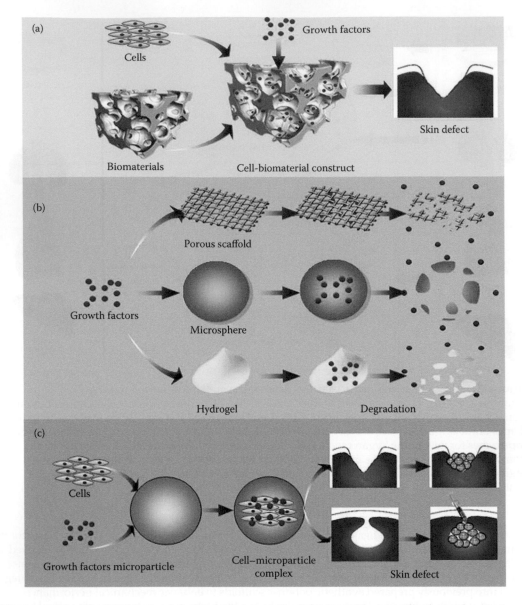

Figure 6.10 The fundamental technologies or methodologies with naturally derived materials in tissue engineering. (a) Naturally derived materials can mimic some features of ECM and thus have the potential to direct the migration, growth, and organization of cells during tissue regeneration and wound healing. Sometimes the biomaterial scaffold with growth factors is also applied to induce *in vivo* tissue regeneration. (b) Different forms of drug delivery vehicles can be designed to incorporate signaling molecules (e.g., growth factors) with naturally derived materials for the regeneration of tissues and organs, which is induced by signaling molecules with in vivo instability. The drug delivery strategies include the encapsulation of growth factors within porous scaffolds, microspheres, and hydrogels. (c) Controlled release of growth factors and cell delivery can be integrated within the same biomaterial, which may provide a novel multifunctional platform able to control and guide the tissue regeneration process. An example of such a strategy is through the formation of microspheres or microparticles. The ability of cell-seeded microparticles to aggregate as living tissue-engineered constructs facilitates their filling of cutaneous or subcutaneous tissue defects.

Table 6.4: Selected Polymeric Biomaterials for Tissue Engineering

Biomaterial

1. Synthetic Polymers			2. Natural Degradable Polymers	
Bulk Biodegradable Polymers	Surface Bioerodible Polymers	Nondegradable Polymers	Polysaccharides	Proteins
Aliphatic polyesters	Poly(ortho ester) (POE)	Poly(tetrafluoroethylene) (PTFE)	Hyaluronan HyA	Collagen
Poly(lactic acid) PLA	Poly(anhydride) (PA)	Poly(ethylene terephthalate) (PET)	Alginate	Gelatin
Poly(D-lactic acid) PDLA	Poly(phosphazene) (PPHOS)	Poly(propylene) (PP)	Chitosan	Fibrin
Poly(L-lactic acid) PLLA	Polyurethane (PU)	Poly(methyl methacrylate) (PMMA)	Starch	Silk
Poly(DL-lactic acid) PDLLA		poly(N-isoproplylacrylamide PNIPAAm		
Poly(glycolic acid) PGA				
Poly(lactic-co-glycolic acid) PLGA				
Poly(ε-caprolactone) PCL				
Poly(hydroxyalkanoate) PHA				
Poly(3- or 4-hydroxybutyrate) PHB				
Poly(3-hydroxyoctanoate) PHO				
Poly(3-hydroxyvalerate) PHV				
Poly(p-dioxanone) PPD or PDS				
Poly(propylene fumarate) PPF				
Poly(1,3-trimethylene carbonate) PTMC				
Poly(glycerol-sebacate) PGS				
Poly(ester urethane) PEU				

Source: Nugent HM, Edelman ER. *Circ Res* 2003;92(10):1068–1078; Seal BL, Otero TC, Panitch A, *Mater Sci Eng R-Rep* 2001;34(4/5):147–230; Atala A, Lanza RP. *Methods of Tissue Engineering*. California: Academic Press; 2002; Gunatillake PA, Adhikari R. *Eur Cell Mater* 2003;5:1–16; Garlotta D. *J Polym Environ* 2001;9:63–84.

Table 6.5: Main Physical Characteristics of Various Biomaterials

Materials	Source	Features	Applications
Collagen	Tendons and ligament	• Acts as a connective tissue • Main protein of sinew, cartilage, bone, and skin • Low immunogenicity and cytotoxicity, reconstructive surgery • Strength blood vessel	• Tissue engineering • Occular surgery • Drug delivery system, orthopedics, and dentistry • Teeth tissue engineering
Silk protein	Extracted from the collagen inside animals' connective tissue	• Strength blood vessel • Biodegradable, biocompatible, and nonimmunogenic • Can be coupled via carbodiimide chemistry to peptides	• Teeth tissue engineering • Useful for bone tissue engineering • Approved by FDA
Alginate	Abundant in the cell walls of brown algae	• Natural polysaccharide obtained from seaweed • Biocompatible, mildness of gelation condition and low immunogenicity • Can degrade by enzymolysis *in vivo* with no cytotoxicity • Alginate beads are usually made by calcium ion crosslinking	• Used in food and pharmaceutical industries • Biomedical, biomaterial, and therapeutic application • Wound dressing • Drug delivery system • Cell culture media • Neural tissue engineering
Hyaluronic acid (HA)	In the ECM of all higher animals	• Can be chemically and structurally modified for different applications • HA sponge has an appropriate structure, biocompatibility, and biodegradation as a scaffold for dental pulp regeneration • Important constituent of ECM	• Tissue engineering • Viscoelastic properties are useful for medical applications
Chitosan	Shells of shrimp and crabs	• Most abundant polymer after cellulose • Biocompatible and biodegradable • Good DNA carrier • Useful for electrospinning • When the degree of deacetylation of chitin reaches 50%, it becomes soluble and is called chitosan • Chitosan is the only pseudo natural cationic polymer	• Tissue engineering • Chitin could serve as replacements for bone, cartilage, arteries, veins, and musculofascial replacement
Peptide	Mouse tumor cells	• Peptides and proteins are replacing polymers as biomaterials • Can be integrated with other organic and inorganic components to form nanocomposites • Plays a key role in activating cellular interactions and tissue regeneration	• Tissue engineering • Bone, cartilage, and dentin

Source: Morsi YS. *Tissue Engineering of the Aortic Heart Valve: Fundamentals and Developments* (Paperback). October 30, 2012 Gazelle Distribution; Atala A, Lanza RP, editors. *Methods of Tissue Engineering.* California: Academic Press; 2002.

Collagen hydrogel fibers are one of the most popular natural polymer-based hydrogel scaffolds in tissue-engineering applications. As shown in Figure 6.11, these collagen hydrogel fibers are formed particularly through self-aggregation and crosslinking (through pyridinium cross-links) of collagen molecules in a hydrated environment. Collagen molecules are composed of tropocollagen triple helixes, where each triple helix results from the self-arranging of three polypeptides strands. Table 6.6 intends to summarize some relevant tissue-engineering applications of collagen-based scaffolds reported as research works.

6.3.1.2 Albumin

Albumin is an abundant water-soluble blood protein comprising almost 50% of total plasma mass in the body. Albumin carries hydrophobic fatty acids in the blood stream and maintains blood pH carefully. As albumin is essentially ubiquitous in the body, nearly all tissues have enzymes that can degrade it making it a promising polymer for biomedical applications. Albumin's solubility allows for the protein to be easily processed into a number of different shapes including fibers,

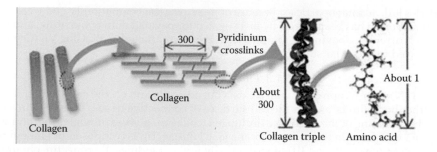

Figure 6.11 Schematic illustration showing the basic structure of collagen hydrogel fibers [57,58].

Table 6.6: Collagen-Based Matrices/Scaffolds for Different Tissue-Engineering Applications

Polymer(s)/Carrier/ Scaffold Structure	Active Biomolecule	Encapsulated/Seeded Cell Type (Source)	Animal Model	TE Application
Collagen/ hydroxylapatite	NGF	–	Calvaria defects	Bone
Collagen sponge s	bFGF	Chondrocyte	Nude mice subcutaneous implantation	Cartilage
Collagen gel	BMP-2 gene	Bone marrow stromal cells	Mouse femoral muscle	Bone/cartilage
Collagen gel	PDGF-A gene PDGF-B gene	–	Rabbit dermal ulcer Swine dermal wound	Skin
Collagen gel	VEGF	–	Chorioallantoic membrane	Vascularization
Collagen gel with gelatin microspheres	FGF-2		Mouse groin	Adipose
Collagen–agarose beads–cells			Adults mesenchymal stem cells	Not defined
Collagen sponge		Alveolar osteoblasts gingival fibroblasts	Critical-size defect in mouse skull	Bone
Collagen sponge and hydrogel		Human intervertebral disc cells		Intervertebral disc
Collagen sponge	–	Porcine third molar cells	Omentum of Immune compromised rats	Tooth
Collagen sponge x	–	Chondrocytes (autologous)	Sheep chondral defects	Cartilage
Collagen sponge	–	Preadipocytes (human)	Nude mice subcutaneous implantation	Adipose
Collagen–GAG scaffold	–	Bone marrow-derived mesenchymal stem cells	Rat myocardial infarction	Cardiovascular
Collagen scaffold (fleece)	–	Smooth muscle cells (human)	Nude mice subcutaneous implantation	Genitourinary tract
Collagen vitrigel	–	Glomerular mesangial cells	Epithelial cells	Renal glomerular tissue

Abbreviations: NGF, nerve growth factor; bFGF, basic fibroblast growth factor; BMP-2, bone morphogenetic protein-2; PDGF, platelet-derived growth factor; VEGF, vascular endothelial growth factor; FGF-2, fibroblast growth factor-2; GAG, glycosaminoglycans. Compiled from References 59 and 60.

microparticles [61], and nanoparticles. Because of its serological compatibility and weak mechanical strength, albumin has been primarily investigated for payload delivery, coating, and suturing applications. Currently, a bovine albumin-based adhesive marketed as BioGlue VR (CryoLife, GA) is FDA approved for vascular surgery [62].

6.3.1.3 Fibronectin and Fibrin

Fibronectin (FN) is a glycoprotein, which exists outside cells and on the cell surface. It also exists in blood, other body fluids, and on the cell surfaces of connective tissue. This protein associates with the other proteins of the ECM like fibrinogen, collagen, glycosaminoglycans, and with suitable receptors which are in the cell membrane [63]. Fibronectin is composed of tandem repeats of three distinct types (I, II, and III) of individually folded modules. Fibronectin, obtained from bovine or human plasma, is a high molecular weight glycoprotein that can bind collagen, fibrin, and heparin. It is found in its soluble form in blood and participates in wound healing process. It can be aggregated to form mats, which can be used as scaffolds for the repair of neural tissue [64]. These mats contain pores that all orient in the same direction to allow for guidance of regenerating neurons, provide cell adhesion sites, and can absorb growth factors, storing them as reservoir.

Fibrin, a complex network formed by polymerization of fibrinogen in the presence of the enzyme thrombin, is not a regular component of the ECM but is found as a temporary matrix that is replaced by the ECM and is currently used as fibrin glue in clinical applications [65]. Similarly, fibrin glue has been used as a carrier for growth factors and is injected into the site that needs repair for enhancing healing and subsequently accelerating repair processes [66]. Fibrin hydrogels have been used widely in various tissue-engineering applications owing to their high tissue-like water content, high biocompatibility in general, mechanical properties that parallel the properties of soft tissues, efficient transport of nutrients and waste, powerful ability to uniformly encapsulate cells, and ability to be injected as a liquid that gels in situ. Fibrin has been used for skin graft fixation, as a sealant to prevent bleeding, and as a vehicle for exogenous growth factors to accelerate wound healing. Fibrin has also been used as delivery vehicles for various cells, including keratinocytes, fibroblasts [67], and mesenchymal stem cells [68]. Injection of the cell–fibrin complex leads to the formation of tissue that is histologically more mature; however, biomechanical measurements will be important for determining the functionality of fibrin for this application [69].

6.3.1.4 Silk and Spider Silk

Unlike the polysaccharides hyaluronan and chitin, silk is a protein-based polymer, produced by insects and spiders. In recent years, silks and silk derivatives have been studied in tissue engineering as lightweight yet tough biomaterials [70]. For this reason, silk has been used to reinforce gelatin scaffolds, resulting in greater tensile and bending strength [71].

Silk proteins are biodegradable, biocompatible, nonimmunogenic, and approved by FDA [72] and can be coupled via carbodiimide chemistry to peptides such as arginine–glycine–aspartic acid (RGD). Moreover, silk-based scaffolds have proved to be useful in bone tissue engineering [73–76].Owing to the effectiveness of the silk properties for hard tissue engineering, four scaffolds with or without RGD peptide were manufactured from biomaterial silk protein with various degrees of pores diameters ranging from 250 and 550 mm diameter, respectively. These scaffolds were subsequently seeded with tooth bud cells and implemented for 4 days postnatal rat tooth. However, it was reported that after implementation in the rat momentum for 20 weeks the harvested scaffolds showed a regeneration of mineralized tissue in all scaffolds. Analyses of harvested implants revealed the formation of bioengineered mineralized tissue that was most robust in 550 mm pore RGD-containing scaffolds and least robust in 250 mm pore-sized scaffolds without RGD [77].

Mandal et al. synthesized gelatin–silk composites that can be loaded with water-soluble drug and fabricated in stackable layers. These constructs were capable of releasing model drug for at least 25 days with release kinetics and degradation tunable by ratio of gelatin to silk [78].

Gelatin–silk hydrogel composites were also synthesized into hydrogels, which gel upon contact with aqueous methanol [79]. This was due to the solution inducing transformation of the silk from random-coil to β-sheet conformation, causing physical crosslinking of the hydrogel. These hydrogels were thermally responsive and, when temperature was increased from 20°C to 37°C, construct swelling greatly increased and the hydrogels experienced greater mass loss due to gelatin release [80].

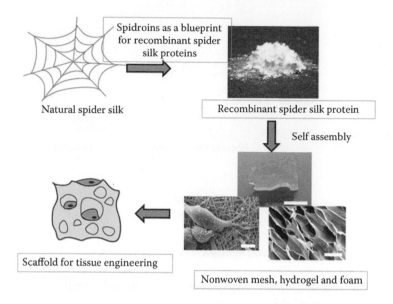

Figure 6.12 Possible application of spider silk materials in tissue engineering.

The properties of silk make it attractive for engineering bone and ligament tissue and extensive research has been done using 3D silk scaffolds in conjunction with mesenchymal stem cells for these applications. Specifically, the Kaplan laboratory has successfully developed such strategies [81,82]. Work from their lab has shown that human mesenchymal stem cells combined with silk scaffolds can be used to engineer bone. One of their first studies demonstrated that the flow conditions around the scaffold as well as the properties of the scaffold influenced the rate of calcium deposition, which is an important consideration for bone tissue engineering [83]. A companion study explored using silk scaffolds modified to contain RGD (arginine–glycine–aspartic acid) peptide sequences for the culture of human mesenchymal stem cells and showed that these scaffolds were appropriate for replacing bone due to the slow scaffold degradation. Other studies have examined the role of pore size to determine its influence on the behavior of the stem cells seeded inside silk scaffolds [84]. A follow-up study showed that macroporous silk scaffolds developed using an aqueous process could also be used for such applications. Overall, the mechanical properties of silk make it an attractive material for engineering bone, cartilage, and ligament tissue from stem cells.

Spider silk fibers fascinate scientists especially due to their extraordinary mechanical properties [85]. Additionally, spider silk is biocompatible, biodegradable, and shows hypoallergenic properties suitable for biomedical applications [72,86] (Figure 6.12). For centuries, spider's webs have been successfully used to stop bleeding and to promote wound healing. Recently, spider silk has been used as an artificial support for nerve regeneration [87,88]. Defects of peripheral nerves can be repaired by a composite nerve graft made of acellularized veins, spider silk fibers, and Schwann cells (SC) mixed with matrigel (a solubilized tissue basement membrane matrix rich in ECM proteins).

6.3.1.4.1 Silk Fibers-Based Hydrogel

The mulberry silkworm, *Bombyx mori*, and nonmulberry silkworm, *Antheraea mylitta*, are sources of the silk for formulation of the hydrogel used in TE and both have diverse morphology and composition with distinct properties for different purpose [89]. Silk fibroin has been used for cell culture, wound dressing, drug delivery, enzyme immobilization, and as a scaffold for bone tissue engineering (Figures 6.13 and 6.14) [90,91]. Silk fibers from the *B. mori* silkworm have a triangular cross section with rounded corners, around 5–10 μm wide. The fibroin heavy chain is composed mostly of beta sheets, due to a 59-mer amino acid repeat sequence with some variations. The flat surfaces of the fibrils reflect light at many angles, giving silk a natural shine [92]. Silk fibers have two main proteins, namely fibroin and sericin. Silk fibroin showed that hydrogel formation and the sol–gel transition were dependent on protein concentration, temperature, and pH [93,94]. The high proportion (50%) of glycine, which is a small amino acid, allows tight

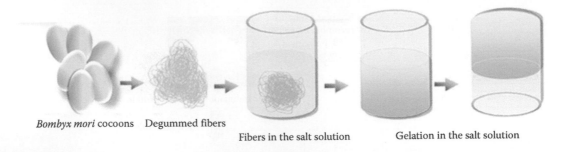

Bombyx mori cocoons   Degummed fibers

Fibers in the salt solution   Gelation in the salt solution

Fabricated hydrogels of Bombyx mori cocoons

Figure 6.13   Processing of cocoons for silk fibers-based hydrogel formation.

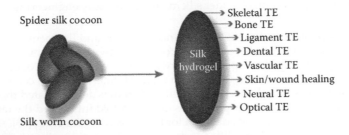

Figure 6.14   Applications of silk hydrogel in tissue engineering.

packing and the fibers are strong and resistant to breaking. Sericin component is important in hydrogel formulation to produce the adhesive properties, which is required for the scaffold support for the cells [95].

6.3.1.5 Self-Assembled Peptides (SAPs)-Based Hydrogels for Tissue Engineering

Peptide-based biomaterials consist of short sequences of amino acids, which can produce self-assembling scaffolds. Hydrogel scaffolds based on self-assembled peptides (SAPs) are one of the main classes in tissue-engineering applications. Self-assembling peptides or peptide amphiphiles are based on principles of protein–protein interactions and protein folding. SAPs are polypeptides that undergo self-assembly under specific conditions, typically a hydrophilic environment, to form fibers or other types of nanostructures [96–100]. Figure 6.15 shows, for instance, a schematic illustration of the self-assembling of amphiphilic peptide molecules. The Stupp Laboratory was one of the first groups to use such self-assembling scaffolds for promoting the differentiation of murine neural progenitor cells into neurons [101]. These scaffolds contained the peptide sequence IKVAV (isoleucine–lysine–valine–alanine–valine) derived from laminin and this sequence had been shown previously to promote neurite outgrowth. This study also illustrates the importance of selecting the appropriate peptide sequence for promoting the survival and differentiation of the stem cells seeded inside such a scaffold. A similar approach was used to develop self-assembling peptide scaffolds seeded with mesenchymal stem cells for bone tissue engineering [102]. These scaffolds incorporated an RGD sequence to allow the cells to adhere to the scaffolds.

These amphiphilic molecules comprise a polypeptide linked to a long chain alkyl tail and also functionalized with cell adhesion ligand (RGD). The polypeptide represents the hydrophilic region of the amphiphilic molecule whereas the long chain alkyl part represents the hydrophobic region. These peptide-based amphiphilic molecules undergo self-assembly into a fibrous

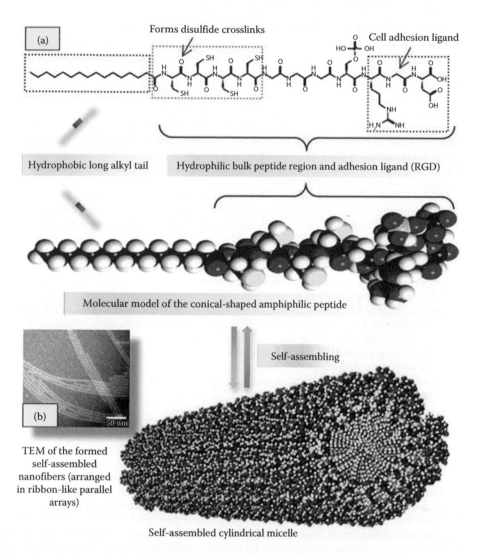

Figure 6.15 (a) Schematic illustration of the self-assembled peptide-amphiphiles (SAPs) functionalized with cell adhesion ligand (RGD) into fibrous cross-linked hydrogel scaffold for bone tissue-engineering applications. (b) TEM of the self-assembled nanofibers in ribbon-like parallel arrays.

cross-linked hydrogel scaffold (arranged in ribbon-like parallel arrays). A variety of amphiphilic SAP-based hydrogels have been used in various tissue-engineering applications [96,103]. These SAP-based hydrogels can also be used to incorporate bioactive molecules and allow their controlled release. SAP-based hydrogels can also be chemically conjugated to different moieties to allow signaling to cell surface receptors and to enhance cellular adhesion. For instance, SAP-based hydrogels have been attached to fibronectin and laminin peptide domains [104]. A further class of SAP-based hydrogels has been developed by Zhang et al. [48,105]. In this class, the synthesized functionalized-peptides were self-assembled into beta sheets, which subsequently converted into hydrogels. The results of the studies showed that these developed SAP-based hydrogels are very promising in generating 3D environments for cell culture and tissue-engineering applications.

In spite of the many superior advantages of using SAPs, such as their effectiveness in forming tissue-like hydrogels, the absence of crosslinking agents to remove, and the relatively easy functionalization, unfortunately they demonstrate poor mechanical characteristics. Consequently, they cannot be used for tissue-engineering applications that require scaffolds with high mechanical integrity.

6.3.1.6 Hyaluronic Acid and Its Derivatives

The name "hyaluronic acid" was invented for the polysaccharide from hyalos, meaning glassy and vitreous, and uronic acid. Hyaluronic acid is an unbranched polysaccharide of repeating disaccharides consisting of D-glucuronic acid and N-acetyl-D-glucosamine [48]. Hyaluronic acid and its derivatives are known to have excellent potential for tissue engineering. This is because hyaluronic acid can be chemically and structurally modified for various applications. It contains sites for cell adhesion and hyaluronan expression is upregulated during embryogenesis, suggesting its suitability as a scaffold material for the culture of ES cells. A recent study from the Langer lab demonstrated that such scaffolds could be used for promoting both self-renewal of human ES cells as well as vascular differentiation [106]. Hyaluronan is also expressed in many different tissues, including cartilage and nerve, suggesting that it could also be used for the culture and differentiation of adult stem cells. Some studies have used mesenchymal stem cells cultured inside hyaluronan scaffolds as a way of repairing cartilage both in vitro and in vivo. Work from the Woodhouse group has also used such approaches to engineer adipose substitutes [106,107]. Other approaches have combined hyaluronan scaffolds with stem cells derived from keratinocytes and adipose for engineering skin and bone, respectively [108]. However, combinations of growth factors with hyaluronic acid sponge are needed for the development of restorative treatment of dental pulp with sound dentin. In addition, hyaluronic acid sponge has the appropriate physical structure, biocompatibility, and biodegradation as an implant for dental pulp regeneration [109]. It was reported that HA shows important roles in some biological processes, including inhibition of inflammation and pain, and differentiation of osteoblastic and osteoclastic cells. In addition, some researchers have reported that intra-articular HA treatment for patients with osteoarthritic knees reduced painful symptoms and improved joint mobility. Dental pulp is a type of connective tissue, and contains large amounts of glycosaminoglycans. Previously, the contribution of HA to the initial development of dentin matrix and dental pulp, *in vivo* application of HA gels on the wound healing processes of dental pulp, and the application of gelatin-chondroitin-hyaluronan tricopolymer scaffold to dental bud cells were reported [110,111].

6.3.1.7 Agarose

Agarose, which is isolated from red algae and seaweed, consists of a galactose-based backbone and is commonly used as a medium for cell culture in the form of agar. One of the attractive properties of agarose is that its stiffness can be altered, allowing for tuning of the mechanical properties of the scaffold. Agarose scaffold have been investigated in combination with stem cells for generating a variety of applications, including cartilage, heart, and nerve. A variety of studies have demonstrated the suitability of agarose scaffolds for promoting stem cells to differentiate into chondrocytes [108]. The different stem cell types used in these studies included bovine mesenchymal stem cells, human mesenchymal stem cells, and adipose-derived stem cells. A different study showed that primate ES cells cultured inside of agarose scaffolds would form aggregates and differentiate into cardiomyocytes that would beat for up to 1 month. Other studies have demonstrated that both mouse and primate ES cells can differentiate into dopaminergic neurons when encapsulated inside agarose microcapsules [112]. This strategy could be used as a potential therapy for Parkinson's disease. Overall, agarose scaffolds provide a versatile platform for tissue engineering. Sakai synthesized a conjugate in which gelatin was covalently cross-linked to agarose that showed a sol-to-gel transition around body temperature. Since the conjugate used in this study did not result in mechanical instability compared to that of an unmodified agarose gel, agarose–gelatin conjugate is a good candidate material for tissue engineering [113].

6.3.1.8 Alginate

Alginate, a natural polysaccharide, ordinarily acquired from brown seaweed and has a number of attractive physical properties such as biocompatibility, mildness of gelation conditions, and low immunogenicity. Alginate contains blocks of (1–4)-linked β-D-mannuronic acid (M) and α-L-guluronic acid (G) monomers (Figure 6.16a). To chelate with divalent cations is the easiest way to prepare alginate hydrogels from an aqueous solution under gentle conditions (Figure 6.16b) [114,115]. The alginate scaffold fabricated by a combination of freeze drying and particulate leaching, showed increased porosity and pore size. Better pore characteristics and swelling properties may permit more cell invasion and nutrient supply. Moreover alginate is thermally stable, noncytotoxic, and biodegradable. Alginate scaffolds have also been used in combination with ES cells to generate hepatocytes and vasculature [116].

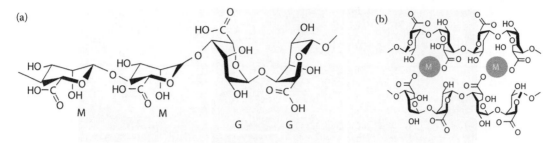

Figure 6.16 (a) Chemical structure of alginate and (b) mechanism of ionic interaction between alginate and divalent cations.

Table 6.7: Key Issues in Alginate Scaffolds

No	Key Issues in Alginate Scaffolds
1	The additions of third component in the alginate-ceramic or alginate-polymer system will be promising biomaterials to improve the properties in osteogenic differentiation
2	Care should be taken regarding alginate purity, viscosity, molecular weight, and percentage used while scaffold fabrication
3	Several studies confirmed that alginate-BMP-2 plays pivotal roles in bone cell proliferation, migration and differentiation, and it is best approach to overcome all the problems
4	Exact amount of BMP-2 should be developed, because excess amount of BMP-2 than required induces bone formation resulting in several side effects that limit its clinical applications
5	Addition of high mechanical strength materials such as carbon nanotube and graphene in alginate composite may mimic the mechanical strength of natural bone

Alginate scaffold seeded with a rat dental-pulp-derived cells and human dental pulp cells was implemented in the back of nude mice. The findings indicated that the seeded cells differentiated into odontoblast-like cells and stimulate calcification in the tooth [117,118]. Moreover, an injectable self-gelling alginate gel with macropores (pores in micrometer range) were constructed by mixing alginate microspheres of calcium with soluble alginate solutions, and then utilized in immuno-therapy in vivo. The results indicated that the soft macroporous gels could encourage cellular penetration and provide ready access to microspheres spreading therapeutic factors implanted in the matrix [119,120] (Table 6.7).

Porous alginate-based scaffolds or sponges with interconnected porous structures and pre-dictable shapes can be easily manufactured by a simple freeze-drying step (Figure 6.17). The mechanical properties and biodegradation rate of freeze-dried scaffolds can be simply modulated by changing the relative parameters of the polymers [121,122]. The mechanical strength mainly depends on porous scaffold forms and structural parameters such as pore size, porosity, and orien-tation. However, the diameter of the pores in freeze-dried scaffolds may not be uniform. The mate-rial components and molecular weight can strongly affect the biodegradation rates of scaffolds.

Kawaguchi et al. fabricated a nanocomposite hydrogel (NC) from sodium alginate and CNTs, and evaluated its mechanical properties and biocompatibility. The NC gel exhibited a mild

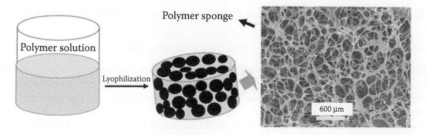

Figure 6.17 Schematic illustration to show the fabricating procedures of alginate-based sponge by the freeze-drying method.

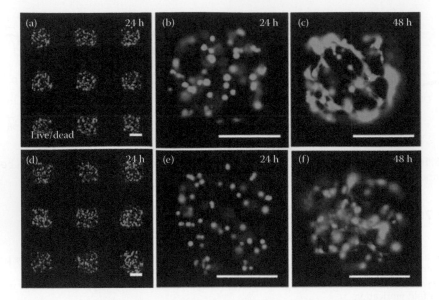

Figure 6.18 Representative images of 3T3 fibroblasts embedded in gelatin gels (a)–(c) and gelatin-CNTs NC gels micropatterns (d)–(f) which were stained with calcein-AM (green)/ethidium homodimer (red). Live/dead assay 24 and 48 h after encapsulation (scale bar = 250μm) [124].

inflammatory response and noncytotoxicity. These results suggested that NC gel was a promising scaffolding material in tissue engineering [123]. CNTs were also incorporated in gelatin gel, and the NC gels proved to be photopatternable and allowed for easy fabrication of microscale structures without harsh processes (Figure 6.18). This NC gel retained good cytocompatibility and tunable stiffness, and can guide osteogenic, neurogenic, and myogenic differentiation of human mesenchymal stem cell (hMSC), which make it suitable for various complex 3D biomimetic tissue-engineering applications [125,124].

6.3.1.9 Chitosan and Carboxymethyl Chitosan

Another polysaccharide that has been explored for tissue-engineering applications is chitosan. It is derived by the deacetylation of chitin and consists of glucosamine units. Chitosan is a cationic polymer obtained from chitin comprising copolymers of β (1 → 4)-glucosamine and N-acetyl-D-glucosamine. Chitin is a natural polysaccharide found particularly in the shell of crustacean, cuticles of insects and cell walls of fungi, and is the second most abundant polymerized carbon found in nature [126]. This polymer has many suitable properties. It can be used for wound dressing, drug delivery, and tissue-engineering (cartilage, nerve, and liver tissue) applications. These properties include the following [127]:

■ Minimal foreign body reaction

■ Mild processing conditions (synthetic polymers often need to be dissolved in harsh chemicals; chitosan will dissolve in water based on pH)

■ Controllable mechanical/biodegradation properties (such as scaffold porosity or polymer length)

■ Availability of chemical side groups for attachment to other molecules

Chitosan has been used extensively as material for regenerating skin, bone, and nerve tissue and has more recently been studied for use in combination with stem cells. Table 6.8 summarizes the applications of polysaccharide-based matrices/scaffolds for tissue-engineering applications.

One of the studies looked at the ability of such 3D scaffolds to promote osteogenic differentiation of mouse mesenchymal stem cells [142]. This study showed that the addition of coraline, another seaweed-derived material, enhanced osteocalcin release over time, which is important for bone formation. Chitosan scaffolds have also been demonstrated to be suitable for mouse

Table 6.8: Polysaccharide-Based Matrices/Scaffolds for Tissue-Engineering Applications

Polymer(s)/Carrier/ Scaffold Structure	Active Biomolecule	Encapsulated/ Seeded Cell Type (Source)	Animal Model	Tissue- Engineering Application
Dextran beads (in Ca–P porous scaffolds)	–	rhBMP-2	Dog class III furcation defect	Bone
Dextran/gelatin hydrogel microspheres	–	IGF-I	Periodontal defect	Bone
Dextran hydrogel porous scaffolds		ECM-derived peptides (adhesion)	Primary embryonic chick dorsal root ganglia cells	Guided cell and axonal regeneration
Carboxymethyl-dextran hydrogel membranes		Lysozyme		Not defined
Agarose film	FGF-2	Periostal explants	Rabbit knee	Cartilage
Agarose gel	BMP-2 gene	Bone marrow stromal cells (transfected)	Mouse femoral muscle	Bone/cartilage
Agarose sponge	Insulin	Pancreatic islets and insulinoma cells	–	Pancreas
Agarose gel	TGF-β1	Human intervertebral disc cells		Intervertebral disc
Agarose gel		Bovine articular chondrocytes		Cartilage
Agarose–fibrin gel		Epithelial, stromal and endothelial cells	Rabbit cornea	Cornea
Gellan gum (Gelrite®)	Antibiotic		Rabbit	Ophthalmology
Gellan gum hydrogel				Eye (vitreous)
Cellulose hollow-fibers	Fibronectin	Bovine coronary artery smooth muscle cells		Not defined
Cellulose porous scaffold		Bovine and human chondrocytes		Cartilage

Abbreviations: rhBMP-2, recombinant human bone morphogenetic protein-2; IGF-1, insulin growth factor-I; ECM, extracellular matrix; FGF-2, fibroblast growth factor-2; BMP-2, bone morphogenetic protein-2; TGF-β1, transforming growth factor-β1. Compiled from References 128 to 141.

ES cell culture as well as for the expansion of stem cells derived from human cord blood [143]. For cartilage tissue engineering, an in vivo study looked at the effects of using chitosan scaffolds seeded with mesenchymal stem cells and transforming growth factor-β as treatment for lesions on the patella of sheep. These cells differentiated into chondrocyte-like cells, demonstrating that such strategies can be effective in vivo. Such studies show that these scaffolds support stem cell differentiation both in vitro and in vivo.

Carboxymethyl chitosan (CMCS) has attracted considerable attention for tissue-engineering application due to its inherent increased bioactivity as compared to chitosan and its ability to promote osteogenesis [144]. Also the capacity of CMCS to chelate calcium from mineralizing solution containing calcium and phosphate to induce calcium phosphate or hydroxyapatite (HAP) formation has made it suitable biopolymer for tissue engineering [145]. Apart from this, it is well known to exhibit excellent biocompatibility, better biodegradability, nontoxicity, and ability to promote cell adhesion, which is desirable in the field of tissue engineering and regenerative medicine. In the past few years, several researchers have utilized CMCS in fabrication of different tissue-engineering biomaterials, which include scaffolds, hydrogels, composites, nanofibers, nanoparticles, dendrimer, and membranes, and for implant functionalization [146–148] due to easy processability of CMCS into these constructs.

Recent advances in the field of tissue engineering and drug delivery have enabled the design and fabrication of scaffolds that can deliver growth factors/therapeutic agents in a more controlled fashion over a defined period of time. In fact, the control over the regenerative and repairing potential of tissue-engineering scaffolds has dramatically improved in recent years, mainly by using drug-releasing scaffolds or by incorporation of drug delivery devices in the tissue-engineering scaffolds [149–151]. Recent strategies of tissue engineering open up the new possibility of constructing scaffolds that can provide the control over the sequestration and delivery of specific bioactive factors to enhance and guide the regeneration process. Figure 6.19 shows the more efficient and effective approach of combining tissue-engineering applications with drug delivery strategy for enhanced repairing and regeneration of damaged and/or diseased tissues/organs.

6.3.1.9.1 Synthetic Biomaterial

PGA, PLA, and their copolymers, poly(lactic acid-*co*-glycolic acid) (PLGA) are a family of linear aliphatic polyesters, which are most frequently used in tissue engineering [152–155]. They have been demonstrated to be biocompatible and degrade into nontoxic components with a controllable degradation rate in vivo and have a long history of use as degradable surgical sutures, having gained FDA (US Food and Drug Administration) approval for clinical use. These polymers degrade through hydrolysis of the ester bonds [156], with degradation products eventually eliminated from the body in the form of carbon dioxide and water; their degradation rates can be tailored to satisfy the requirements from several weeks to several years by altering chemical composition, crystallinity, molecular-weight value, and distribution.

PGA is widely used as polymer for scaffold, due to its relatively hydrophilic nature; it degrades rapidly in aqueous solutions or in-vivo, and loses mechanical integrity between 2 and 4 weeks. PGA has been processed into nonwoven fibrous fabrics as one of the most widely used scaffolds in tissue engineering. The extra methyl group in the PLA repeating unit (compared with PGA) makes it more hydrophobic, reduces the molecular affinity to water, and leads to a slower hydrolysis rate. PLA is degraded by hydrolytic de-esterification into lactic acid. The morphology and crystallinity strongly influence PLA rate of biodegradation and mechanical properties; therefore PLA scaffold degrades slowly in vitro and in vivo, maintaining mechanical integrity until several months [157]. To achieve intermediate degradation rates between PGA and PLA, various lactic and glycolic acid ratios are used to synthesize PLGA [158].

PLGA copolymers, with different PGA/PLA ratio (50:50, 65:35, 75:25, 85:15, and 90:10), are currently applied in skin tissue regeneration and generally for suture applications [159]. These polymers (PLA, PGA, and PLGA) are among the few synthetic polymers approved by the FDA for certain human clinical applications. PLGA has been fabricated into scaffolds by a number of different techniques to create unique nanostructured and microstructured materials that can facilitate tissue development (Figure 6.20).

Polymer printing in particular is a novel technique that holds great promise in the design of tissue-engineering scaffolds. Dr. James Dunn's group has demonstrated the capacity of 3D printing with PLGA [160]. As shown in Figure 6.20, very complex designs with controllable features can be generated to mimic structured tissue like villi for smooth muscle tissue engineering. The ability to utilize this technology with other degradable polymers holds promise in allowing for the design of organ-like structures that until now have been impossible to replicate. PLGA scaffolds have been used in the engineering of bone, cartilage, tendon, skin, liver, and nerve tissue [161–163].

6.4 CONCLUSIONS AND FUTURE PROSPECTS

In this chapter, efficacious biomaterials (natural and synthetic) for scaffolds in tissue engineering and cell seeding were discussed. Considering results using such materials and the mentioned criteria for an appropriate scaffold, it is proved that the selection of materials and method of fabrication depends on the cells and their characteristics. The reason is that the scaffold candidates should mimic the structure and biological activity of the native ECM proteins, which provide adequate mechanical support and regulate cellular activates. In addition, scaffolds must support and define the 3D structure of the tissue-engineered space and maintain the normal state of differentiation within the cellular compartment.

Increasing evidence suggests that biomaterials are yielding an ever growing list of products and successful clinical approaches to maintain, enhance, or restore tissues and organs. These "raw materials" continue to demonstrate great potential and will have an increasingly remarkable impact on synthetic biology, tissue engineering, and clinical regenerative therapies in the future. Stem cells respond to these biomaterials containing native ECM information via self-recognition and interplay, which are very unlikely to elicit severe negative immune responses upon medical application.

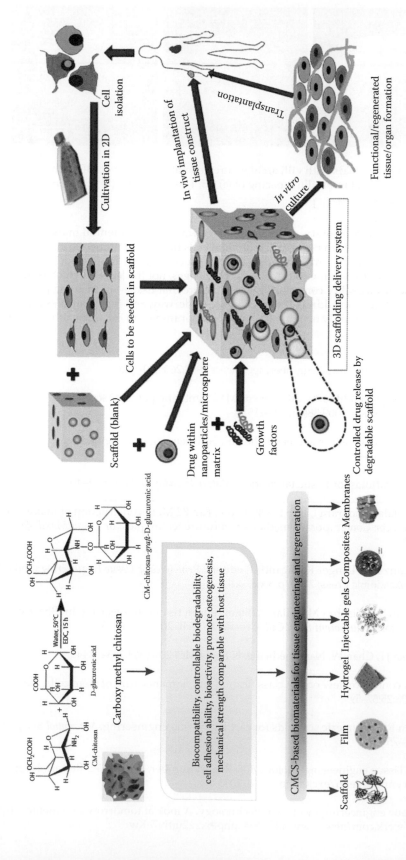

Figure 6.19 More efficient and effective schematic approach of combining tissue-engineering applications with drug delivery strategy for enhanced repairing and regeneration of damaged and/or diseased tissues/organs.

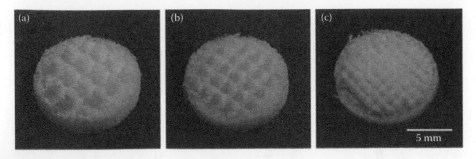

Figure 6.20 PLGA scaffolds with villi architecture generated by indirect 3D printing with villus diameter, height, and intervillus spacing of (a) 0.5, 1, and 0.5 mm; (b) 0.5, 1, and 1 mm; and (c) 1, 1, and 1 mm, respectively.

Tissue engineering is emerging as a vibrant industry with a huge potential market. The biomaterials, scaffolds, artificial organs, and differentiating cells that are combined to create a tissue-engineering product address significant medical needs, such as major tissue and organ damage or failure. The industry faces numerous technical challenges, not the least of which is the establishment of a consensus quality control program to ensure that tissue-engineering products work and are safe to use. Efforts to address these issues are underway, and if past success is any indication, this technology is certainly one that will have a major impact in future healthcare practice.

REFERENCES

1. Langer R, Vacanti JP. Tissue engineering. *Science* 1993;260:920–926.

2. Place ES, George JH, Williams CK, Stevens MM. Synthetic polymer scaffolds for tissue engineering. *Chem Soc Rev* 2009;38(4):1139–1151.

3. Williams DF. To engineer is to create: The link between engineering and regeneration. *Trends Biotechnol* 2006;24:4–8.

4. Peter X. Ma. Scaffolds for tissue fabrication. *Materials Today* 2004;7(5):30–40.

5. Payne KFB, Bala Sundaram I, Deb S, DiSilvio L, Fan KFM. Reconstruction of maxillofacial bone defects: Contemporary methods and future techniques. *Br J Oral Maxillofac Surg* 2014;52:7–15.

6. Bell E. In: Lanza RP, Langer R, Vacanti JP, editors. *Principles of Tissue Engineering* (2nd ed.). California: Academic Press; 2000. p. xxxv–xli.

7. Mashayekhan S, Hajiabbas M, Fallah A. Stem cells in tissue engineering. In: Bhartiya D, Lenka N, editors. *Pluripotent Stem Cell*. Croatia: InTech; 2013. p. 567–579.

8. Kim B, Rutka JT, Chan W. Nanomedicine. *N Engl J Med* 2010;363:2434–2443.

9. Alp Can. A concise review on the classification and nomenclature of stem cells. *Turk J Hematol* 2008;25:57–59.

10. Li W-J, Tuan RS. Polymeric scaffolds for cartilage tissue engineering. *Macromol Symp* 2005;227:65–75.

11. Barrera N. Tissue engineering. Biology 103. Report number: Third Web Report. http://serendip.brynmawr.edu/exchange/node/2083

12. Dvir T. Tissue engineering meets nanotechnology: A look at tomorrow's medicine. http://www.nanowerk.com/news/newsid519690.php#ixzz2ujfN7eKw

13. Mano JF. Evaluating biomaterial- and microfluidic-based 3D tumor models. *Mater Lett* 2015;141:198–202.

14. Sokolsky PM, Agashi K, Olaye A, Shakesheff K, Domb AJ. Polymer carriers for drug delivery in tissue engineering. *Adv Drug Deliv Rev* 2007;59:187–206.

15. Gunatillake PA, Adhikari R. Biodegradable synthetic polymers for tissue engineering. *Eur Cell Mater* 2003;5:1–16.

16. Ikada Y. Challenges in tissue engineering. *J R Soc Interface* 2006;3:589–601.

17. Haigang GU, Zhilian Y, Leong WS, Bramasta N, Tan JP. Control of *in vitro* neural differentiation of mesenchymal stem cells in 3D macroporous, cellulosic hydrogels. *Regenerat Med* 2010;5:245–253.

18. Fallahiarezoudar E, Pourroudposht MA, Idris A, Yusof NM. A review of: Application of synthetic scaffold in tissue engineering heart valves. *Mater Sci Eng C* 2015;48:556–565.

19. Bruder SP, Caplan AI. Bone regeneration through cellular engineering. In: Lanza RP, Lannger R, Vacanti JP, editors. *Principles of Tissue Engineering* (2nd ed.). California: Academic Press; 2000. p. 683–696.

20. Bryant SJ, Anseth KS, Lee DA, Bader DL. Crosslinking density influences the morphology of chondrocytes photoencapsulated in PEG hydrogels during the application of compressive strain. *J Orthop Res* 2004;22(5):1143–1149.

21. DeLong SA, Moon JJ, West JL. Covalently immobilized gradients of bFGF on hydrogel scaffolds for directed cell migration. *Biomaterials* 2005;26:3227–3234.

22. Kapur TA, Shoichet MS. Immobilized concentration gradients of nerve growth factor guide neurite outgrowth. *J Biomed Mater Res A* 2004;68(2):235–243.

23. Ilkhanizadeh S, Teixeira AI, Hermanson O. Inkjet printing of solid-phase growth factor patterns to direct cell. *Biomaterials* 2007;28:3936–3943.

24. Spector M, Michno MJ, Smarook WH, Kwiatkowski GT. A high-modulus polymer for porous orthopedic implants: Biomechanical compatibility of porous implants. *J Biomed Mater Res* 1978;12:665–677.

25. Klawitter JJ, Hulbert SF. Application of porous ceramics for the attachment of load bearing internal orthopedic applications. *J Biomed Mater Res A Symp* 1971;2:161–229.

26. Holly CE, Schoichet MS, Davies JE. Engineering three-dimensional bone tissue in vitro using biodegradable scaffolds: Investigating initial cell-seeding density and culture period. *J Biomed Mat Res* 2000;51(3):376–382.

27. Zandparsa R. Latest biomaterials and technology in dentistry. *Dent Clin N Am* 2014;58:113–134.

28. Hoshiba T, Lu H, Kawazoe N, Chen G. Decellularized matrices for tissue engineering. *Expert Opin Biol Ther* 2010;10:1717–1728.

29. Lange R, Luthen F, Beck U, Rychly J, Baumann A, Nebe B. Cell-extracellular matrix interaction and physico-chemical characteristics of titanium surfaces depend on the roughness of the material. *Biomol Eng* 2002;19(2–6):255–261.

30. He W, Gonsalves KE, Batina N, Poker DB, Alexander E, Hudson M. Micro/nanomachining of polymer surface for promoting osteoblast cell adhesion. *Biomed Dev* 2003;5(2):101–108.

31. Hetal P, Minal B, Ganga S. Biodegradable polymer scaffold for tissue engineering. *Trends Biomater Artif Organs* 2011;25(1):20–29.

32. Ehrbar M, Rizzi SC, Hlushchuk R, Djonov V, Zisch AH, Hubbell JA et al. Enzymatic formation of modular cell-instructive fibrin analogs for tissue engineering. *Biomaterials* 2007;28:3856–3866.

33. Badylak SF, Weiss DJ, Caplan A, Macchiarini P. Engineered whole organs and complex tissues. *Lancet* 2012;379:943–952.

34. Chen F-M, Liu X. Advancing biomaterials of human origin for tissue engineering. *Progr Polym Sci* 2016;53:86–168.

35. Halperin A, Fragneto G, Schollier A, Sferrazza M. Primary versus Ternary Adsorption of Proteins onto PEG Brushes. *Langmuir* 2007;23(21):10603–10617.

36. Kim BS, Baez CE, Atala A. Biomaterials for tissue engineering. *World J Urol* 2000;18:2–9.

37. Huang S, Fu X. Naturally derived materials-based cell and drug delivery systems in skin regeneration. *J Controlled Release* 2010;142:149–159.

38. Yannas IV, Ratner BD, Hoffman AS, Schoen FJ, Lemons J, editors. San Diego, CA, USA: Elsevier Academic Press; 2004. p. 127–136.

39. Guo XD, Zheng QX, Du JY, Yang SH, Wang H, Shao ZW et al. Molecular tissue engineering: Concepts, status and challenge. *Univ Technol* 2002;17:30–34.

40. Lee CH, Singla A, Lee Y. Biomedical applications of collagen. *Int J Pharmacogn* 2001;221:1–22.

41. Lavik E, Langer R. Tissue engineering: Current state and perspectives. *Appl Microbiol Biotechnol* 2004;65:1–8.

42. Yaylaoglu MB, Yildiz C, Korkusuz F, Hasirci V. A novel osteochondral implant. *Biomaterials* 1999;20(16):1513–1520.

43. Brown CD, Hoffman AS. In: Atala A, Lanza RP, editors. *Methods of Tissue Engineering*. California: Academic Press; 2002. p. 565–574.

44. Badylak SF. The extracellular matrix as a biologic scaffold material. *Biomaterials* 2007;28(25):3587–3593.

45. Nugent HM, Edelman ER. Tissue engineering therapy for cardiovascular disease. *Circ Res* 2003;92(10):1068–1078.

46. Seal BL, Otero TC, Panitch A. Polymeric biomaterials for tissue and organ regeneration. *Mater Sci Eng R-Rep* 2001;34(4/5):147–230.

47. Garlotta D. A literature review of poly(lactic acid). *J Polym Environ* 2001;9:63–84.

48. Morsi YS. Tissue Engineering of the Aortic Heart Valve: Fundamentals and Developments (Paperback). October 30, 2012 Gazelle Distribution.

49. Chen Q-Z, Harding SE, Ali NN, Lyon AR, Boccaccini AR. Biomaterials in cardiac tissue engineering: Ten years of research survey. *Mater Sci Eng R* 2008;59:1–37.

50. Klein B, Schiffer R, Hafemann B, Klosterhalfen B, Zwadlo-Klarwasser G. Inflammatory response to a porcine membrane composed of fibrous collagen and elastin as dermal substitute. *J Mater Sci Mater Med* 2001;12:419–424.

51. Marston WA, Usala A, Hill RS, Mendes R, Minsley MA. Initial report of the use of an injectable porcine collagen-derived matrix to stimulate healing of diabetic foot wounds in humans. *Wound Repair Regen* 2005;13:243–247.

52. Chunlin Y, Hillas PJ, Buez JA, Nokelainen M, Balan J, Tang J et al. The application of recombinant human collagen in tissue engineering. *BioDrugs* 2004;18(2):103–119.

53. Chen GP, Ushida T, Tateishi T. Hybrid biomaterials for tissue engineering: A preparative method for PLA or PLGA-collagen hybrid sponges. *Adv Mater* 2000;12:455–467.

54. Pieper J, Hafmans T, Van Wachem P, Van Luyn M, Brouwer L, Veerkamp J et al. Loading of collagen-heparan sulfate matrices with bFGF promotes angiogenesis and tissue generation in rats. *J Biomed Mater Res* 2002;62:185–194.

55. Martins A, Araújo JV, Reis RL, Neves NM. Electrospun nanostructured scaffolds for tissue engineering applications. *Nanomedicine* 2007;2(6):929–942.

56. Ulery BD, Nair LS, Laurencin CT. Biomedical applications of biodegradable polymers. *J Polym Sci Part B: Polym Phys* 2011;49:832–864.

57. Buehler MJ. Molecular nanomechanics of nascent bone: Fibrillar toughening by mineralization. *Nanotechnology* 2007;18:295102.

58. El-Sherbiny IM, Yacoub MH. Hydrogel scaffolds for tissue engineering: Progress and challenges. *Global Cardiology Science and Practice* 2013:38:317–342.

59. Letic-Gavrilovic A, Piattelli A, Abe K. Nerve growth factor β(NGFβ) delivery via a collagen hydroxyapatite (Col/Hap) composite and its effects on new bone ingrowth. *J Mater Sci Mater Med* 2003;14:95–102.

60. Wang PC, Takezawa T. Reconstruction of renal glomerular tissue using collagen vitrigel scaffold. *J Biosci Bioeng* 2005;99:529–540.

61. Okoroukwu ON, Green GR, D'Souza MJ. Development of albumin microspheres containing Sp H1-DNA complexes: A novel gene delivery system. *J Microencapsul* 2010;27:142–149.

62. Shen Z, Li Y, Kohama K, Oneill B, Bi J. Improved drug targeting of cancer cells by utilizing actively targetable folic acid-conjugated albumin nanospheres. *Pharmacol Res* 2011;63:51–58.

63. Ebner R, Lackner JM, Waldhauser W, Major R, Czarnowska E, Kustosz R et al. Biocompatibile TiN-based novel nanocrystalline films. *Bull Polish Acad Sci* 2006;54(2):167–173.

64. Malafaya PB, Silva GA, Reis RL. Natural-origin polymers as carriers and scaffolds for biomolecules and cell delivery in tissue engineering applications. *Adv Drug Deliv Rev* 2007;59:207–233.

65. Le Nihouannen D, Guehennec LL, Rouillon T, Pilet P, Bilban M, Layrolle P et al. Microarchitecture of calcium phosphate granules and fibrin glue composites for bone tissue engineering. *Biomaterials* 2006;27:2716–2722.

66. Oju J, Soo Hyun R, Ji Hyung C, Kim B-S. Control of basic fibroblast growth factor release from fibrin gel with heparin and concentrations of fibrinogen and thrombin. *J Controlled Release* 2005;105:249–259.

67. Jimenez PA, Jimenez SE. Tissue and cellular approaches to wound repair. *Am J Surg* 2004;187:56S–64S.

68. Bensaid W, Triffitt JT, Blanchat C, Oudina K, Sedel L, Petite H. A biodegradable fibrin scaffold for mesenchymal stem cell transplantation. *Biomaterials* 2003;24:2497–2502.

69. Wechselberger G, Russell R, Neumeister M, Schoeller T, Piza-Katzer H, Rainer C. Successful transplantation of three tissue-engineered cell types using capsule induction technique and fibrin glue as a delivery vehicle. *Plastic Reconst Surg* 2002;110:123–129.

70. Wang Y, Kim HJ, Vunjak-Novakovic G, Kaplan DL. Stem cell-based tissue engineering with silk biomaterials. *Biomaterials* 2006;27(36):6064–6082.

71. Shubhra QT, Alam A, Beg M. Mechanical and degradation characteristics of natural silk fiber reinforced gelatin composites. *Mater Lett* 2011;65(2):333–336.

72. Altman GH, Diaz F, Jakuba C, Calabro T, Horan RL, Chen JS et al. Silk-based biomaterials. *Biomaterials* 2003;24:401–416.

73. Kim J, Kim U, Kim H, Li C, Wada M, Leisk G et al. Bone tissue engineering with premineralized silk scaffolds. *Bone* 2008;42:1226–1234.

74. Uebersax L, Hagenmüller H, Hofmann S, Gruenblatt E, Müller R, Vunjaknovakovic G et al. Effect of scaffold design on bone morphology in vitro. *Tissue Eng* 2006;12:3417–29.

75. Hofmann S, Hagenmuller H, Koch AM, Muller R, Vunjak-Novakovic G, Kaplan DL et al. Control of in vitro tissue-engineered bone-like structures using human mesenchymal stem cells and porous silk scaffolds. *Biomaterials* 2007;28:1152–1162.

76. Meinel L, Karageorgiou V, Hofmann S, Fajardo R, Snyder B, Li C et al. Engineering bone-like tissue in vitro using human bone marrow stem cells and silk scaffolds. *J Biomed Mater Res* 2004;71A:25–34.

77. Xu WP, Zhang W, Asrican R, Kim HJ, Kaplan DL, Yelick PC. Accurately shaped tooth bud cell-derived mineralized tissue formation on silk scaffolds. *Tissue Eng Part A* 2008;14:549–557.

78. Mandal BB, Mann JK, Kundu SC. Silk fibroin/gelatin multilayered films as a model system for controlled drug release. *Eur J Pharm Sci* 2009;37(2):160–171.

79. Gil ES, Spontak RJ, Hudson SM. Effect of beta-sheet crystals on the thermal and rheological behavior of protein-based hydrogels derived from gelatin and silk fibroin. *Macromol Biosci* 2005;5(8):702–709.

80. Gil ES, Frankowski DJ, Spontak RJ, Hudson SM. Swelling behavior and morphological evolution of mixed gelatin/silk fibroin hydrogels. *Biomacromolecules* 2005;6(6):3079–3087.

81. Mauney JR, Nguyen T, Gillen K, Kirker-Head C, Gimble JM, Kaplan DL. Engineering adipose-like tissue in vitro and in vivo utilizing human bone marrow and adipose-derived mesenchymal stem cells with silk fibroin 3D scaffolds. *Biomaterials* 2007;28:5280–5290.

82. Mehlhorn AT, Niemeyer P, Kaschte K, Muller L, Finkenzeller G, Hartl D et al. Differential effects of BMP-2 and TGF-1 on chondrogenic differentiation of adipose derived stem cells. *Cell Prolif* 2007;40:809–823.

83. Meinel L, Karageorgiou V, Fajardo R, Snyder B, Shinde-Patil V, Zichner L et al. Bone tissue engineering using human mesenchymal stem cells: Effects of scaffold material and medium flow. *Ann Biomed Eng* 2004;32:112–122.

84. Meinel L, Fajardo R, Hofmann S, Langer R, Chen J, Snyder B et al. Silk implants for the healing of critical size bone defects. *Bone* 2005;37:688–698.

85. Gerritsen VB. The tiptoe of an airbus. *Protein Spotlight Swiss Prot* 2002;24:1–2.

86. Vollrath F, Barth P, Basedow A, Engström W, List H. Local tolerance to spider silks and protein polymers in vivo. *In Vivo* 2002;16:229–234.

87. Allmeling C, Jokuszies A, Reimers K, Kall S, Choi CY, Brandes G et al. Spider silk fibres in artificial nerve constructs promote peripheral nerve regeneration. *Cell Prolif* 2008;41:408–420.

88. Allmeling C, Jokuszies A, Reimers K, Kall S, Vogt PM. Use of spider silk fibres as an innovative material in a biocompatible artificial nerve conduit. *J Cell Mol Med* 2006;10:770–777.

89. Silva SS, Popa EG, Gomes ME, Oliveira MB, Nayak S, Subia B et al. Silk hydrogels from non-mulberry and mulberry silkworm cocoons processed with ionic liquids. *Acta Biomater* 2013;9(11):8972–8982.

90. Murphy AR, Kaplan DL. Biomedical applications of chemically-modified silk fibroin. *J Mater Chem* 2009;19(36):6443–6450.

91. Vlierberghe SV, Dubrue P, Schacht E. Biopolymer-based hydrogels as scaffolds for tissue engineering applications: A review. *Biomacromolecules* 2011;12(5):1387–1408.

92. Matsumoto A, Kim HJ, Irene Y, Wang TX, Cebe P, Kaplan DL. Silk. In: Lewin M, editor. *Handbook of Fiber Chemistry*, vol. 3. Northwest: CRC Press; 2006. p. 383–401.

93. Kim UJ, Park JY, Li CM, Jin HJ, Valluzzi R, Kaplan DL. Structure and properties of silk hydrogels. *Biomacromolecules*. 2004;5(3):786–792.

94. Yucel T, Cebe P, Kaplan DL. Vortex-induced injectable silk fibroin hydrogels. *Biophys J* 2009;97(7):2044–2050.

95. Jun Z, Chen GQ. The study of the structures of silk fibers grafted with hexaflurobutyl methacrylate. *International Forum of Textile and Engineering for Doctoral Candidates*, China; 2006.

96. Gutowska A, Bae YH, Feijen J, Kim SW. Heparin release from thermosensitive hydrogels. *J Controlled Release* 1992;22:95–104.

97. Adams DJ, Holtzmann K, Schneider C, Butler MF. Self-assembly of surfactant-like peptides. *Langmuir* 2007;23:12729–12736.

98. Guler MO, Stupp SI. A self-assembled nanofiber catalyst for ester hydrolysis. *J Am Chem Soc* 2007;129:12082–12083.

99. Williams BAR, Lund K, Liu Y, Yan H, Chaput JC. Self-assembled peptide nanoarrays: An approach to studying protein–protein interactions. *Angew Chem Int Ed* 2007;46:3051–3054.

100. Guler MO, Soukasene S, Hulvat JF, Stupp SI. Presentation and recognition of biotin on nanofibers formed by branched peptide amphiphiles. *Nano Lett* 2005;5:249–252.

101. Silva GA, Czeisler C, Niece KL, Beniash E, Harrington DA, Kessler JA et al. Selective differentiation of neural progenitor cells by high-epitope density nanofibers. *Science* 2004;303:1352–1355.

102. Hosseinkhani H, Hosseinkhani M, Tian F, Kobayashi H, Tabata Y. Osteogenic differentiation of mesenchymal stem cells in self-assembled peptide-amphiphile nanofibers. *Biomaterials* 2006;27:4079–4086.

103. Hwang JJ, Lyer SN, Li LS, Claussen R, Harrington DA, Stupp SI. Self-assembling biomaterials: Liquid crystal phases of cholesteryl oligo(L-lactic acid) and their interactions with cells. *Proc Natl Acad Sci USA* 2002;99:9662–9667.

104. Davis ME, Motion JPM, Narmoneva DA, Takahashi T, Hakuno D, Kamm RD et al. Injectable self-assembling peptide nanofibers create intramyocardial microenvironments for endothelial cells. *Circulation* 2005;111:442–450.

105. Zhang S. Fabrication of novel biomaterials through molecular self assembly. *Nat Biotechnol* 2003;21:1171–1178.

106. Gerecht S, Burdick JA, Ferreira LS, Townsend SA, Langer R, Vunjak-Novakovic G. Hyaluronic acid hydrogel for controlled self-renewal and differentiation of human embryonic stem cells. *Proc Nat Acad Sci USA* 2007;104:11298–11303.

107. Flynn L, Prestwich GD, Semple JL, Woodhouse KA. Adipose tissue engineering with naturally derived scaffolds and adipose-derived stem cells. *Biomaterials* 2007;28:3834–3842.

108. Flynn LE, Prestwich GD, Semple JL, Woodhouse KA. Proliferation and differentiation of adipose-derived stem cells on naturally derived scaffolds. *Biomaterials* 2008;29(12):1862–1871.

109. Inuyama Y, Kitamura C, Nishihara T, Morotomi T, Nagayoshi M, Tabata Y et al. Effects of hyaluronic acid sponge as a scaffold on odontoblastic cell line and amputated dental pulp. *J Biomed Mater Res* 2010;92B:120–128.

110. Kuo TF, Huang AT, Chang HH, Lin FH, Chen ST Chen RS et al. Regeneration of dentin-pulp complex with cementum and periodontal ligament formation using dental bud cells in gelatin-chondroitin-hyaluronan tri-copolymer scaffold in swine. *J Biomed Mater Res A* 2008;86:1062–1068.

111. Kitamura C, Nishihara T, Terashita M, Tabata Y, Jimi E, Washio A et al. Regeneration approaches for dental pulp and periapical tissues with growth factors, biomaterials, and laser irradiation. *Polymers* 2011;3:1776–1793.

112. Ando T, Yamazoe H, Moriyasu K, Ueda Y, Iwata H. Induction of Dopamine-Releasing Cells from Primate Embryonic Stem Cells Enclosed in Agarose Microcapsules. *Tissue Eng* 2007;13:2539–2547.

113. Sakai S, Hashimoto I, Kawakami K. Synthesis of an agarose-gelatin conjugate for use as a tissue engineering scaffold. *J Biosci Bioeng* 2007;1309:22–26.

114. Narayanan RP, Melman G, Letourneau NJ, Mendelson NL, Melman A. Photodegradable iron(III) cross-linked alginate gels. *Biomacromolecules* 2012;13:2465–2471.

115. Skjak-Braerk G, Grasdalen H, Smidsrod O. Inhomogeneous polysaccharide ionic gels. *Carbohydr Polym* 1989;10:31–54.

116. Maguire T, Novik E, Schloss R, Yarmush M. Alginate-PLL microencapsulation: Effect on the differentiation of embryonic stem cells into hepatocytes. *Biotechnol Bioeng* 2006;93:581–591.

117. Fujiwara S, Kumabe S, Iwai Y. Isolated rat dental pulp cell culture and transplantation with an alginate scaffold. *Okajimas Folia Anat Jpn* 2006;83:15–24.

118. Kumabe S, Nakatsuka M, Kim GS, Jue S, Aikawa F, Shin JW et al. Human dental pulp cell culture and cell transplantation with an alginate scaffold. *Okajimas Folia Anat Jpn* 2006;82:147–156.

119. Hori Y, Winans A, Irvine D. Modular injectable matrices based on alginate solution/microsphere mixtures that gel in situ and co-deliver immunomodulatory factors. *Acta Biomater* 2009;5:969–982.

120. Venkatesan J, Bhatnagar I, Manivasagan P. Alginate composites for bone tissue engineering: A review. *Int J Biol Macromol* 2015;72:269–281.

121. Bhardwaj N, Kundu SC. Electrospinning: A fascinating fiber fabrication technique. *Biotechnol Adv* 2010;28:325–347.

122. Sapir Y, Kryukov O, Cohen S. Integration of multiple cell-matrix interactions into alginate scaffolds for promoting cardiac tissue regeneration. *Biomaterials* 2011;32:1838–1847.

123. Kawaguchi M, Fukushima T, Hayakawa T, Nakashima N, Inoue Y, Takeda S et al. Preparation of carbon nanotube-alginate nanocomposite gel for tissue engineering. *Prep Dent Mater J* 2006;25:719.

124. Bajpai AK, Gupta R. Magnetically mediated release of ciprofloxacin from polyvinyl alcohol based superparamagnetic nanocomposites. *J Mater Sci Mater M* 2011;2:357.

125. Shin SR, Bae H, Cha JM, Mun JY, Chen YC, Tekin H et al. Carbon nanotube reinforced hybrid microgels as scaffold materials for cell encapsulation. *ACS Nano* 2012;6:362.

126. Khor E, Lim LY. Implantable applications of chitin and chitosan. *Biomaterials* 2003;24(13):2339–2349.

127. Willerth S, Sakayama-Elbert Sh. Approaches to neural tissue engineering using scaffolds for drug delivery. *Adv Drug Delivery Rev* 2007;59(4–5):325–338.

128. Xu XL, Lou J, Tang TT, Ng KW, Zhang JH, Yu CF et al. Evaluation of different scaffolds for BMP-2 genetic orthopedic tissue engineering. *J Biomed Mater Res B: Appl Biomater* 2005;75B:289–303.

129. Gruber HE, Hoelscher GL, Leslie K, Ingram JA, Hanley EN. Three-dimensional culture of human disc cells within agarose or a collagen sponge: Assessment of proteoglycan production. *Biomaterials* 2006;27:371–376.

130. Gruber HE, Leslie K, Ingram J, Norton HJ, Hanley EN. Cell-based tissue engineering for the intervertebral disc: In vitro studies of human disc cell gene expression and matrix production within selected cell carriers. *Spine J* 2004;4:44–55.

131. Mouw JK, Case ND, Guldberg RE, Plaas AHK, Levenston ME. Variation in matrix composition and GAG fine structure among scaffolds for cartilage tissue engineering. *Osteoarthr Cartil* 2005;13:828–836.

132. Stevens MM, Marini RP, Martin I, Langer R, Shastri VP. FGF-2 enhances TGF-beta1-induced periosteal chondrogenesis. *J Orthop Res* 2004;22:1114–1119.

133. Suri S, Banerjee R. In vitro evaluation of in situ biopolymeric gels as short term vitreous substitutes. *J Biomed Mater Res A* 2006;79A:650–664.

134. Sultana Y, Aqil M, Ali A. Ion-activated, Gelrite®-based in situ ophthalmic gels of pefloxacin mesylate: Comparison with conventional eye drops. *Drug Deliv* 2006;13:215–219.

135. Chen FM, Wu ZF, Wang QT, Wu H, Zhang YJ, Nie X, Jin Y. Preparation of recombinant human bone morphogenetic protein-2 loaded dextran-based microspheres and their characteristics. *Acta Pharmacol Sin* 2005;26:1093–1103.

136. Chen FM, Zhao YM, Wu H, Deng ZH, Wang QT, Zhou W et al. Enhancement of periodontal tissue regeneration by locally controlled delivery of insulin-like growth factor-I from dextran-co-gelatin microspheres. *J Controlled Release* 2006;114:209–222.

137. Levesque SG, Shoichet MS. Synthesis of cell-adhesive dextran hydrogels and macroporous scaffolds. *Biomaterials* 2006;27:5277–5285.

138. Zhang RS, Tang MG, Bowyer A, Eisenthal R, Hubble J. A novel pH- and ionic-strengthsensitive carboxy methyl dextran hydrogel. *Biomaterials* 2005;26:4677–4683.

139. Bloch K, Lozinsky VI, Galaev IY, Yavriyanz K, Vorobeychik M, Azarov D et al. Functional activity of insulinoma cells (INS-1E) and pancreatic islets cultured in agarose cryogel sponges. *J Biomed Mater Res A* 2005;75A:802–809.

140. Alaminos M, Sanchez-Quevdo MD, Munoz-Avila JI, Serrano D, Medialdea S, Carreras I et al. Construction of a complete rabbit cornea substitute using a fibrin-agarose scaffold. *Invest Ophthalmol Visual Sci* 2006;47:3311–3317.

141. Svensson A, Nicklasson E, Harrah T, Panilaitis B, Kaplan DL, Brittberg M et al. Bacterial cellulose as a potential scaffold for tissue engineering of cartilage. *Biomaterials* 2005;26:419–431.

142. Gravel M, Gross T, Vago R, Tabrizian M. Responses of mesenchymal stem cell to chitosan-coralline composites microstructured using coralline as a gas forming agent. *Biomaterials* 2006;27:1899–1906.

143. Cho CH, Eliason JF, Matthew HW. Application of porous glycosaminoglycan-based scaffolds for expansion of human cord blood stem cells in perfusion culture. *J Biomed Materials Res A* 2008;86(1):98–107.

144. Muzzarelli RAA. Chitins and chitosans for the repair of wounded skin, nerve, cartilage and bone. *Carbohydr Polym* 2009;76:167–182.

145. Budiraharjo R, Neoh KG, Kang ET, Kishen A. Bioactivity of novel carboxymethyl chitosan scaffold incorporating MTA in a tooth model. *Int Endod J* 2010;43:930–939.

146. Zhu AP, Zhao F, Fang N. *J Biomed Mater Res A* 2008;86:467–476.

147. Hu X, Neoh K-G, Shi Z, Kang E-T, Poh C, Wang W. An in vitro assessment of titanium functionalized with polysaccharides conjugated with vascular endothelial growth factor for enhanced osseointegration and inhibition of bacterial adhesion. *Biomaterials* 2010;31:8854–8863.

148. Lin Q, Lan X, Li Y, Yu Y, Ni Y, Lu C. Anti-washout carboxymethyl chitosan modified tricalcium silicate bone cement: Preparation, mechanical properties and in vitro bioactivity. *J Mater Sci Mater Med* 2010;21:3065–3076.

149. Chen R, Mooney D. Polymeric growth factor delivery strategies for tissue engineering. *Pharm Res* 2003;20:1103–1112.

150. Tessmar JK, Göpferich AM. Matrices and scaffolds for protein delivery in tissue engineering. *Adv Drug Deliv Rev* 2007;59:274–291.

151. Holland T, Mikos A. *Tissue Engineering I*. Berlin Heidelberg: Springer; 2006. p. 161–185.

152. Chu C, Lu A, Liszkowski M, Sipehia R. Enhanced growth of animal and human endothelial cells on biodegradable polymers. *Biochim Biophys Acta* 1999;1472:479e85.

153. Zhang R, Ma PX. *Methods of Tissue Engineering*. San Diego: Academic Press; 2001. p. 715.

154. Pachence JM, Kohn J. Biodegradable polymers. In: Lanza RP, Langer R, Chick WL, editors. *Principles of Tissue Engineering* (2nd ed.). San Diego: Academic Press; 2000. p. 263.

155. Bolland Benjamin JRF, Kanczler Janos M, Ginty Patrick J, Howdle Steve M, Shakesheff Kevin M, Dunlop Douglas G et al. The application of human bone marrow stromal cells and poly(DL-lactic acid) as a biological bone graft extender in impaction bone grafting. *Biomaterials* 2008;29:3221–3227.

156. Lin ASP, Barrows TH, Cartmell SH, Guldberg RE. Microarchitectural and mechanical characterization of oriented porous polymer scaffolds. *Biomaterials* 2003;24:481–489.

157. Wie G, Ma PX. Structure and properties of nano-hydroxyapatite/polymer composite scaffolds for bone tissue engineering. *Biomaterials* 2004;25:4749–4757.

158. Park GE, Pattison MA, Park K, Webster TJ. Accelerated chondrocyte functions on NaOH-treated PLGA scaffolds. *Biomaterials* 2005;26:3075–3086.

159. Bendix D. Chemical synthesis of polylactide and its copolymers for medical applications. *Polym Degrad Stab* 2008;59:129–135.

160. Perron JK, Naguib HE, Daka J, Chawla A, Wilkins R. A study on the effect of degradation media on the physical and mechanical properties of porous PLGA 85/15 scaffolds. *J Biomed Mater Res Part B: Appl Biomater* 2009;91:876–886.

161. Bhang SH, Lim JS, Choi CY, Kwon YK, Kim BS. The behavior of neural stem cells on biodegradable synthetic polymers. *J Biomater Sci Polym Ed* 2007;18:223–239.

162. He L, Zhang Y, Zeng C, Ngiam M, Liao S, Quan D et al. Manufacture of PLGA multiple-channel conduits with precise hierarchical pore architectures and in vitro/vivo evaluation for spinal cord injury. *Tissue Eng Part C Methods* 2009;15:243–255.

163. Olson HE, Rooney GE, Gross L, Nesbitt JJ, Galvin KE, Knight A et al. Neural stem cell- and Schwann cell-loaded biodegradable polymer scaffolds support axonal regeneration in the transected spinal cord. *J Tissue Eng Part A* 2009;15:1797–1805.

7 Ocular Implants

7.1 INTRODUCTION

The human eye is the most interesting complex organ of the central nervous system composed of several different structures and layers, with specific physiological roles (protects the ocular globe against external aggressions), which responds to a great deal of internal and external stimuli throughout its normal function. Its smaller anterior portion is able to receive and focus light and the larger posterior portion is responsible for detecting light. The eye transmits it as pulse to brain where it is recognized as an image. The main physiological structure of the eye with key ocular components is shown in Figure 7.1a. The eye is a nearly spherical hollow globe (diameter of 24 mm and a mass of about 7.5 g) filled with fluids (humors), is transparent at the front portion and opaque (or nearly so) over the remaining 80% of its surface, and housed in an eye socket, or orbit, within the skull. The optical path is composed of two anatomical regions (transparent liquids and solids): anterior segment and posterior segment. Cornea and conjunctiva are part of the anterior segment, whereas retina, which translates the light entering the eye into nervous signals, is the part of the posterior segment. In between the anterior and posterior segments is the lens that is a 4 mm thick transparent biconvex structure, having an average diameter of 9 mm and high refractive index 1.36 at the periphery and 1.42 on the visual axis (due to the synthesis of specialized proteins called as crystallins). The lens can control the focal distance accurately by changing its shape by an automatic nervous system through a process known as accommodation. It is situated just behind the iris and the pupil, consists of a capsule (outer elastic envelope, consisting of type IV collagen containing approximately 10% glycosaminoglycans, which can mold the lens during accommodation), an epithelium (can produce a wide range of macromolecules, i.e., nondividing, enucleate, lens fiber cells) and an internal lens substance. It is attached to the ciliary body via a network of elastic fibers, the zonules, which are responsible for further refracting, that is, bending and focusing the light that enters the eye. Tenon's capsule is a sheet of connective tissue that fills the space between globe and orbit with fat and provides a smooth socket permitting the free movement of the globe [1–5].

The walls of the eye are composed of three distinct tissue layers: an outer *scleral/corneal* layer, that is, a collagenous layer (the anterior portion is transparent to visible light and focuses the light on the retina called the anterior sclero-corneal layer, i.e., cornea, whereas the posterior portion is opaque and called the sclera that covers approximately five-sixth of the eye surface) that encircles the eye and provides it with mechanical strength, an intermediate *vascular/choroidal* layer termed the uvea, , a pigmented layer that comprises the iris (a small pigmented disk formed of muscular tissue acting as a biological aperture to control the amount of light entering the eye by controlling the size of the pupil through a combination of contraction and relaxation of radial and circular muscle fibers), a ciliary body (secretes aqueous humor, which provides nutrients to the avascular tissues in the anterior segment and maintains the intraocular pressure) in the anterior portion and the vascular choroid in the posterior portion (a vast network of capillaries that supplies the retina with nutrients), and an inner *retina* layer (a complex enervated structure covering approximately two-third of the internal posterior surface of the globe, consisting of nervous cells connected to receptors sensitive to light, the photoreceptors, arranged on a layer of a pigmented tissue that detects and transduces light signals to the brain). The clear aqueous humor crudely resembles a filtrate of plasma (composed of fibrinogen, plasma fibronectin, growth factors such as epidermal growth factor (EGF) and insulin-like growth factor 1 (IGF-1) and serum albumin, and novel protease, active against IGF-1 binding proteins, lower levels of urea and glucose but much higher concentrations of pyruvate, lactate, bicarbonate, and ascorbate, secreted by active processes from the ciliary epithelial cells), is filled into the anterior segment that separates the cornea from the anterior side of the lens, whereas gelatinous vitreous humor referred to as the vitreous body (a gel that is composed of water (over 98 wt%), hyaluronic acid, collagen and plasma proteins, imparts stability to the posterior components of the eye, attenuates the stresses imposed on the retina by sudden movement, and is bounded by the retina, the ciliary body, and the posterior capsule of the lens) is filled into the posterior segment. The macula lutea, a small dot, is located at the bottom of the eye, on the axis of the pupil is the highest visual accuracy zone of the eye [6–10].

Cornea is a five layered nonvascularized collagenous structure of about 500-μm thickness, makes clear transparent surface of the outer eye, provides protection from infection and physical damage to the eye, and acts as a clear window for light to pass into the eye, is composed of the epithelium (a major hydrophilic barrier), Bowman's membrane, the stroma (a major lipophilic barrier),

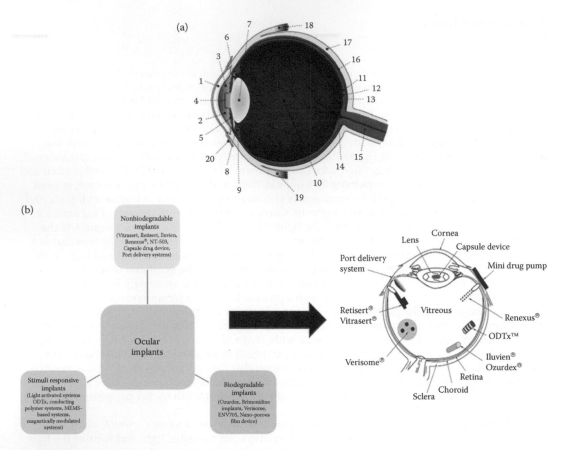

Figure 7.1 (a) The structure of the eye with its essential elements: 1, cornea; 2, anterior chamber; 3, aqueous humor; 4, pupil; 5, iris; 6, posterior chamber; 7, crystalline lens; 8, zonule; 9, ciliary body; 10, vitreous body; 11, retina; 12, macula; 13, fovea; 14, head of the optic nerve; 15, optic nerve; 16, choroid; 17, sclera; 18, lateral rectus muscle; 19, medial rectus muscle; and 20, conjunctiva [17]. (b) A schematic representation of types of ocular implants approved by FDA and their locations in the eye.

Descemet's membrane, and the endothelium (a minor lipophilic barrier) [11]. On the other hand, the conjunctiva is a thin clear vascularized mucus membrane, composed of stratified columnar epithelium which covers the anterior part of the sclera up to the cornea and lines the inside of the eyelids, that acts as a lubricant, hydration and cleaning agent by producing mucus and tears (secrete approximately 2–3 µL of mucus per day), and prevents the entrance of pathogenic agents and foreign bodies into the eye [11–14].

The sclera is commonly referred to as the "white of the eye" visible at the surface of the globe (thickness ranging from 1 mm at the posterior pole to 0.3 mm just behind the rectus muscle insertions), is an opaque fibrous slightly elastic protective outer layer of the eye, and is composed of collagen that maintains the shape of the globe, internal and external intraocular pressure, and serves as the attachment site for the extraocular muscles insertions [14–16].

7.2 NEED FOR EYE REMOVAL: ETIOLOGY AND SURGERY

The eye is a highly protected vital organ of vision that plays an important role in facial expression of living organisms and its visibility needs to be maintained, which is a key determinant of healthy aging. It is protected by various anatomical and physiological barriers. However, an eye of a person may be damaged due to injury or diseases, such as infection due to uveitis, diabetic retinopathy, macular edema, endophthalmitis, proliferative retinopathy, age related macular degeneration and glaucoma, a tumor or malignancy, leading to partial or complete blindness, if left untreated. Blindness is the second most dreaded disease in the world because around 285 million

Table 7.1: Five Generations of Lens Implants

Generation	Date	Intraocular Lens	Materials Used	Advantages	Disadvantages
First-generation IOLS	1950	Ridley posterior chamber IOL (biconvex PMMA PC IOL)	Heavy PMMA	Optical	Uveitis Secondary glaucoma Hyphema Decentration/dislocation
Second-generation IOLS	1952–1962	Anterior chamber IOLs (AC IOLs)	PMMA, rigid design, closed loop	Do not require posterior capsule Capsule usually removed therefore no PCO	Corneal complications (decompensation, edema, pseudophakic bullous, keratopathy, IOL corneal touch), CMO, uveitis, UGH, subluxation, dislocation
Third-generation IOLS	1953–1973	Iris-supported IOLs (Phakic IOL)	PMMA	Do not require posterior capsule	Iris complications: (iris chafing and erosion, pupil changes, pupillary block, PAS—peripheral anterior synechiae)
Fourth-generation IOLS	1970 to present day	Modified AC IOLs like Choyce Mark VIII and Mark IX lens, flexible loop AC IOL, etc.	PMMA, flexible haptics, open loop	Do not require posterior capsule, better fixation, corneal complications rare	CMO retinal detachment
Fifth-generation IOLS	1975 to present day	Modern posterior chamber IOL (PC IOL)	Standard PMMA designs Foldable lenses—silicone, hydrogel, acrylic Scleral-sutured IOL Multifocal IOLs	Less corneal problems	Require intact zonules and posterior capsule Less CMO Less retinal detachment Less UGH Less pupil block Optical

people are suffering from partial or full blindness and every year seven million new cases are being reported [18]. It is assumed that out of the total debilitating ocular diseases, more than 50% are posterior segment ocular diseases including age-related macular degeneration (AMD), diabetic macular edema, proliferative vitreoretinopathy, posterior uveitis, retinal vascular occlusions, choroid neovascularization (CNV), and diabetic retinopathy, that impact on the patients' vision loss and therefore their quality of life if left untreated [19]. However, the treatment of the posterior eye segment disease is limited due to some structural and physiological barriers. Surgery is the most common treatment option for posterior segment ocular disorders. In the last decade, there is an improvement in surgical techniques, anesthesia, and implant materials for patient's satisfaction [20]. In surgery, eyeball is removed from the orbit and mechanically replaced by an ocular implant to achieve better cosmesis and rehabilitation of the anophthalmic patient. Moreover, they only provide modest relief and generally result in low patient adherence to the therapy [21].

Recently, stimuli responsive polymer-based implants have gain considerable attention in the biomedical field due to their responsive nature toward external stimuli [22–27] (Table 7.1). Therefore, ocular implants are synthesized from stimuli responsive either biodegradable or nonbiodegradable polymers for treatment of eye disease. Such implants are generally divided into closed-loop (self-regulating in internal stimulus) and open-loop systems (require an external stimulus) [28]. Currently, FDA approved ocular implants namely Vitrasert®, Retisert® (two being nonbiodegradable systems anchored to the sclera), and Ozurdex® (a biodegradable rod injected into the vitreous) are used in treatment of eye defects. A nonbiodegradable implant, Iluvien®, which had been applied in EU countries, now recently received FDA approval [29–34] (Figure 7.1b).

7.3 OCULAR IMPLANTS

In last decade, a large number of ocular implants and biomaterials devices have been developed and employed with mainly cosmetic intent for correcting the functional deficiencies of disease, age and ocular trauma, uveitis and rubeotic glaucoma as well as for sustained release of drugs from either biodegradable or nonbiodegradable polymeric systems over several months to years. It is necessary for a surgeon to fill some solid implant after removal of the globe or its internal contents to maintain the orbital volume and socket motility. Artificial eye has two major components: orbital implant (placed at the time of enucleation or evisceration to reduce contracture and volume deficit) and ocular prosthesis (placed 6–8 weeks after enucleation/evisceration and inserted anterior to the orbital implant to make the artificial eye appear life-like). Some ocular implants are discussed below.

7.3.1 Orbital Implants

When an eye of patient is removed permanently or partially, that is, enucleation is done due to some reason such as infection, disease, or trauma, orbitals implants have been used as a surgical implant into the scleral and shell and conjuctival closure to fill the space in order to maintain the orbital volume, repair the fractured eye orbit bone, lift the ocular globe into its correct position (avoid enophthalmos), discourage bacterial colonization of the surface, and release systemic antibiotics for the treatment of infection [35–37]. Evidence from thousand years ago supports that Sumerians and Egyptians were able to surgically remove the ocular globe as well as to make artificial eyes and replace with precious stones, bronze, copper, and gold. However, in the last 60 years, with the advancement of science, many biomaterials have been used to design orbital implants to reduce the complication rate and improved the patient's clinical outcomes and satisfaction [38] (Figure 7.2).

Currently, there are two main surgical approaches, namely evisceration and enucleation, carried out for the removal of diseased eye of patient in the cases of intraocular malignancy (e.g., retinoblastoma, which can develop especially in children), blind painful eye, prevention of sympathetic ophthalmia in a blind (or even seeing) eye, severe trauma, cosmesis, and infections not responsive to pharmaceutical therapy. Out of the two approaches, evisceration (used in the treatment of active, uncontrolled endophthalmitis) is superior to enucleation with regard to motility and cosmetic appearance, less invasive and less surgically complex, because it involves the removal of the intraocular contents of the eye while the sclera, Tenon's capsule, conjunctiva, extraocular muscles, and optic nerve are left intact, whereas entire globe with surrounding structures and tissues is removed from the orbital socket, together with the scleral envelope and a portion of the optic nerve in enucleation (apply if infection has spread to the sclera, extraocular tissues and structures, tumors that are confined to the ocular globe) [39–42]. However, modern enucleation procedures maintain the motility of artificial eye and cosmesis outcomes by careful attachment of extraocular muscles to the silicone or acrylic custom-made prosthetic implants with various types of adhesives [43].

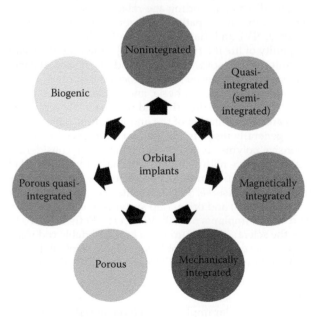

Figure 7.2 Types of various orbital implants.

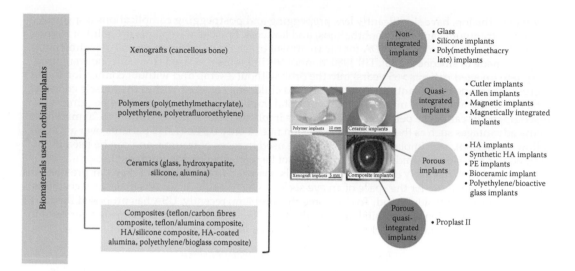

Figure 7.3 Types of materials used in synthesizing orbital implants.

The materials that can be used as orbital implant (properly designed, reproducible, manmade device is placed at the time of enucleation or evisceration and fills the anophthalmic socket, i.e., replace orbital volume and maintain adequate motility to an artificial eye) should be biocompatible, strong to support the orbital contents and maintain orbital volume, available in sufficient quantities, easy to graft into proper shape and size (replacing the anophthalmic socket volume and restoring an acceptable esthetic appearance to the patient's face), easily fixable in situ, on degradation its by product produces minimal foreign-body reaction, osteoconductive and osteoinductive (Figure 7.3). At present glass, gold, silver, platinum, stainless steel, cork, ivory, wool, aluminum-based materials, and rock-derived materials (asbestos) have been used to manufacture orbital implants [44] (Figure 7.3).

It is recognized that porosity of orbital plays an important role in clinical success, that is, porous implant shows less fibroblast ingrowth and a chronic inflammatory response (overall failure rate of approximately 10% for porous implants). Therefore, scientists are giving more attention for synthesizing porous orbital implants based upon hydroxyapatite or porous polyethylene [45–48].

7.3.1.1 Nonintegrated Implants

Nonintegrated implants are the orbitals devices that are nonporous implants, have no direct attachment to the ocular prosthesis, are made of silicone and poly(methylmethacrylate) (PMMA), and do not allow fibrovascular in-growth as well as do not contain any specific apparatus for attachment to the extraocular muscles. Some nonintegrated implants are discussed below.

7.3.1.1.1 Glass

Till World War II (WWII), glass eyes were used as the most popular materials for replacement of damaged eyes of patients. Mules implant was a hollow blown glass sphere applied as first orbital implant until WWII in different sizes during evisceration and enucleation surgeries to reduce socket retraction, intraorbital fat redistribution, and superior sulcus deformity [49,50]. Mostly lighter Mules implants were used to decrease stress on the lower lid and associated ectropion formation. However, Mules implants as orbital implants have been almost totally abandoned due to major drawback of high extrusion rates (50%–90%) to decreased stress on the lower lid and associated ectropion formation, brittleness, and the risk of implosion due to sudden temperature changes [51].

7.3.1.1.2 Silicone Implants

From the last 60 years, silicone implants (proposed in the late 1960s by Soll) have gain attraction as suitable material for orbital implants in various surgical applications due to their remarkable properties such as biological/chemical inertness, flexibility, ease of handling, wrapped within a sclera foil or other suitable biomaterial, can be placed into the orbit and Tenon's capsule and conjunctiva sewn over the top, have significantly less prepegging and postpegging complications (especially pyogenic granuloma and hypo-ophthalmos) and low cost. Episcleral implants are solid or porous implants that are approved by FDA for the treatment of scleral buckling in retinal detachment surgery, made of silicone [52,53]. Till 1980, nonporous implants prepared from silicone were used as sphere (in aged patients >65 years) into the orbit without a wrap and without connection to the rectus, or wrapped (in infants and preschool-aged children), centered within the muscle cone and attached to the four rectus muscles placed as orbital implants in those cases where pegging is discouraged or cannot be performed [54]. Silicone implants (sizes ranging from 14 to 20 mm) have many advantages such as they have low extrusion rate of only 0.84% (1/119 patients over a 10-year follow-up period), zero implant migration, can be used in cases of trauma, and can be used if extraocular muscles are unidentifiable and will not be reattached to the implant [55].

It is found that inevitably contract and deform is observed in an eye socket if ocular prosthesis is not able to compensate for the space of an eye socket, which results in an unsatisfactory cosmesis and can continue into adulthood. To overcome this problem, recently, USA has proposed the use of silicone for preparation of an orbital device called the "Flexiglass eye" actually made to expand to fill the pediatric patient's eye socket, whose clinical trial is going on from 2005 [56].

7.3.1.1.3 Poly(methylmethacrylate) Implants

PMMA is an excellent biocompatible transparent polymer used in various biomedical fields as a substituent of orbital implants for damaged eyes and recently proposed for the repair of extensive orbito-facial defects due to trauma. It is used for the fabrication of intraocular lenses [57], as well as rigid and semi-rigid contact lenses [8], and also used in oculoplasty. Frueh and Felker were the first scientists who designed the baseball implant from PMMA. In 1985, during a 2 years case study of 35 secondary and six primary baseball implants in patients, Tyers and Collin found complications, that is, postoperative edema in 59% of cases, but most of them were resolved by pharmaceutical treatment [58]. They found that baseball implants have excellent motility and volume correction as compared with that of quasi-integrated implants and might be recommended as a safe and convenient secondary implant in the volume deficit anophthalmic socket.

In Pakistan, Sahaf implants type I were implanted by Kamal-Siddiqi et al. in 60 enucleated patients from 2003 to 2006 in various sizes to restore different ocular volumes, which were made of solid PMMA, that is characterized by a two-piece design wherein the posterior hemispherical portion gave support to hold recti muscles and the anterior convex curvature supported the ocular prosthesis. Authors found that implant has satisfactory socket filling property [59]. From 2006 to 2009, Sahaf type II nonintegrated implant made of pear-shaped PMMA was implanted in Pakistani patients who underwent enucleation or in cases of exenterated socket, rested on the orbital floor and projected up to fill the orbit [60]. On the basis of their review, Agahan and Tan reported that hollow PMMA implants by fusing two hemispherical elements, made from medical-grade PMMA powder, are more stable as compared to a solid implant because they show less implant migration due to less gravitational force [61]. However, multicenter clinical trials with an adequate patient sample size and a longer follow-up are needed to establish the long-term stability of the implant.

7.3.1.2 Quasi-Integrated Implants

Quasi-integrated orbital implant was introduced in about 70 years ago during WWII to provide adequate motility without interrupting the conjunctival lining, with minimum discharge and infections due to their irregularly shaped anterior surfaces that create an indirect coupling mechanism between implant and ocular prosthesis. During implantation, the posterior surface is modified to fit it with the anterior surface of the implant, although it remains buried beneath the conjunctiva.

7.3.1.2.1 Cutler Implants

The Cutler implant so-called basket implants was ocular motility implants, introduced in the late 1940s and early 1950s, and made from 14-mm sphere of acrylic and tantalum mesh with a short cylinder tube 14 mm (had four openings through which the rectus muscles were pulled through and sutured) in diameter extending forward from its anterior surface with a tantalum male peg, which was embedded in the posterior surface of the prosthesis [62]. Similarly, Whitney and Olson's acrylic implant with tantalum mesh belt (for attachment of recti and Tenon's capsule), and Rudemann's famous (or infamous) modified acrylic eye implant, with tantalum mesh for attachment of tissues [63]. However, such plants suffer from excess mucus drainage and eventual migration, which proved a nuisance to patients.

7.3.1.2.2 Allen Implants

Prof. James Allen and ocularist Lee Allen improved the cutler implants and developed new quasi-integrated implant so-called Allen implant, by incorporating a thin rod (peg) to PMMA implant in which each rectus muscle was passed through a peripheral tunnel, split lengthwise to straddle the gold peg and sutured to its antagonist. However, due to early stage problems such as infections due to bacterial colonization, it was modified by removing peg. The modified Allen implants were implanted by suturing the muscles through a central 6 mm opening and Tenon's capsule and conjunctiva were completely closed over the flat PMMA surface of the implant. However, its flat surface did not support the weight of the ocular prosthesis against gravity and causes migration. Therefore, in 1959, the first next generation implants so-called Iowa implant I were introduced by Lee Allen and 1 year later modified implant named as Iowa implant II was introduced which had the same shape but nearly one-third larger in volume than Iowa Implant I. Both implants were made of PMMA, had four peripheral mounds (height 5 mm) on the anterior surface designed to integrate with four depressions on the back of the ocular prosthesis that supported the ocular prosthesis and reduced the gravitational effect on the lower lid [64–66]. The central anterior depression of both implants was overlapped and tied by the rectus muscles brought together through the valleys between the mounds. During implantation, holes were made in implants to promote fibrovascular tissue in-growth. In the late 1980s, these implants were further modified called universal implants which had lower, more rounded mounds [67,68].

7.3.1.2.3 Magnetic Implants

Magnetic implants introduced in 1950s by Roper-Hall, which were modified Allen implants, consist of a 21 mm PMMA hemisphere with a flat anterior face into which a magnet was embedded; a ring of the same material stood forward of the face and had tunnels through which the four rectus muscles might pass. These implants showed better horizontal movement than vertical by means of the action of magnets with opposite poles incorporated on the posterior surface of the prosthesis and within the anterior region of the implant [69,70], and could be increased in all directions if additional magnets were placed in the ocular prosthesis but strong magnets compressed conjunctiva and Tenon's capsule tissue between implant and prosthesis, thereby leading to breakdown and exposure along the outer edges [71]. These implants suffer from problems such as local toxicity related to the accumulation of iron ions within the conjunctival tissues, magnet rusting, and can be potentially hazardous during magnetic resonance imaging (MRI) because of the movement or dislodgement of the foreign metal object [72].

7.3.1.2.4 Mechanically Integrated Implants

Mechanically integrated implants were developed in the late 1940s not only for enucleation but also for evisceration. These implants had satisfactory movement, were made of PMMA, had square (female) receptacle at exposed face and gold square (male) pegs attached to ocular prosthesis, and tantalum wires were used to maintain the device passing through the sclera and the peg passed through a hole in the cornea. However, these implants also suffer from infection due to bacterial colonization of peg/tissues [73,74].

7.3.1.3 Porous Implants

Porous implants were developed by scientist to overcome the complications related to noninte-grated implants and quasi-integrated implants. However, porous implants do not show movement as the irregular anterior surface of quasi-integrated implants do. But they show fibrovascularization when scleral windows were produced by the surgeon, less infection as well as the capability of more effective treatment of infections via an antibiotic systemic therapy. Some examples of clinically used porous orbital implants are collected in Figure 7.3. In 1899, Guist's implant was prepared by heating spheres of cancellous bone containing predominantly of ultramicroscopic crystals of HA with small amounts of calcium carbonate and calcium citrate [75,76] which was widely used orbital implant before WWII [77].

In the 1960s, Molteno et al. [78] reported that the biodegradable microcrystalline HA matrix has superiority than a smooth-surfaced polymeric implant because it does not migrate through the tissues, the mass of host connective tissue incorporating the bone mineral implant would likely persist unchanged for the patient's whole life, and small exposures of the implant during the postoperative period frequently healed spontaneously. The early model used deproteinized (antigen-free) bone from calf fibulae which were more porous and fragile than other available HA implants, costly, and unable to support a peg [79–81].

Due to high cost of HA-based implants, in 1970s, Lyall developed [82] the hemispherical orbital porous implants by using Proplast, an inert felt-like composite material composed of polytetrafluoroethylene (Teflon) and carbon fibers. The implant showed good motility and less rate of extrusion and rejection after implantation. Now the use of Proplast has declined because of long-term postoperative complications, primarily late infections, associated with its use [83].

Hydroxyapatite (HA) formally belongs to the class of calcium orthophosphates has been widely used for more than 50 years in orthopedics and dentistry for bone repair. Due to its similarities with hard tissues, in the mid-1980s, the first porous implant made from coralline hydroxyapatite (HA) (Bio-Eye® Orbital Implants or Integrated Orbital Implants, Inc., San Diego, CA) has revolutionized anophthalmic socket surgery, which showed less rate of migration, extrusion, and infection because its interconnected porous structure allows host fibrovascular in-growth and also allows the treatment of ocular infection by antibiotic therapy [84]. Such implants show better motility because extraocular muscles can be securely attached to the HA implant [85].

The wide range of movement of HA-based porous implants can be improved by placing a peg into the HA implant, which can subsequently be coupled to the posterior surface of the ocular prosthesis imparting a more life-like quality to the artificial eye. Besides these advantages, porous HA implants have some drawbacks such as their high cost, brittle nature that makes difficult suturing the extraocular muscles directly to the implant, rough surface adversely impacts on biocompatibility, and implant involves damage to marine life ecosystems due to the harvesting of natural corals. Therefore, it is generally recommended that the HA implants should be placed within a wrapping material (Figure 7.3d) before being introduced into the orbit [86–88].

These drawbacks can be reduced by using Synthetic HA implants (FCI, Issy-Les-Moulineaux, Cedex, France, have similar composition to Bio-Eye® and less expensive, but have lower porosity), Chinese HA implant (H + Y Comprehensive Technologies, Philadelphia, PA; contain some CaO impurities that, after hydration in host tissues, may form $Ca(OH)_2$), Brazilian HA implant (high weight, lower porosity, and lower pore interconnectivity, consequently enhanced risk of implant migration and limited fibrovascularization), India synthetic HA implants (75 vol% porosity, pore sizes ranging from 100 to 300 µm) [89–92]. However, in last two decades, a large number of low cost materials have been developed to act as an "ideal" porous orbital implant with a reduced complication profile.

Medpor® implant (Porex Surgical, Inc., Newnan, GA) is a synthetic orbital implant made of polyethylene, has porous nature and used in the orbit as well as for the surgical repair of orbital floor fractures with or without a wrapping material because they can be directly attached with extraocular muscles. Many studies have reported that it is a better alternative to the Bio-Eye® HA because it is smooth, malleable, easy to implant, induces less inflammation and fibrosis, and less irritation of the overlying conjunctiva following placement than HA, can be used in the pediatric population with satisfactory outcomes and relatively low complications rates [93–97]. However, these porous implants show lesser rate of vascularization that depends on their pore size (implants with a 400 lm pore size vascularize more rapidly than those having a 200 lm pore size), higher exposure rates, and higher overall complication rates as compared to those of HA implants, and most surgeons find difficulties during implantation due to the absence of holes [98]. These problems of implants were overcome by next generation PE implants having a complex shape and advanced functionalities; these include SST™, Porex Surgical Inc. (have more porous posterior surface to facilitate fibrovascular in-growth, nonporous anterior surface to prevent abrasion of the overlying tissue with suture tunnels for easier muscle attachment) and Medpor Quad™ Motility Implant, Porex Surgical, Inc. (standard porous sphere) [99,100]. In the late 1990s, polytetrafluoroethylene-based porous implants such as ePTFE or Gore-Tex, W.L. Gore & Associates, Flagstaff, AZ, were investigated as porous orbital implants. These implants showed induced inflammatory reactions due to nonbiomaterial nature [101].

From long time, aluminum oxide (Al_2O_3) is widely used in orthopedic applications due to its good biocompatibility and high mechanical strength. In 2000, it is approved by the US Food and Drug Administration as "Bioceramic implant," a porous orbital implant for ophthalmoplasty because it is biocompatible, bio-inert, less expensive, has finely crystalline microstructure, do not induce infections, and its manufacturing did not involve any damage to marine life ecosystems [102]. However, later studies suggested that alumina devices were associated with higher exposure rates and higher overall complication rates as compared to HA implants. These problems can be reduced by a standard enucleation process [103,104]. These problems of alumina implants were removed by composite porous HA-coated porous alumina implants with different multiple interconnected pores sizes (300, 500, and 800 μm) developed by Korean researchers in the early 2000s, which have porous Al_2O_3 skeleton acted as a load-bearing member, whereas the 20-μm-thick HA coating layer was advocated to provide biocompatibility and long-term stability in the eye, showed fibrovascularization, low price and easy manufacture [105,106].

Polyethylene/bioactive glass-based porous implants were investigated by Choi et al. [107] as manufacture of orbital implants due to its bio-inertness and ability to form a stable interface and stimulating bone tissue regeneration. They found that inclusion of BG particulate did not significantly increase the rate of fibrovascular in-growth into porous PE orbital implants.

7.3.1.4 Porous Quasi-Integrated Implants

The porous quasi-integrated implants were developed to incorporate advantages of both porous and quasi-integrated implants for more comfort of patients. The first such implants (Proplast II, Vitek, Inc., Houston, TX) were developed by Girard and coworkers, were composed of Teflon and alumina, and had a siliconized nonporous posterior surface to allow smoother movements, together with a porous anterior portion to facilitate fibrovascular in-growth, and had a nipple on its anterior surface that could integrate with a depression on the posterior surface of the ocular prosthesis. However, such implants had poor motility and biocompatibility. This problem was overcome by next generation implants having a semispherical anterior part, made of synthetic porous HA to guarantee tissue integration, joined to a posterior part that was manufactured using a silicone rubber; the horizontal and vertical eye muscles were sutured crosswise in front of the implant to ensure better stability and motility [108,109].

7.3.1.5 Complications in Orbital Implants Replacement

An ideal orbital implant must be biocompatible, easy to implant, cost effective, nonbiodegradable, have adequate volume replacement to support the ocular prosthesis as well as good motility transmitted to the ocular prosthesis. With the advancement of science, a large number of materials have been developed as orbital implants to incite minimal host response, characterized by walling off the implant by a pseudocapsule. However, they suffer from many complications during replacement of damaged eye of patients. These complications can be categorized as early complications (occurring within 6 months of the procedure) and late complications (occurring more than 6 months after the procedure) or implant-related, host- (or patient-) related, and related to the surgery (Figure 7.4).

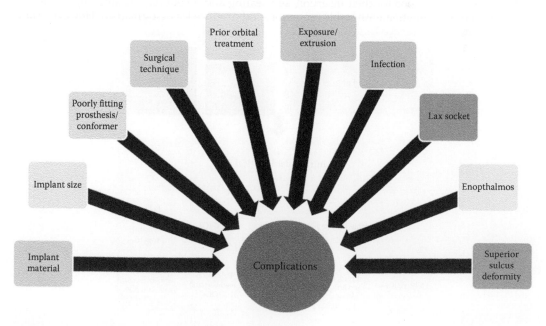

Figure 7.4 A schematic representation of complications in orbital implants.

7.3.2 Intraocular Lenses

Cataract is the most common world-leading cause of blindness which affect either the crystalline lens (lenticular), or the anterior or posterior part of the lens capsule (capsular), or both of them (capsulolenticular), and causes the cloudiness and the opacification of the lens by interrupting the proper transmission of light through the lens. There are two ophthalmic surgical procedures namely cataract extraction and intraocular lens implantation being performed to compensate for the loss of the natural crystalline lens [110].

The first intraocular lens implantation was reported in the eighteenth century, Italian oculist Tadini was the first who implanted first artificial lens made of a small glass into the eye of his patient to replace the crystalline lens after cataract extraction. Nearly at the same time, Casamata developed and inserted his lenses made of glass, which sank posteriorly [111].

The first generation of intraocular lens was made of Perspex (rigid polymethylmethacrylate, diameter 8.32 mm and power +24 D), and implanted by ophthalmologist Harold Ridley behind the iris after an extracapsular cataract surgery of 45-year-old lady in 1950 at St. Thomas' Hospital. However, the first-generation IOLs suffer from inferior decentration and posterior dislocation, inflammation, secondary glaucoma, etc., and led to high myopia and astigmatism. With the advancement of science, the field of IOLs has developed and presently we are using the fifth-generation IOLs (Table 7.1) [112].

On the basis of position of IOLs in the eye, they can be categorized into three types, anterior chamber IOL, iris slip IOL, and posterior chamber IOL. The anterior chamber IOL sits in front of the iris but behind the cornea. The iris slip IOL is implanted to straddle the pupil whereas the posterior chamber IOL is implanted behind the iris or on the capsular bag to correct aphakia [8] (Figure 7.5 and Table 7.2). During the last 50 years, a large number of materials such as PMMA, silicone, esters of poly(meth)acrylic acid, and hydrogels of poly(meth)acrylic acid have been developed to synthesize ideal biomaterials for intraocular lens. However, the selection of IOL materials depends on biocompatibility of materials because it affects the blood aqueous barrier, the cellular reaction on the anterior surface of the lens, and the effect on the lens capsule.

PMMA was the first material used due to its biocompatibility, smooth surface, high refractive index, chemical inertness, and minimal intraocular inflammatory reaction. But it has one disadvantage that it is rigid in nature. Therefore, it requires a larger incision for insertion. Patients suffering from uveitics, that is, more precipitation, can be cured by heparin-coated PMMA IOLs [113,114].

Foldable IOLs have been developed to overcome the problem of larger incision for insertion of PMMA IOLs. Now a large range of foldable IOLs are available for cataract extraction because they require small incision for their insertion, self-sealing and do not require suturing, allow quicker visual rehabilitation with stable refraction, and produce less astigmatism. However, they

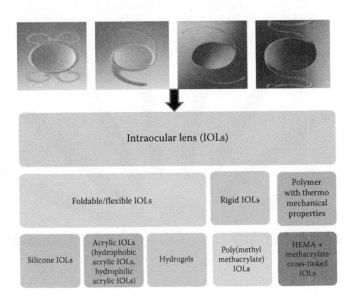

Figure 7.5 Types of intraocular lenses.

Table 7.2: Properties, Advantages, and Disadvantages of the IOL Types

IOLs Types	Properties	Advantages	Disadvantages
Silicone–elastomer polydimethylsiloxane	Capable of large and reversible deformations • Good memory • Surface deposits are common • Additives in silicone IOL are • UV chromophore • Phenyl group to increase refractive index from 1.41 to 1.46	Foldable—small incision, fairly low incidence of PCO	Low refractive index–thicker IOLs (first-generation silicone), high refractive index—thinner IOLs (second-generation silicone), pits with YAG laser, rapid unfolding in the eye Dislocation after YAG More decentration More anterior capsule contraction Slippery when wet Cannot use with silicone oil
Hydrogels	Hydrate to farm soft, swollen, rubbery mass • Hydrophilic hence repel cells and microbes • Refractive index 1.43–1.48	Foldable—small incision Good biocompatibility • Low inflammatory cell reaction Fewer pits with YAG laser Controlled unfolding Less endothelial cell damage with cornea touch	LECs on anterior IOL surface high incidence of PCO
Flexible acrylic	Good viscoelastic and 3D stability • Viscoelasticity is temperature dependent with increase elasticity at higher temperature	Foldable—small incision High refractive index—thin IOLs Very low incidence of PCO LEC regression Biocompatible Fewer pits with YAG laser Slow uncontrolled folding	Short experience Tacky surface—sticks to forceps More difficult to fold Glistenings Glare
PMMA	Hard and rigid • Inert and nonautoclavable • Causes mechanical irritation and ethothelial loss if touched • Endothelium while insertion • Hydrophobic—so causes adherence of cell and bacteria • Refractive index 1.47 and 1.55	Long-term experience Good biocompatibility Cheap	Rigid so need large incision Pits with YAG laser High incidence of PCO
Polymer with thermo mechanical properties	Hydrated with water content of 20% • Rigid below 250°C and flexible at higher temperature • RI 1.47	Avoids the rapid, explosive opening which can be seen with three-piece silicone IOLs which may cause iatrogenic damage to the capsule or other anterior segment structures	Tacky surface—sticks to forceps

are more expensive than PMMA IOLs and have a higher incidence of decentration if a continuous curvilinear capsulorhexis is not used. Silicone is used to synthesize foldable IOLs. Silicone IOLs are transparent homogeneous, heat-resistant, autoclavable, moldable, and compressible flexible lens coated with a liquid hydrophobic film (silicone oil), made of highly cross-linked elastic polymers of polysiloxane chains, having 1.41–1.46 refractive index. The refractive index of silicone IOLs can be improved by incorporating phenyl groups as methyl substitute. Due to hydrophobic nature of silicone IOLs, they provoke cellular reaction on the surface as well as become slippery when wet and, as a result, become difficult to handle. Now old silicone IOLs has been modified with collagen and named as Collamer IOLs with better biocompatibility and less postoperative complications [114–116].

The ideal materials for IOLs must fulfill the requirements such as easy insertion, slow unfolding, and absence of crease marks. These requirements are better fulfilled by acrylic IOLs because they have high refractive index which allows making thinner lens and as consequence requiring smaller incisions for implantation and faster eye restoration together with minimal postoperative complications. Acrylic IOLs can be classified as hydrophilic (e.g., PHEMA hydrogel which is soft and resembles living tissue like materials that swell extensively in water but insoluble in water (38% water content), causes low interfacial tension and reduces the tendency of biological rejection mechanisms) and hydrophobic acrylic IOLs (e.g., AcrySof [Alcon], esters of poly(meth)acrylic acid, mainly poly(2-phenethyl (meth)acrylate) [poly(PE(M)A)], absorb less water but have high refractive index, undergo less damage during YAG laser capsulotomy), on the basis of their composition [114,115].

Recently, ARRAY multifocal IOLs, that is, multifocal IOLs and bifocal IOLs, are developed in an attempt to provide both distance and near vision without additional spectacle correction, as they form separate images of near and distance objects and enable patients to be less dependent on spectacles following surgery. However, such patients found night driving more difficult than the patients with monofocal IOLs due to "halo-effect," and also multifocal IOLs reduce contrast sensitivity and the patient is not able to see shape of image under poor visibility conditions such as low light or fog [117].

7.3.3 Contact Lenses

Contact lenses are thin lenses most widely used for cosmetic or therapeutic reasons to correct vision and mild ametropia in people because they provide better peripheral vision, and do not collect moisture such as rain, snow, condensation, or sweat. There are many reasons to use contact lens such as esthetics and cosmetics or functional or optical reasons (severe ametropia or aniso-metropia, regular postoperative astigmatismor irregular astigmatism). Different types of contact lenses are available in market to change the appearance of the eye (cosmetic contact lens), for correcting vision (corrective contact lenses), for constant viewing (multifocal contact lenses), for severely compromised eyes (therapeutic scleral lenses), and for treatment and management of nonrefractive disorders of the eye (therapeutic soft lenses) as well as according to their modulus of elasticity (soft and hard contact lenses) (Figure 7.6).

The concept of contact lenses was clinically used first time in 1880s, which were made from glass shells that covered the whole of the front of the eye to provide correct vision but they were uncomfortable to wear. In 1940s, with the advancement of polymer science, PMMA was used as an ideal material for manufacturing the contact lenses because of its unique properties such as biocompatibility, transparent nature and chemical inertness. It is estimated that there are approximately 35 million contact lens wearers in the United States and over 1.65 million in the United Kingdom. Rigid or hard contact lenses were made from PMMA which are durable, light in weight, have acceptable surface wettability and good optical properties, and are able to replace the natural

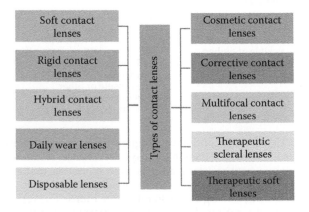

Figure 7.6 A schematic representation of types of contact lenses.

shape of the cornea with a new refracting surface, that is, can be used for astigmatism. However, the use of PMMA-based hard lenses was limited due to their poor oxygen permeability as they do not permit flow of oxygen to cornea.

This problem of rigid contact lenses was overcome by designing rigid gas permeable (RGP) contact lenses in the 1970s. These contact lenses had higher oxygen permeabilities (Dk = 10–30), were made by copolymerizing methyl methacrylate (MMA) with methacrylate-functionalized siloxanes such as methacryloxypropyltris(trimethyl siloxy silane) (TRIS), and their crosslinking ratio affected the oxygen permeability, modulus of elasticity, hardness, and wettability. Recently developed rigid contact lenses (composed of fluoromethacrylates such as hexa-fluoroisopropyl methacrylate (HFIM) with TRIS, MMA) have long time application due to their high oxygen permeability.

Rigid contact lenses are good for providing better vision but they mainly suffer from problems such as low oxygen permeability, lens wettability, and overall comfort to patient. Therefore, in 1961, Otto Wichterle brought a concept of soft contact lenses which were either hydrogels or silicone-based elastomers. These were synthesized by PHEMA that had 38% water content, more oxygen permeability, excellent wettability, and offered instant wearer comfort. Now, a large number of hydrophilic monomers such as N-vinylpyrrolidinone (NVP) and glyceryl methacrylate (GMA) are used to prepare soft contact lenses. They can be weared for period of 30 days but their long use can cause infection and inflammation to the eyes [118].

Now with the advancement in polymer science, soft contact lenses are prepared from silicon elastomer to extend wear time of lenses because they possess good optical properties with excellent oxygen permeability, good mechanical properties, and tear resistance. Silicon-based soft contact lenses have low surface energy that results in very poor tear wetting, a propensity to bind tear lipids and contact lens adhesion to the cornea. The wettability of silicone-based contact lenses can be improved either by plasma treatment, use of high surface energy molds in the manufacturing processes in order to encourage the orientation of the polar components at the lens surface, or by grafting hydrophilic polymers such as polyethylene glycols to the lens surface [119].

Recently, scientists are working to improve oxygen permeability of contact lenses with less inflammatory response to long-term wear because surface of contact lenses affects the adhesion and activation of neutrophils that will in turn influence the inflammatory response to the lens. Therapeutic contact lenses may be used as a drug delivery device for the treatment of ocular diseases; colored contact lenses may serve to disguise damaged or unsightly eyes [120].

7.3.4 Ocular Drug Delivery

The diseases in the posterior segment of eye directly impact the patient's vision and quality of life and are the major cause of blindness in the world. Therefore, biopharmaceuticals are making increasing impact on medicine for treatment of anterior and posterior diseases of eyes. Conventional ophthalmic drugs delivery system include eye drops, ointments, and gels, which are suitable for treatment of the anterior segment of the eye (cornea, conjunctiva, sclera, and anterior uvea) but not able for treatment of posterior segment of the eyes due to defense mechanisms of the ocular globe as well as anatomical and physiological barriers, static and dynamic barriers in place (Figure 7.7). It is found that only a small amount (1%–3%) reaches the intraocular tissue by conventional ocular drug delivery systems (DDSs) [19–122]. Therefore, surgery is opted for the treatment for diseases of the posterior segment as transport of drugs applied by traditional dosage forms cannot be maintained in concentrations in the target tissues for a long duration. Now, with the advancement in science, surgery is less applied by an eye surgeon [121].

For the treatment of posterior eye diseases, various novel techniques using biodegradable or nonbiodegradable polymer technology system implanted or injected directly into the vitreous, to obtain long-term sustained release of drugs, have been introduced in the market (Figure 7.8).

Two types of strategies have been developed for the treatment of anterior and posterior diseases namely known as anterior DDSs and posterior DDSs. Anterior DDSs include eye drops (AzaSite® for bacterial conjunctivitis; AzaSite Plus™ for blepharoconjunctivitis; Rysmon® TG for glaucoma; Betoptic S® for glaucoma; TobraDex® ST for blepharitis, Timoptic-XE® for glaucoma; and Cationorm® for mild dry eye), soft contact lenses (developed by Vistakon Pharmaceuticals, LLC, Philadelphia, PA; and SEED Co., Ltd., Tokyo, Japan, with Senju Pharmaceutical Co., Ltd., Osaka, Japan which are in clinic trial), Cul-de sac Inserts (Ocusert®, consists of two outer layers of ethylene-vinyl acetate copolymer (EVA), and an inner layer of pilocarpine in alginate gel within di-(ethylhexyl)phthalate for uniform controlled release of pilocarpine drug; Lacrisert®, water soluble rod-shaped insert composed of hydroxypropyl cellulose for dry eyes; and Ocufit SR®, minidisc ocular DDS clinically failure), Punctal Plugs (used for retention time and increase absorption

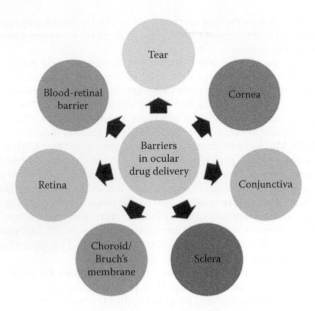

Figure 7.7 A schematic representation of barriers in conventional ocular drug delivery systems.

and efficacy of drugs developed by QLT, Inc., Vancouver, Canada; and Vistakon Pharmaceuticals, LLC for latanoprost and bimatoprost, respectively), and subconjunctival/episcleral implants (LX201, composed of silicone for release of cyclosporine A for long time; 3T Ophthalmics, a tiny bathtub composed of silicone under clinical trial developed by Irvine, CA; Latanoprost SR insert, composed of a poly(DL-lactide-*co*-glycolide) (PLGA) tube containing a latanoprost-core and ends are capped with silicon and PVA for release of latanoprost developed by Pfizer, Inc., New York) [123–135].

Diseases affecting the posterior eye segment are presently increasing and the treatment of these diseases requires a direct and local application of the agent to the posterior eye segment via topical, subtenon, subconjunctival, scleral, and intravitreal routes. However, the subconjunctival, scleral, and intravitreal routes are effective for controlled prolong release of drug via implants for the posterior eye treatment as they offer direct drug delivery to the target site with minimal systemic loss and can be implanted at the site of vitreous, sclera and subconjunctiva [136].

Posterior DDSs may be classified as nonbiodegradable, biodegradable, and stimuli-responsive polymeric systems on the basis of polymer used (Figure 7.9). Nonbiodegradable polymeric implants are mostly synthesized by polyvinyl alcohol (PVA), ethylene vinyl acetate (EVA), and silicon. Nonbiodegradable polymeric implant-based posterior DDSs follow zero order drug release path for effective concentrations release of drug for extended periods of time because they show diffusion controlled release. Due to the hydrophobic nature of silicon and ethylene vinyl acetate-based implants they can be applied for limited drugs whereas PVA-based implants are hydrophilic in nature and can be used for broader range of drugs [137–140].

Recently, stimuli-responsive polymer-based implants have been developed for drug delivery to the posterior segment of the eye because they show abrupt changes in structure, solubility, charge, volume, and hydrophobic–hydrophilic balance in response to physical or chemical changes in the environment, and release drug at a constant rate on the individual requirements and the disease state [141,142].

Traditionally they suffer from problems of the low therapeutic response and efficacy. Therefore, nanocarriers-based strategies have been introduced for improving the residence time and the corneal penetration of ocular drugs because they allow for an increased bioavailability and therapeutic efficacy of ophthalmic drugs, and enhance the permeability of ocular tissues to drugs, provide a specific drug targeting over several hours, reduce or prevent side effects, decrease the frequency of administration, and increase the patient's adherence to therapy [143–146].

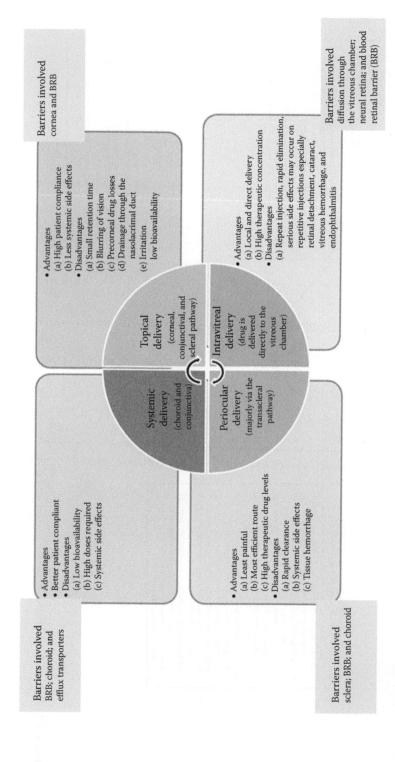

Barriers involved
cornea and BRB

• Advantages
  (a) High patient compliance
  (b) Less systemic side effects
• Disadvantages
  (a) Small retention time
  (b) Blurring of vision
  (c) Precorneal drug losses
  (d) Drainage through the
       nasolacrimal duct
  (e) Irritation
      low bioavailability

Barriers involved
diffusion through
the vitreous chamber;
neural retina; and blood
retinal barrier (BRB)

• Advantages
  (a) Local and direct delivery
  (b) High therapeutic concentration
• Disadvantages
  (a) Repeat injection, rapid elimination,
       serious side effects may occur on
       repetitive injections especially
       retinal detachment, cataract,
       vitreous hemorrhage, and
       endophthalmitis

Topical
delivery
(corneal,
conjunctival, and
scleral pathway)

Intravitreal
delivery
(drug is
delivered
directly to the
vitreous
chamber)

Systemic
delivery
(choroid and
conjunctiva)

Periocular
delivery
(majorly via the
transscleral
pathway)

Barriers involved
BRB; choroid; and
efflux transporters

• Advantages
  • Better patient compliant
• Disadvantages
  (a) Low bioavailability
  (b) High doses required
  (c) Systemic side effects

Barriers involved
sclera; BRB; and choroid

• Advantages
  (a) Least painful
  (b) Most efficient route
  (c) High therapeutic drug levels
• Disadvantages
  (a) Rapid clearance
  (b) Systemic side effects
  (c) Tissue hemorrhage

Figure 7.8   Features of various routes of administration for posterior eye delivery.

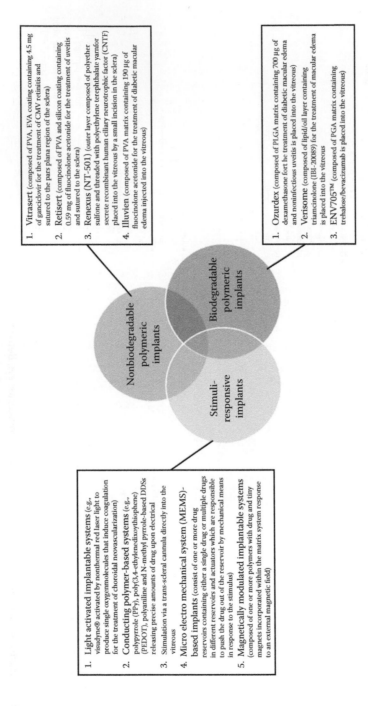

Figure 7.9 Types of drug delivery systems used for posterior segment drug infections.

7.4 CONCLUSIONS AND FUTURE PERSPECTIVES

The successful treatment of ocular pathologies depends upon the bioavailability of ophthalmic formulations. Therefore, there are many strategies to improve the bioavailability and the therapeutic response of drugs applied in the ocular globe. The extensive range of biomaterials has been investigated for use in the development of indwelling ocular implants selected primarily on the basis of their mechanical properties and biofunctionality without full consideration of their ocular compatibility. Therefore, uveal and capsular biocompatibility of materials must be studied and adopted at a regulatory level to enable the biological challenges to be addressed. Porous ceramics such as HA and alumina have been shown to allow fibrovascular ingrowth, which is a fundamental characteristic to ensure a safe stability of orbital implants *in situ* and to reduce the risk of postoperative infection. The reverse strategy that consists in modulating the surface properties of an appropriate bulk polymer is by far more realistic. As already discussed, the surface coating should not affect the bulk performances of the lens, while being nontoxic, nonimmunogenic, and stable upon sterilization and long-term application.

Delivering drug in appreciable amount to the posterior eye segment necessitates direct but invasive delivery, which needs to be repeated regularly over a period of several months to years. The use of nanocarrier systems preferably as ocular drops, with a potential to overcome highly protective anatomical barriers and physiological constraints or as periocular, or intravitreal injections, which can deliver the drug for a prolonged period of time requiring less frequent administration, may be an answer to this problem. The nano-ocular drops combine the benefits of conventional delivery systems, that is, self-administration, patient compliance, convenience, and minimized side effects with enhanced ocular bioavailability, low frequency of administration, and prolonged action without being invasive or harmful to the tissue integrity. However, a majority of these systems are still in a nascent stage of development and are yet to see the pharmaceutical market due to issues related to the cost of development and manufacture, ability for scale up, and approval by the regulatory authorities.

REFERENCES

1. Bayliss J, Shore N. In: McCord Jr. CD, editor. *Ophthalmic Surgery*. New York: Raven Press, 1981. p. 313–147.

2. Geroshi DH, Matsuda M, Yee RW. Pump function of the human corneal endothelium. *Ophthalmology* 1995;92:1.

3. Joyce NC, Navon SE, Sayon R, Zieske JD. Expression of cell cycle associated proteins in human and rabbit corneal endothelium *in situ*. *Invest Ophthalmol Vis Sci* 1996;37:1566.

4. Faragher RGA, Mulholland B, Tuft SJ, Sandeman S, Khaw PT. Ageing and the cornea. *Br J Ophthal* 1997;81:814–7.

5. Intraocular lens implantation. NIH Consensus Statement 1979;2:37–42.

6. Mutlu B. *Course: Intraocular Lenses*. Middle East University, Biotechnology Research Unit, Dubai, 2002.

7. Dumaine L. *Corré lation entre les proprié té s physico-chimiques de polymé res permettant de moduler la prolifé ration cellulaire et celles permettant de favoriser le glissement de lentilles intraoculaires. Thesis*. Ecole Centrale de Lyon, Lyons, France, 2004, pp. 79–85.

8. Lloyd AW, Faragher RGA, Denyer SP. Ocular biomaterials and implants. *Biomaterials* 2001;22:769–785.

9. Linnola R. *The Sandwich Theory: A Bioactivity Based Explanation for Posterior Capsular Opacification after Cataract Surgery with Intraocular Lens Implantation*. Academic dissertation. Finland: Faculty of Medicine, University of Oulu, 2001.

10. Linnola RJ, Werner L, Pandey SK, Escobar-Gomez M, Znoiko SL, Apple DJ. Adhesion of fibronectin, vitronectin, laminin, and collagen type IV to intraocular lens materials in

pseudophakic human autopsy eyes. Part 1: Histological sections. *J Cataract Refract Surg* 2000;26:1792–1806.

11. Troy DB, Beringer P. *Remington: The Science and Practice of Pharmacy* (21st ed.) Philadelphia, USA: Lippincott Williams & Wilkins, 2006.

12. Eperjesi DF, Liu J, Gan Y. Recent advances in topical ophthalmic drug delivery with lipid-based nanocarriers. *Drug Discov Today* 2013;18(5–6):290–297.

13. Almeida H, Amaral MH, Lobão P, Sousa Lobo JM. Applications of poloxamers in ophthalmic pharmaceutical formulations: An overview. *Expert Opin Drug Deliv* 2013;10(9):1223–1237.

14. De la Fuente M, Raviña M, Paolicelli P, Sanchez A, Seijo B, Alonso MJ. Chitosan-based nanostructures: A delivery platform for ocular therapeutics. *Adv Drug Deliv Rev* 2010;62(1):100–117.

15. Presland A, Myatt J. Ocular anatomy and physiology relevant to anaesthesia. *Anaesth Intensive Care Med* 2010;11(10):438–443.

16. Malhotra A, Minja FJ, Crum A, Burrowes D. Ocular anatomy and cross-sectional imaging of the eye. *Semin Ultrasound CT MRI* 2011;32(1):2–13.

17. Francesco B. Biomaterials and implants for orbital floor repair. *Acta Biomater* 2011;7:921–935.

18. Pascolini D, Mariotti SP. Global estimates of visual impairment: 2010. *Br J Ophthalmol* 2012;96:614–618.

19. Janoria KG, Gunda S, Boddu SH, Mitra AK. Novel approaches to retinal drug delivery. *Expert Opin Drug Deliv* 2007;4:371–388.

20. Mules PH. Evisceration of the globe, with artificial vitreous. *Trans Ophthalmol Soc UK* 1885;5:200–6.

21. Wyatt J, Rizzo J. Ocular implants for the blind. *IEEE Spectrum* 1996;33:47–53.

22. Ariga K, Kawakami K, Ebara M, Kotsuchibashi Y, Ji Q, Hill JP. Bioinspired nanoarchitectonics as emerging drug delivery systems. *New J Chem* 2014;38:5149–5163.

23. Patel GC, Dalwadi CA. Recent patents on stimuli responsive hydrogel drug delivery system. *Recent Pat Drug Deliv Formul* 2013;7:206–215.

24. Buwalda SJ, Boere KW, Dijkstra PJ, Feijen J, Vermonden T, Hennink WE. Hydrogels in a historical perspective: From simple networks to smart materials. *J Control Release* 2014;190:254–273.

25. Tomatsu I, Peng K, Kros A. Photoresponsive hydrogels for biomedical applications. *Adv Drug Deliv Rev* 2011;63:1257–1266.

26. Sortino S. Photoactivated nanomaterials for biomedical release applications. *J Mater Chem* 2012;22:301–318.

27. Neffe AT, Wischke C, Racheva M, Lendlein A. Progress in biopolymer-based biomaterials and their application in controlled drug delivery. *Expert Rev Med Devices* 2013;10:813–833.

28. Shiino D, Murata Y, Kataoka K, Koyama Y, Yokoyama M, Okano T, Sakurai Y. Preparation and characterization of a glucose-responsive insulin-releasing polymer device. *Biomaterials* 1994;15:121–128.

29. Jabs DA. Treatment of cytomegalovirus retinitis, *Arch Ophthalmol* 1992; 110:185–187.

30. Jaffe GJ, Martin D, Callanan D, Pearson PA, Levy B, Comstock T. Fluocinolone acetonide implant (Retisert) for noninfectious posterior uveitis: thirty-four-week results of a multicenter randomized clinical study. *Ophthalmology* 2006;113:1020–1027.

31. Musch DC, Martin DF, Gordon JF, Davis MD, Kuppermann BD, Heinemann MH et al. Treatment of cytomegalovirus retinitis with a sustained release ganciclovir implant. *N Engl J Med* 1997;337:83–90.

32. Wang J, Jiang A, Joshi M, Christoforidis J. Drug delivery implants in the treatment of vitreous inflammation. *Mediat Inflamm* 2013;2013: 780634.

33. Haghjou N, Soheilian M, Abdekhodaie MJ. Sustained release intraocular drug delivery devices for treatment of uveitis. *J Ophthal Vis Res* 2011;6:317–329.

34. http://www.psivida.com/products-iluvien.html (accessed 09.06.14. Perma link: http://perma.cc/4WYV-AA5D).

35. Rubin PAD. Enucleation, evisceration and extenteration. *Curr Opin Ophthalmol,* 1988;4:39–48.

36. Perry AC. Integrated orbital implants. *Adv Ophthal Plast Reconstr Surg* 1988;8:75–81.

37. Rubin PAD, Popham JK, Bilyk JR, Shore JW. Comparison of brovascular ingrowth into hydroxyapatite and porous polyethylene orbital implants. *Ophthal Plast Reconstr Surg* 1994;10:96–110.

38. Kelley JJ. History of ocular prostheses. *Int Ophthalmol Clin* 1970;10:713–719.

39. Levine MR, Pou CR, Lash RH. Evisceration: Is sympathetic ophthalmia a concern in the new millennium? *Ophthal Plast Reconstr Surg* 1999;15:4–8.

40. Moshfeghi DM, Moshfeghi AA, Finger PT. Enucleation. *Surv Ophthalmol* 2000;44:277–301.

41. Custer PL. Enucleation: Past, present, and future. *Ophthal Plast Reconstr Surg* 2000;16:316–321.

42. Deacon BS. Orbital implants and ocular prostheses: A comprehensive review. *J Ophthal Med* 2008;42:1–11.

43. Nerad JA, Carter KD, LaVelle WE, Fyler A, Branemark PI. The osseointegration technique for the rehabilitation of the exenterated orbit. *Arch Ophthalmol* 1991;109:1032–1038.

44. Sami D, Young S, Petersen R. Perspective on orbital enucleation implants. *Surv Ophthalmol* 2007;52:244–265.

45. Dutton JJ. Coralline hydroxyapitate as an ocular implant. *Ophthalmology* 1991;98:370–377.

46. Sutula FC, Rodgers IR. Hydroxyapatite in orbital reconstruction. *Ophthalmol Clin North Am* 1991;4:183–188.

47. Shields CL, Shields JA, De Potter P. Hydroxyapatite orbital implant after enucleation. Experience with initial 100 consecutive cases. *Arch Ophthalmol* 1992;110:333–338.

48. Bilyk JR, Rubin PAD, Shore JW. Correction of enophthalmos with porous polyethylene implants. *Int Ophthalmol Clin* 1992;32:151–156.

49. Luce CM. A short history of enucleation. *Int Ophthalmol Clin* 1970;10:681–687.

50. Gougelmann HP. The evolution of the ocular motility implant. *Int Ophthalmol Clin* 1970;10:689–711.

51. Christmas NJ, Gordon CD, Murray TG, Tse D, Johnson T, Garonzik S. et al. Intraorbital implants after enucleation and their complications: A 10-year review. *Arch Ophthalmol* 1998;116:1199–1203.

52. Baino F. Scleral buckling biomaterials and implants for retinal detachment surgery. *Med Eng Phys* 2010;32:945–956.

53. Shoamanesh A, Pang NK, Oestreicher JH. Complications of orbital implants: A review of 542 patients who have undergone orbital implantation and 275 subsequent PEG placement. *Orbit* 2007;26:173–182.

54. Jordan DR, Klapper SR. Controversies in enucleation technique and implant selection: Whether to wrap, attach muscles and peg? In: Guthoff RF, Katowitz JA. editors. *Oculoplastics and Orbit*. Berlin, Germany: Springer-Verlag; 2010. p. 195–211.

55. Nunnery WR, Cepela MA, Heinz GW, Zale D, Martin RT. Extrusion rate of silicone spherical anophthalmic socket implants. *Ophthal Plast Reconstr Surg* 1993;9:90–95.

56. Baino F, Perero S, Ferraris S, Miola M, Balagna C, Verne E, Vitale-Brovarone C, Coggiola A, Dolcino D, Ferraris M. Biomaterials for orbital implants and ocular prostheses: Overview and future prospects. *Acta Biomater* 2014;10:1064–1087.

57. Bozukova D, Pagnoulle C, Jerome R, Jerome C. Polymers in modern ophthalmic implants—Historical background and recent advances. *Mater Sci Eng R* 2010;69:63–83.

58. Frueh BR, Felker GV. Baseball implant—A method of secondary insertion of an intraorbital implant. *Arch Ophthalmol* 1976;94:429–430.

59. Kamal-Siddiqi Z, Lal G, Hye A. Outcome of Sahaf enucleation implants in 60 patients. *Pak J Ophthalmol* 2008;24:34–36.

60. Kamal Z, Rizwan-Ullah M, Lal G, Hye A, Akram-Sahaf I. Reconstruction of empty sockets with Sahaf's orbital implant. *Pak J Ophthalmol* 2010;26:128–132.

61. Agahan ALD, Tan AD. Use of hollow polymethylmethacrylate as an orbital implant. *Philippine J Ophthalmol* 2004;29:21–25.

62. Guyton JS. Enucleation and allied procedures. *Am J Ophthalmol* 1949;(32);1517; passim.

63. Guyton JS. Enucleation and allied procedures: A survey of semiburied implants. *Am J Ophthalmol* 1949;(32):1725–1734.

64. Allen L, Ferguson EC, Braley AE. A quasi-integrated buried muscle cone implant with good motility and advantages for prosthetic fitting. *Trans Am Acad Ophthalmol Otolaryngol* 1960;64:272–286.

65. Allen L, Spivey BE, Burns CA. A larger Iowa implant. *Am J Ophthalmol* 1969;68:397–400.

66. Spivey BE, Allen L, Burns CA. The Iowa enucleation implant—A 10-year evaluation of technique and results. *Am J Ophthalmol* 1969;67:171–188.

67. Jordan DR, Anderson RL, Nerad JA, Allen L. A preliminary report on the universal implant. *Arch Ophthalmol* 1987;105:1726–1731.

68. Jordan DR. Anophthalmic orbital implants. *Ophthalmol Clin North Am* 2000;13:587–608.

69. Roper-Hall MJ. Orbital implants. *Trans Ophthalmol Soc UK* 1954;74:337–346.

70. Roper-Hall MJ. Magnetic orbital implant. *Br J Ophthalmol* 1956;40:575.

71. Soll DB. Evolution and current concepts in the surgical treatment of the anophthalmic orbit. *Ophthal Plast Reconstr Surg* 1986;2:163–171.

72. Kotzé DJ, De Vries C. A quick guide to safety and compatibility of passive implants and devices in an MR environment. *SA J Radiol* 2004;8:6–12.

73. Cutler NL. A ball and ring implant for use in enucleation. *Trans Ophthalmol Soc UK* 1947;67:423–425.

74. Young JH. A new ocular prosthetic aid: The intra-ocular implant. *Br J Ophthalmol* 1951;35:623–627.

75. Klement R, Tromel G. Hydroxylapatit, der Hauptbestandteil der anorganischen Knochen- und Zahnsubstanz. *HoppeSeyler's Z Physiol Chem* 1932;230:263–269.

76. Bredig MA. Zur Apatitstruktur der anorganischen Knochen- und Zahnsubstanz. *HoppeSeyler's Z Physiol Chem* 1933;260:239–243.

77. Spaeth EB. *The Principles and Practice of Ophthalmic Surgery*. London: Henry Kimpton; 1939.

78. Molteno ACB, Van Rensberg JHJ, Van Rooyen B, Ancker E. Physiological orbital implant. *Br J Ophthalmol* 1973;57:615–621.

79. Molteno ACB. Antigen-free cancellous bone implants after removal of an eye. *Trans Ophthalmol Soc NZ* 1980;32:36–39.

80. Jordan DR, Hwang I, Brownstein S, McEachren T, Gilberg S, Grahovac S et al. The Molteno M-sphere. *Ophthal Plast Reconstr Surg* 2000;16:356–362.

81. Perry JD, Goldberg RA, McCann JD, Shorr N, Engstrom R, Tong J. Bovine hydroxyapatite orbital implant: A preliminary report. *Ophthal Plast Reconstr Surg* 2002;18:268–274.

82. Lyall MG. Proplast implant in Tenon's capsule after excision of the eye. *Trans Ophthalmol Soc UK* 1976;96:79–81.

83. Whear NM, Cousley RR, Liew C, Henderson D. Post-operative infection of proplast facial implants. *Br J Oral Maxillofac Surg* 1993;31:292–295.

84. Nunnery WR, Heinz GW, Bonnin JM, Martin RT, Cepela MA. Exposure rate of hydroxyapatite spheres in the anophthalmic socket: Histopathologic correlation and comparison with silicone sphere implants. *Ophthal Plast Reconstr Surg* 1993;9:96–104.

85. Dutton JJ. Coralline hydroxyapatite as an ocular implant. *Ophthalmology* 1991;98:370–377.

86. Gayre GS, Lipham W, Dutton JJ. A comparison of rates of fibrovascular ingrowth in wrapped versus unwrapped hydroxyapatite spheres in a rabbit model. *Ophthal Plast Reconstr Surg* 2002;18:275–280.

87. Babar TF, Hussain M, Zaman M. Clinico-pathologic study of 70 enucleations. *J Pak Med Assoc* 2009;59:612–614.

88. Owji N, Mosallaei M, Taylor J. The use of mersilene mesh for wrapping of hydroxyapatite orbital implants: Mid-term result. *Orbit* 2012;31:155–158.

89. Jordan DR, Bawazeer A. Experience with 120 synthetic hydroxyapatite implants (FCI3). *Ophthal Plast Reconstr Surg* 2001;17:184–190.

90. Mawn LA, Jordan DR, Gilberg S. Scanning electron microscopic examination of porous orbital implants. *Can J Ophthalmol* 1998;33:203–209.

91. Jordan DR, Hwang I, Gilberg S, Brownstein S, McEachren T, Grahovac S et al. Brazilian hydroxyapatite implant. *Ophthal Plast Reconstr Surg* 2000;16:363–369.

92. Kundu B, Sinha MK, Mitra S, Basu D. Synthetic hydroxyapatite-based integrated orbital implants: A human pilot trial. *Indian J Ophthalmol* 2005;53:235–241.

93. Baino F. Biomaterials and implants for orbital floor repair. *Acta Biomater* 2011;7:3248–3266.

94. Blaydon SM, Shepler TR, Neuhaus RW, White WL, Shore JW. The porous polyethylene (Medpor) spherical orbital implant: A retrospective study of 136 cases. *Ophthal Plast Reconstr Surg* 2003;19:364–371.

95. Goldberg RA, Dresner SC, Braslow RA, Kossovsky N, Legmann A. Animal model of porous polyethylene orbital implants. *Ophthal Plast Reconstr Surg* 1994;10:104–109.

96. Jordan DR, Brownstein S, Dorey M, Yuen VH, Gilberg S. Fibrovascularization of porous polyethylene (Medpor) orbital implant in a rabbit model. *Ophthal Plast Reconstr Surg* 2004;20:136–143.

97. Thakker MM, Fay AM, Pieroth L, Rubin PA. Fibrovascular ingrowth into hydroxyapatite and porous polyethylene orbital implants wrapped with acellular dermis. *Ophthal Plast Reconstr Surg* 2004;20:368–373.

98. Rubin PA, Popham JK, Bilyk JR, Shore JW. Comparison of fibrovascular ingrowth into hydroxyapatite and porous polyethylene orbital implants. *Ophthal Plast Reconstr Surg* 1994;10:96–103.

99. Woog JJ, Dresner SC, Lee TS, Kim YD, Hartstein ME, Shore JW et al. The smooth surface tunnel porous polyethylene enucleation implant. *Ophthal Surg Lasers Imaging* 2004;35:358–362.

100. Rubin PA, Popham J, Rumelt S, Remulla H, Bilyk JR, Holds J et al. Enhancement of the cosmetic and functional outcome of enucleation with the conical orbital implant. *Ophthalmology* 1998;105:919–925.

101. Mortemousque B, Leger F, Velou S, Graffan R, Colin J, Korobelnik JF. S/e-PTFE episcleral buckling implants: An experimental and histopathologic study. *J Biomed Mater Res* 2002;63:686–691.

102. Rahaman MN, Yao A, Sonny Bal B, Garino JP, Ries MD. Ceramics for prosthetic hip and knee joint replacement. *J Am Ceram Soc* 2007;90:1965–1988.

103. Wang JK, Lai PC, Liao SL. Late exposure of the bioceramic orbital implant. *Am J Ophthalmol* 2009;147:162–170.

104. Wang JK, Lai PC. Bioceramic orbital implant exposure repaired by a retroauricular myoperiosteal graft. *Ophthalmic Surg Lasers Imaging* 2008;39:399–403.

105. You CK, Oh SH, Kim JW, Choi TH, Lee SY, Kim SY. Hydroxyapatite coated porous alumina as a new orbital implant. *Key Eng Mater* 2003;240–242:563–566.

106. Jordan DR, Brownstein S, Gilberg S, Coupal D, Kim S, Mawn L. Hydroxyapatite and calcium phosphate coatings on aluminium oxide orbital implants. *Can J Ophthalmol* 2002;37:7–13.

107. Choi HY, Lee JE, Park HJ, Oum BS. Effect of synthetic bone glass particulate on the fibrovascularization of porous polyethylene orbital implants. *Ophthal Plast Reconstr Surg* 2006;22:121–125.

108. Girard LJ, Eguez I, Soper JW, Soper M, Esnaola N, Homsy CA. Buried quasiintegrated enucleation implant of Proplast II: A preliminary report. *Ophthalmic Plast Reconstr Surg* 1990;6:141–143.

109. Guthoff R, Vick HP, Schaudig U. Prevention of postenucleation syndrome: The hydroxyl-apatite silicone implant. Preliminary experimental studies and initial clinical experiences. *Ophthalmology* 1995;92:198–205.

110. Hiratsuka Y, Ono K, Kanai A. The present state of blindness in the world. *Nippon Ganka Gakkai Zasshi* 2001;105(6):369–373.

111. Marcher A. *Memoirs of Giacomo Casanova de Seingalt* (vol. 8). R&R Clarke for Limited Editions Club; 1940. pp. 45–50.

112. Spalton DJ. Harold Ridley's first patient. *J Cataract Refract Surg* 1999;25:156.

113. Scholtz S. History of Ophthalmic Viscosurgical Devices. *Cataract Refract Surg Today Eur* 2006; I (September/November):61–62.

114. Kecová H, Necăs A. Phacoemulsification and Intraocular Lens Implantation: Recent Trends in Cataract Surgery. *Acta Vet Brno* 2004;73:85–92.

115. Seward HC. Folding intraocular lenses: Materials and methods. *Br J Ophthalmol* 1997;81:340–341.

116. McLoone E, Mahon G, Archer D, Best R. Silicone oil-intraocular lens interaction: Which lens to use? *Br J Ophthalmol* 2001;85:543–545.

117. Javitt MD, Wang F, Trentacost DJ, Rowe M, Tarantino N. Outcomes of cataract surgery with multifocal intraocular lens implantation: Functional status and quality of life. *Ophthalmology* 1997;104:589–599.

118. Williams TJ, Willcox MDP, Schneider RP. Interactions of bacteria with contact lenses: The effect of soluble protein and carbohydrate on bacterial adhesion to contact lenses. *Optometry Vis Sci* 1998;75:266–271.

119. Taylor RL, Willcox MDP, Williams TJ, Verran J. Modulation of bacterial adhesion to hydrogel contact lenses by albumin. *Optometry Vis Sci* 1998;75:23–29.

120. McDonald MB, McCarey BE, Storie B, Beurman RW, Salmeron B, Jan RIJ et al. Assessment of the long term corneal response to hydrogel intrastromal lenses implanted in monkey eyes for up to five years. *J Cataract Refract Surg* 1993;19:213–222.

121. Edelhauser HF, Rowe-Rendleman CL, Robinson MR, Dawson DG, Chader GJ, Grossniklaus HE et al. Ophthalmic drug delivery systems for the treatment of retinal diseases: Basic research to clinical applications. *Invest Ophthalmol Vis Sci* 2010;51:5403–5420.

122. Maurice DM, Mishima S. Ocular pharmacokinetics. In: Sears ML, editor. *Handbook of Experimental Pharmacology*. Berlin, Heidelberg, Germany: Springer; 1984. pp. 16–119.

123. InSite Vision DuraSite®. Available online: http://www.insitevision.com/durasite.

124. InSite Vision AzaSite®. Available online: http://www.insitevision.com/marketed_products.

125. Wade A, Weller P. Methylcellulose. In: *Handbook of Pharmaceutical Excipients*. Washington, DC, USA: American Pharmaceutical Association; 1994. pp. 306–309.

126. Purslow C, Wolffsohn JS. Ocular surface temperature: A review. *Eye Contact Lens* 2005;31:117–123.

127. Alcon, Inc. Alcon launches TobraDex® ST suspension. Available online: http://invest. alconinc.com/phoenix.zhtml?c=130946&p=RssLanding&cat=news&id=1474062.

128. Scoper S, Kabat A, Owen G, Stroman D, Kabra B, Faulkner R et al. Ocular distribution, bactericidal activity and settling characteristics of TobraDex® ST ophthalmic suspension compared with TobraDex® ophthalmic suspension. *Adv Ther* 2008;25:77–88.

129. Peterson RC, Wolffsohn JS, Nick J, Winterton L, Lally J. Clinical performance of daily disposable soft contact lenses using sustained release technology. *Contact Lens Anterior Eye* 2006;29:127–134.

130. SEED. Available online: http://jds.jasdaq.co.jp/documents/tekiji/TD0SCJ2MWUUBKDAA.PDF.

131. Aton Pharma, Inc. Lacrisert® (Hydroxypropylcellulose ophthalmic insert). Available online: http://www.lacrisert.com/ECP/pdfs/Lacrisert_PI.pdf.

132. Bawa R. Ocular inserts. In: Mitra AK, editor. *Ophthalmic Drug Delivery Systems*. New York, USA: Marcell Dekker, Inc.; 1993. pp. 223–260.

133. Bartlett JD, Boan K, Corliss D, Gaddie IB. Efficacy of silicone punctal plugs as adjuncts to topical pharmacotherapy of glaucoma—A pilot study. Punctal plugs in glaucoma study group. *J Am Optom Assoc* 1996;67:664–668.

134. ClinicalTrials.gov. Study to assess LX201 for prevention of corneal allograft rejection or grant failure in subjects who have experienced one or more rejection episodes following penetrating keratoplasty. Available online: http://clinicaltrials.gov/ct2/show/NCT00447642?term=LX-201 &rank=2.

135. ClinicalTrials.gov. Safety study of latanoprost slow release insert (Latanoprost SR). Available online: http://clinicaltrials.gov/ct2/show/NCT01180062.

136. Urtti A. Challenges and obstacles of ocular pharmacokinetics and drug delivery. *Adv Drug Deliv Rev* 2006;58:1131–1135.

137. Bourges JL, Bloquel C, Thomas A, Froussart F, Bochot A, Azan F et al. Intraocular implants for extended drug delivery: Therapeutic applications. *Adv Drug Deliv Rev* 2006;58:1182–1202.

138. da Silva R, Fialho SL, Siqueira RC, Jorge R, da Silva Cunha Jr A. Implants as drug delivery devices for the treatment of eye diseases. *Braz J Pharm Sci* 2010;46:585–595.

139. Rahimy MH, Peyman GA, Chin SY, Golshani R, Aras C, Borhani H et al. Polysulfone capillary fiber for intraocular drug delivery: *In vitro* and *in vivo* evaluations. *J Drug Target* 1994;2:289–298.

140. http://www.neurotechusa.com/ect-platform.html (accessed 09.06.14. Perma link: http://perma.cc/R5R3-Y4YC).

141. Kost J, Langer R. Responsive polymeric delivery systems. *Adv Drug Deliv Rev* 2012;64:327–341.

142. Ong FS, Kuo JZ, Wu W, Cheng C, Blackwell WB, Taylor BL et al. Personalized medicine in ophthalmology: From pharmacogenetic biomarkers to therapeutic and dosage optimization. *J Pers Med* 2013;3:40–69.

143. Achouri D, Alhanout K, Piccerelle P, Andrieu V. Recent advances in ocular drug delivery. *Drug Dev Ind Pharm* 2013;39(11):1599–1617.

144. Zimmer A, Kreuter J. Microspheres and nanoparticles used in ocular delivery systems. *Adv Drug Deliv Rev* 1995;16(1):61–73.

145. Nagarwal RC, Kant S, Singh PN, Maiti P, Pandit JK. Polymeric nanoparticulate system: A potential approach for ocular drug delivery. *J Control Release* 2009;136(1):2–13.

146. Luo Q, Zhao J, Zhang X, Pan W. Nanostructured lipid carrier (NLC) coated with chitosan oligosaccharides and its potential use in ocular drug delivery system. *Int J Pharm* 2011;403(1–2):185–191.

8 Polymers in Cardiovascular Implants

8.1 INTRODUCTION

In the past 10 decades, there has been a tremendous growth in new medical devices and related innovations based on biomaterial to replace, assist, and repair some parts of the body and its functions. Biomaterials are either natural or manmade materials used in therapeutic or diagnostic systems (permanent replacement of defective organs and tissues, temporary support of defective or normal organs in form of implants, and medical devices such as enamels, orthodontics, heart valves, catheters, fracture fixation, bone grafts, artificial hips, knees, pacemakers, etc.) in direct contact with biological systems for any period of time, as a whole or part of a system, which interacts with human tissue and body fluids to treat, improve, or replace anatomical element(s) (tissue, organ, or function of the body) in a reliable, safe, and physiologically acceptable manner. One of the prime requirements of medical implants, which are used in contact with blood, like heart valves or vascular slants, is biocompatibility; that means, they should show only minimum induction of blood clot formation so that in vivo the fibrinolytic system can compete the fibrinogenic system. As a consequence, both the blood platelets as well as the blood clotting cascade in the plasma should be minimally activated by the surface [1].

Cardiovascular diseases (CVDs) cover a range of conditions affecting both the heart and the blood vessels, and are a major health problem that results in substantial morbidity and death worldwide due to dysfunctional or diseased valve, atherosclerosis, narrowing of the arteries and small blood vessels by plaque deposition, and aging of the population [2–5]. Therefore, the improved healthcare has become a great need of the hour. Currently, there are several treatment options for blocked blood vessels such as angioplasty, stenting, thrombolysis, and surgical bypass. While these treatments are well established, they have their inherent limitations and complications and also typically do not regenerate the damaged organs. Therefore, there is a need to develop new strategies for regenerating tissue following ischemia [6]. Although various commercial cardiovascular implants include processed biological substances (collagen and heparin), metals (titanium, stainless steel, nitinol, cobalt–chrome alloys, etc.) and polymeric biomaterials (polytetrafluorethylene, polyethylene terephthalate, polyurethane, polyvinyl chloride, etc.) have been approved by Food and Drug Administration (FDA) as effective implants and graft materials and millions of patients benefit from these products. Both synthetic and natural polymers have been trialed, though each has its own limitations. While the former allows easy processing and modifications, the later offers better cyto- and biocompatibility [3]. However, there is still need for an ideal device that can help patients who are suffering from CVDs because cardiovascular system consists of the heart and all the blood vessels, and cardiovascular biomaterials may contact blood (both arterial and venous), vascular endothelial cells, fibroblasts, and myocardium, as well as a number of other cells and a cellular matrix material that make up all biological tissue and may provoke coagulation and platelet activation. Therefore, the foremost requirements for biomaterials used in contact with blood include prevention of the coagulation cascade and platelet activation. Now, most permanently implanted cardiovascular devices are designed to treat underlying medical conditions or provide enhanced functions. However, the main causes of failure of cardiovascular devices are excessive growth of the tissues surrounding the device, thrombosis (clots may occlude the device or may occlude small blood vessels, resulting in heart attacks, strokes, paralysis, failures of other organs, etc.), damage blood cells, and hemolysis (occur as a reaction to the material surface and the blood) that necessitate reoperation or cause morbidity or death. Cardiovascular biomaterials may also in contact with other tissues. Cardiovascular biomaterials, either temporary or permanent devices, can be divided into three categories: temporary external devices (simple tubing for bypass or hemodialysis, oxygenators, arterial filters, and hemodialysis equipment), temporary internal devices (catheters, guide wires, and cannulae used in bypass circuits), and permanent internal devices (pacemakers, defibrillators, stents, left ventricular assist devices, and artificial hearts) [7–11].

8.2 BLOOD–BIOMATERIAL INTERFACIAL INTERACTION MECHANISM AND BIOCOMPATIBILITY OF CARDIOVASCULAR BIOMATERIALS

Cardiovascular biomaterials may be classified as temporary and permanent devices as well as internal or external devices on the basis of their use. In general they come in contact of blood during their uses and their contact duration may be limited (<24 h), prolonged (>24 h to 30 days), and permanent (>30 days). It is found that major cause of failure of cardiovascular biomaterials is nonbiocompatibility, that is, the initiation of thrombosis formation by the blood-contacting devices, which arises due to unfavorable blood–material interface, which is the initial factor for the implant failure [12–15]. When cardiovascular biomaterials come in contact of blood, it leads to a number of unfavorable reactions namely adsorption of protein on the materials, initiation of coagulation cascade and the formation of fibrin, activation of the complement cascade as part of the innate immune system and local inflammation, and dysfunction of the endothelium caused by the damage of endothelial cells (ECs) and hyperplasia of smooth muscle cells (SMCs). Thrombus formation on biomaterial surfaces is a complex network of processes that depends on the surface chemistry of the biomaterial and on characteristics of blood flow in which the biomaterial is immersed [16]. Collectively, this ensemble of reactions is known as the coagulation cascade, which culminates in the production of thrombin (Factor IIa), a crucial end product of the coagulation process. Thrombin acts as a powerful accelerator of proximal coagulation reactions and at the same time converts fibrinogen into strands of fibrin.

The coagulation cascade is considered as a complex physiological response system and consists of two separate initial pathways: intrinsic (adsorption of proteins on the surface of implanted cardiac biomaterial) and extrinsic (release of tissue factor from the damaged cells at the site of injury) as shown in Figure 8.1 [17]. When a foreign body comes in contact of blood, plasma proteins adsorb on the surface within few minutes [18]. This process transforms the configuration of the adsorbed

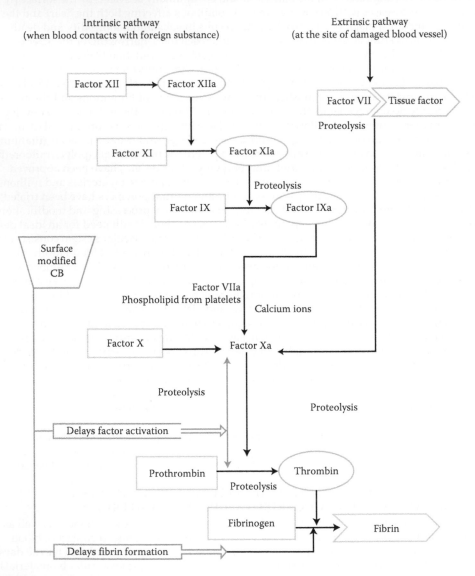

Figure 8.1 A schematic representation of extrinsic and intrinsic pathways of coagulation cascade.

proteins and lead to the activation of coagulation factor XII and activates the intrinsic pathway, that is, adsorbed protein forms a complex comprising collagen, high-molecular-weight kininogen (HMWK), prekallikrein, and factor XII [19]. Afterward, this complex got cleaved by contact activation and activates various immune responses like kinin system, coagulation, fibrinolytic, and complement system. To start with, activated factor XII activates factor XI, which thereby activates factor IX and activated factor IX in turn activates factor X. Upon activation of factor X, it results in the cleavage of prothrombin to thrombin in the presence of other supporting cofactors. Activated thrombin converts fibrinogen to fibrin, which eventually gets stabilized as a red thrombus or clot. Tissue factors act as cofactor to activate factor X. There is also a possibility for factor VII to activate factor IX, which in turn activates factor X. Except for factor VII, all factors of extrinsic pathway are similar to intrinsic pathway leading to the formation of thrombus [18,19]. While protein adsorption to the surface occurs within seconds of blood–biomaterial contact, the activation of the clotting cascade to thrombin and fibrin formation takes 10–15 min, followed by the activation of platelets shortly thereafter. The complement activation and associated inflammatory reactions occur in parallel, playing the dominant role in body's defense mechanisms against foreign materials [18]. Therefore, regulation of complement pathway in order to control coagulation system is also a fascinating method to obtain new-generation blood-contacting surface with excellent hemocompatibility.

In addition to this, some toxic effects may also occur such as cytotoxicity, genotoxicity, mutagenicity, and carcinogenicity, which may produce local (adverse effects emerge only in the affected areas) and systemic effects (effects occur even far away from the distance of the application of the implant). Therefore, care should be taken to evaluate the biocompatibility of the cardiac device. As shown above, protein adsorption on biomaterial surfaces increased both blood contact activation and platelet activation causing thrombotic and thromboembolic complications. Therefore, cardiovascular tissue engineering focused on surface modifications to prevent blood protein adsorption, that is, surface modification of cardiovascular biomaterials to provide hydrophobic, chemically inert surface or coating as it reduces protein-binding capacity. Another strategy is the development of stable "membranemimetic" films using the protein-repelling properties of the phospholipid monolayer (phosphorylcholine), the main component of biological membranes, via attachment of biochemically active molecules such as heparin or thrombomodulin that displayed prolonged stability and activity in high shear environment, and immobilization of platelet inhibitors [20–24]. Promising materials such as polyethylene oxide, pyrolytic carbon coating, phosphorylcholine surfaces, elastin-inspired polymer surface, heparin, thrombomodulin, and antiplatelet drugs can be used in cardiovascular biomaterials to improve biomaterial hemocompatibility by inhibiting protein and cell adsorbtion, thrombin and fibrin formation, and platelet activation. Selection criteria for materials used in cardiovascular biomaterials is discussed below:

1. *Biocompatibility.* Thrombus formation is caused both by exposing blood to a foreign surface and by flow instabilities and depends on the mechanical and surface properties. Therefore, biomaterials surface must not be thrombus resistant.

2. *Ability to deliver and foster cells.* The material should not only be biocompatible (i.e., nontoxic) but also foster cell attachment, differentiation, and proliferation.

3. *Biodegradability.* The composition of the material should lead biodegradation in vivo at rates appropriate to tissue regeneration.

4. *Mechanical properties.* The substrate should provide mechanical support to cells until sufficient new extracellular matrix (ECM) is synthesized by cells.

5. *Porous structure.* The scaffold should have an interconnected porous structure for cell penetration, tissue in growth and vascularization, and nutrient delivery.

6. *Fabrication.* The material should possess desired fabrication capability, for example, being readily produced into irregular shapes of scaffolds that match the defects in bone of individual patients.

7. *Commercialization.* The synthesis of the material and fabrication of the scaffold should be suitable for commercialization.

8.3 CARDIOVASCULAR BIOMATERIALS

Heart disease is the leading cause of death and disability in both industrialized nations and the developing world caused by a variety of underlying diseases, including ischemic heart disease with or without an episode of acute myocardial infarction, hypertensive heart disease, valvular heart disease, and primary myocardial disease, accounting for approximately 40% of all human mortality [25]. There are two types of strategies, that is, pharmacological therapy and interventional therapy employed to treat the heart diseases. Drug therapy focuses on reduction of work load (utilizing diuretics, nitrates) and protection from the toxic humoral factors while interventional therapy uses surgery or implantation of pacing devices to control electrical/mechanical asynchrony [26–31]. However, both methods are inappropriate at later stage to control disease progression [32]. Eventually, heart transplantation is the ultimate treatment option to end-stage heart failure but it also associated with problems such lack of organ donors and complications associated with immune suppressive treatments. Now scientists are developing new strategies to repair the injured heart [33] (Figure 8.2a and b).

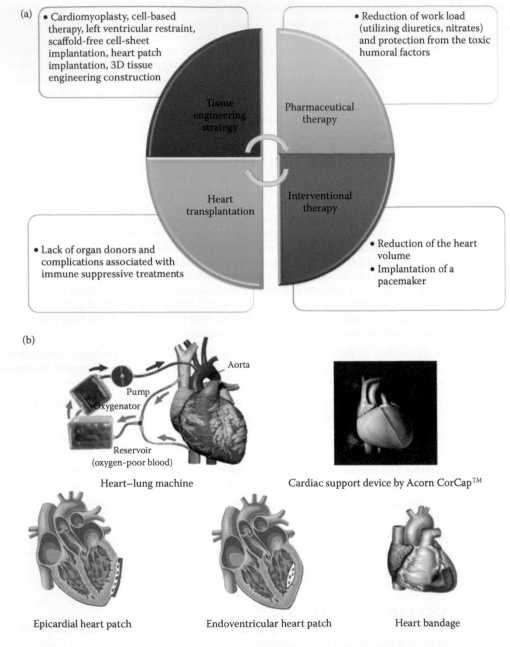

Figure 8.2 (a) Currently applied or potential strategies for the treatment of heart failure. (b) Schematic representation of various heart failure treatment devices.

In the early stage of surgical therapy, heart–lung machine was developed to perform the functions of the heart and lungs during an open-heart surgery [34], such as coronary bypass surgery and valve replacement [35,36]. In cardiomyoplasty, a preprepared skeletal muscle was wrapped around the heart, and paced to contract with the heart, to improve cardiac pumping power, that is, left ventricular performance, reduce cardiac dilation, and interrupt disease progression [37–40]. Marlex mesh (polypropylene) [41], Merselene mesh (knitted polyester) [42], Acorn CorCap™ heart mesh (knitted polyester), and Myocor TM Myosplint1 [37] are four representative cardiac support devices that have been under investigation. None of these devices has received approval of the FDA [43].

In the cell-based therapy, isolated cells are injected to the infarct region via the pericardium, coronary arteries, endocardium, or by 3D implant bandage onto the infarct heart, which is populated in vitro with cells and implanted later in vivo [44–47]. There are two types of patches, that is, the ring- or sheet-shaped heart patch used to deliver cell, reduction of elevated myofibril stresses, as well as histological and functional changes to clinical left ventricular metrics and provide mechanical support [48].

A more ambitious strategy is 3D tissue regeneration strategy in which myocardial tissue generated ex vivo and implanted on heart to replace and repair tissue and maintain and enhance its function [49–51] because they can produce in vitro healthy cells for cell-based therapy, as well as for organ development, functional cell differentiation from stem cells, environment–cell interaction, cancer biology, new drug treatment, and could ultimately be used for the repair of injured or diseased tissues.

8.4 CLASSIFICATION OF CARDIOVASCULAR BIOMATERIALS

Cardiovascular biomaterials include metals and their alloys, polymers, and some biological materials. In this subtitle, a brief discussion of these cardiovascular biomaterials for various applications will be highlighted.

8.4.1 Hydrogel-Based Cardiovascular Biomaterials

Vasculogenesis and angiogenesis are the commonly used methods that are responsible in the formation of blood vessels. Angiogenesis is a complex process that involves outgrowth of new blood vessels from preexisting ones. It consists of four chronological steps: (i) the stimulation of ECs by angiogenic factors (fibroblast growth factor1 [bFGF] and vascular endothelial growth factor [VEGF]), (ii) degradation of the surrounding capillary basal lamina by activated ECs via extracellular proteinases (matrix metalloproteinases [MMPs]), (iii) capillary sprout formation and migration of ECs mediated by their integrins, and (iv) vessel maturation due to growth factors such as angiopoietin-1 (Ang-1) or platelet-derived growth factor (PDGF). In this process various types of biomaterials have been used as ECM loaded with growth factors to improve the localized delivery of growth factors for therapeutic angiogenesis in ischemic tissues as well as to stimulate morphogenesis and tissue repair. Out of them, hydrogels have attracted much attention as scaffold biomaterials due to their unique properties such as structurally similar to the tissue ECM, biocompatible, biodegradable, can be processed under relatively mild conditions, and can be delivered in a minimally invasive manner. Currently, many types of natural and synthetic hydrogels have been used for therapeutic angiogenesis (Table 8.1) (Figure 8.3) [52].

8.4.2 Silk-Based Cardiovascular Biomaterials

Proteins, such as collagen, elastin, elastin-like-peptides, albumin, and fibrin, being one of the components of natural tissues, are widely used as cardiovascular biomaterials [53]. Silk fibroin of silkworms is a commonly available natural biopolymer, which is used in lips, eyes, oral surgeries, and in the treatment of skin wounds [54] due to its properties like mechanical strength, elasticity, biocompatibility, excellent (ca. 95%) optical transparency throughout the visible range with remarkable surface smoothness and water-based processing, less risk of infection, the presence of easy accessible chemical groups for functional modifications, and controllable biodegradability [54–56].

Silk possesses large molecular weight (200–350 kDa or more) with bulky repetitive modular hydrophobic domains, consisting of the repeated amino acid sequence, which are assembled into nanocrystals which are interrupted by small hydrophilic groups consisting of bulky and polar side chains and forming the amorphous part of the secondary structure [57–59]. The chain conformation in amorphous blocks is random coil, which gives elasticity to silk [60,61]. Silk-based biomaterials are clinically used as flow-diverting devices and stents (employed in the reconstruction of an intracranial aneurysm artery) [62,63], and its composites with collagen or poly (ethylene glycol

Table 8.1: Summary of Biomaterials Used to Deliver Growth Factors in Diseased Animal Models

Biomaterial	Growth Factors Used	Diseased Animal Model	Results
Alginate	VEGF and PDGF-BB	Rodent myocardial infarction, mouse hindlimb ischemia	More mature vessels with improved cardiac function
Chitosan	FGF-2	Chronic rabbit myocardial infarction	Improvement in systolic pressure at the left ventricle, larger amount of viable myocardium and blood vessels
Fibrin	Engineered variant of VEGF164; α2-PI1-8-VEGF-A164	Rodent hindlimb ischemia and wound healing, rabbit hindlimb ischemia	Stable and functional angiogenesis with improved perfusion, augmentation of collateral vessel development and improved limb perfusion
PEG-fibrinogen hydrogel	VEGF	Rodent myocardial infarction	Enhanced vascularization in the ischemic myocardium and improved cardiac function observed
PLG	VEGF	Murine hindlimb ischemia	Improved lower extremity perfusion, greater degree of mature vasculature
PLGA polymer scaffold	VEGF and PDGF	Mouse hindlimb ischemia	High proportions of mature blood vessels and increased number of collaterals
Heparin-conjugated fibrin	bFGF	Murine hindlimb ischemia	Enhanced neovascularization and significant reduction in muscle fibrosis and inflammation

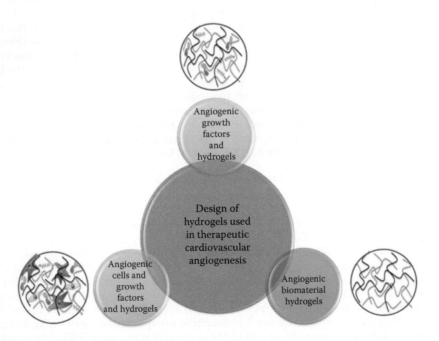

Figure 8.3 Design of hydrogels used in therapeutic cardiovascular angiogenesis. Hydrogel can be made using angiogenic biomaterials such as fibrin, or combined with angiogenic growth factors and/or endothelial progenitor cells.

diglycol diglycidyl ether) are successfully used to develop vascular constructs [64]. In a study, silk stents are also employed in the reconstruction of an intracranial aneurysm artery (tubular ~3 mm with a thickness of 0.15 mm and average tensile strength of 2.42 MPa) [65].

8.4.3 Polymers Used in Soft-Tissue Engineering

Natural or synthetic polymers are widely used in tissue engineering as substrates to deliver cell and provide mechanical support to damaged part, and for cellular attachment, proliferation, and differentiation in its native state. Table 8.2 shows advantages and disadvantages of polymeric biomaterials for tissue engineering.

8.4.3.1 Naturally Occurring Polymers

Natural polymers possess many advantages over synthetic such as biocompatibility, biodegradability, and not cause foreign materials response when implanted in humans. Table 8.3 presents major naturally occurring polymers, their sources, and applications. Among them, collagen, fibrin, gelatin, and alginate have been extensively investigated for myocardial tissue engineering [66,67]. Collagen is the major component of natural ECMs of soft tissue. Therefore, in early stage, mostly collagens and chitosan were used for tissue-engineering applications.

8.4.3.2 Synthetic Polymers

Natural polymers are biocompatible and nontoxic but their use in implants is limited because they suffer from many problems such as stimulate an immune response, source to source variability of properties, possibility of bacterial or viral contamination, and possible antigenicity. Due to these reasons, synthetic polymers have historically been the material of choice for implants as they possess superior properties such as nonimmunogenic, ease of production, control over properties of the polymer, ready availability, and versatility of manipulation. For these reasons, synthetic polymers are used in many biomedical implants such as poly(methyl methacrylate) (PMMA) for ocular implants, ultrahigh MW polyethylene in artificial hip joints, poly(lactide) and poly(glycolide) polymers as sutures, and silicone polymers as breast implants.

8.4.3.2.1 Synthetic Polymer-Based Fiber

In vascular vessel substitute or device, used materials must possess certain degree of porosity needed for cellular in growth from surrounding tissue but at the same time do not allow

Table 8.2: Advantages and Disadvantages of Polymeric Biomaterials for Tissue Engineering

Biomaterial	Positive Effect	Negative Effect
Naturally occurring polymers	Excellent biocompatibility (nor foreign body reactions) Biodegradable (with a wide range of degradation rates) Bioresorbable	1. Poor processability 2. Poor mechanical properties
Bulk biodegradable synthetic polymers, for example, poly(lactic acid), poly(glycolic acid), poly(lactic-co-glycolic acid), poly(propylene fumarate)	1. Good biocompatibility 2. Biodegradable (with a wide range of degradation rates) 3. Bioresorbable 4. Off-the-shelf availability 5. Good processability 6. Good ductility	1. Inflammatory caused by acid degradation products 2. Accelerated degradation rates cause collapse of scaffolds
Surface bioerodible synthetic polymers, for example, Poly(phosphazene), Poly(ortho esters), Poly(anhydrides)	1. Good biocompatibility 2. Retention of mechanical integrity over the degradative lifetime of the device 3. Significantly enhanced tissue in growth into the porous scaffolds, owing to the increment in pore size 4. Good processability 5. Off-the-shelf availability	1. They cannot be completely replaced by new tissue 2. Concern associated with the long-term effect
Nondegradable synthetic polymers	1. No foreign body reactions 2. Tailorable mechanical properties 3. Good processability 4. Off-the-shelf availability	1. Second surgery is required 2. Concern associated with the long-term effect if they have to stay in the host organ for a lifetime

Table 8.3: Naturally Occurring Polymers, Their Sources, and Applications

Polymer	Source	Applications
Chitosan, collagen–GAG (alginate) copolymer	Shells of shrimps and crabs	Multiapplications, including cardiac tissue engineering, artificial skin graft for skin replacement
Collagen	Tendon and ligaments	Multiapplications, including cardiac tissue engineering
Albumin	In blood	Transporting protein, used as coating to form a thromboresistant surface
Hydaluronic acid	In ECM of higher animals	Biocompatible and biodegradable polymer synthesis for cardiac tissue engineering
Fibrinogen-fibrin	Purified from plasma in blood	Multiapplications, including cardiac tissue engineering
Gelatin	Extracted from the collagen inside animals' connecting tissue	Multiapplications, including cardiac tissue engineering
Matrigel TM (gelatinous protein mixture	Mouse tumor cells	Myocardial tissue engineering
Alginate	Abundant in the cell wall of brown algae	Multiapplications, including cardiac tissue engineering
Polyhydroxyalkanoate	By fermentation	Cardiovascular and bone tissue engineering

blood leakage. Synthetic vessel substitutes can be broadly classified into two categories, fibrous and contiguous, on the basis of porous nature of materials. Polyester (Dacron®) woven or knitted fabrics belong to fibrous synthetic vessel substitute in cardiovascular applications whose degree of porosity is controlled by weft and warp-type knit as well as by a bewildering number of coatings of materials such as fluoropolymer [68], collagen and heparin-bound polymer [69], fibrin [70], FGF [71], silicone elastomer [72], gelatin. The failure of Dacron-based materials arises due to protein adsorption on to the surface, followed by platelet adhesion, inflammatory cell penetration, and EC/SMC migration. In most of the cases, platelet-containing fibrin coagulum is deposited on lumen-facing side, whereas a dense layer of foreign body cells is formed on the outer surface. Currently, ePTFE coating is preferred to avoid the clot formation on the Dacron-based materials.

8.4.3.2.2 *Expanded PTFE (ePTFE) Grafts*

Polytetrafluoroethylene (PTFE) is a synthetic fluorocarbon polymer commonly named as Teflon developed by Dupont Co., and used in cardiovascular engineering in vascular grafts and heart valves. PTFE sutures are used in the repair of mitral valve for myxomatous disease and also in surgery for prolapse of the anterior or posterior leaflets of mitral valves. PTFE is particularly used in implantable prosthetic heart valve rings. Small-diameter vascular grafts are required when there is no saphenous vein in cardiosystem. In such condition, expanded PTFE-based materials are used for peripheral vessel bypass, particularly for the femoropopliteal artery because of its small pore size (30 to ~100 μm), low coefficient of friction, mechanically relatively stable, and easily manufactured in many sizes and shapes, including the crimped variety and much stiffer than arteries or veins, good moduli (~3–6 MPa) [73,74]. A study showed that the patency of ePTFE Goretex® grafts is lower than heparinized Dacron [66] and gelatin-coated, double velour Dacron graft [75] by involving ATK femoropopliteal. The events leading to the low patency are predominantly thrombotic; in turn it appears that none of these grafts ever develops a full coverage of ECs on their lumen-facing side.

In another study, it was found that ePTFE grafts with a mean pore size (internodal distance) of 90 μm showed higher EC coverage at 18 weeks (75%) versus the standard PTFE graft (30 μm internodal distance; EC coverage 23%). In another study involving aortoiliac grafting in dogs [76] with 60 μm ePTFE, the higher porosity did not show higher patency rate compared to the 30 μm ePTFE. In human trial, ePTFE grafts with 60 and 30 μm showed virtually no endothelialization at 3 months [77]. Recently, carbon coating or carbon impregnation [76,78,79], fibrin glue with growth factors are used to improve the patency rate of ePTFE grafts but none of these treatments have been tested in humans.

8.4.3.2.3 Polyurethane Grafts

It is found that both thrombus formation and intimal hyperplasia are cause of the loss of patency. The loss in patency cannot be estimated with precision because it, occurring over a longer time frame (6 months upward), is likely to be caused by compliance mismatch. Polyurethane is a polymer formed by repeating units of urethane monomer containing average two or more functional groups because they are synthesized by the reaction between isocyanates with a polyol. Polyurethane is highly elastic synthetic polymer and it is applied in cardiovascular grafts for short-term applications due to good physiochemical and mechanical properties, highly biocompatible, and high shear strength, elasticity, and transparency, and also due to its instability under enzymatic and oxidative attack. Moreover, the surface of polyurethane has good resistance for microbes and the thrombosis formation by PU is almost similar to the versatile cardiovascular biomaterial like PTFE. Earlier polyester urethanes, such as Estane® grafts, are hydrolytically unstable because they hydrolyze under water or by enzymatic attack or both. Polyether PU (PEEU) are next-generation graft materials used in cardiovascular implants due to their hydrolytic stability than polyester urethanes under both acidic and alkaline conditions but they show degradation in enzymatic condition, or under degrades as well as in oxidative environments [80]. Mitrathane® is a PEEU-based graft developed by US Company, Mitral [81], by phase inversion from solutions in dimethyl acetamide, has microporosity but not interconnected, and shows low occlusion due to various factors, including poor attachment at the anastomotic site [82,83].

Newtec Vascular Products (UK) developed PEEU Pulse-Tec® graft. Vectra® graft of Thoratec Laboratories (USA), used for short-term application such as vascular access during hemodialysis, was approved by the FDA in 2000 [84].

The instability of PEU and PEEU was improved by introduction of microporous polycarbonate urethanes (PCUs) (trade-named Vascugraft®) by Braun-Melsungen AG and tested as early as 1983 in animals [85]. Later it was found that it contained a polycarbonate segment. An animal study suggested that Vascugraft had faster endothelialization rates, as well as lower amount of neo-intima formation, compared to ePTFE. Many studies reported the inferior nature of PU than ePTFE. Therefore, scientist tried to prepare materials by combining PU (as the weft, running circumferentially) and Dacron (as the warp, running longitudinally) to match the entire stress–strain curve for the human common carotid artery (CCA) [86]. In another approach, graft was prepared by the combination of Dacron and stretched PU fibers in both the warp and the weft, allowing for "stretchability" in both directions. Bench measurements showed the first construction to mimic the CCA stress–strain curves more closely, although the match was by no means exact.

8.4.3.2.4 Synthetic Biodegradable Polymers

In cardiovascular applications, synthetic biodegradable polymers can be used as an implantable graft (short time period, which then degrades while tissue remodeling occurs around it and inside it), or as a scaffold for growing vascular tissue ex vivo, followed by implantation of cell-containing polymeric structure. Fully biodegradable coronary or peripheral stents must satisfy the following requirements: biocompatible, structural integrity, biodegradable, degradation product piece not to be released into the lumen, and radio-opaque to enable its safe and facile deployment. Polyglactin 910 is a highly degradable polymer, which is prepared from copolymerization of poly(lactide) and poly(glycolide) (90% glycolide, also known as PLGA), used as a biodegradable suture [87]. The reasons for selection of polyglactin 910 as biodegradable suture were faster rate of erosion (disappearance) of the mesh or graft enabling easier ingression and growth of tissues into the mesh as well as degradation of polymer stimulates endothelialization via an intermediary, the macrophages [88,89]. However, fast degradable polymer-based vascular graft suffers from poor burst strength, unable to withstand blood pressure surges, and shows extensive dilation or even developing aneurysms. This problem was resolved by using poly(dioxanone) that is a polyether-ester, had the absorption rate in the body longer than Vicryl® or polyglactin 910 (90/10 PGLA), as well as had lesser thickness than polyglactin 910. However, these slower rates of degradation also slow down cell growth within the mesh. Consequently dilation effects are expected to be less significant and cell in growth rate is also slower for PDS. After that, binary system was synthesized consisting of 74% PGLA and 26% PDS as superior cell in growth materials and good burst strength [90]. These degradable materials are good for cardiovascular stent but there is a finite possibility that pieces of the graft could break off and float in the bloodstream.

When biodegradable polymers are used as scaffolds materials, it is necessary that autologous cells must be there to avoid host rejection. This necessitates a longer processing time, enhances likelihood of infections and a planned surgical procedure, and is clearly not indicated for emergency situations. Currently, synthetic biodegradable scaffold-based materials are used in cardiovascular tissue engineering. Considerable innovation has gone into trying to shorten the time required to grow a functioning artery ex vivo; even greater advances are expected in the future. In 2002, Japanese researchers synthesized synthetic biodegradable scaffold for the reconstruction of a larger (10-mm diameter) pulmonary artery in a 4-year-old patient [91]. In this scaffold, autologous cells were cultured for a month and designed for erosion in 2 months. After that, it was implanted into 20 patients by 2002 containing autologous cells seeded onto a PGA/PCL–PLA copolymer mesh.

8.4.3.2.5 Bio-Inspired Materials

Artificial or synthetic proteins are better option for cardiovascular application due to their better batch-to-batch reproducibility of structure, not contaminated by microbials. They need no complicated extraction procedure that may destroy some structural features; these are less immunogenic because they are synthesized by biosynthetic route which gives them better chemical and physical properties as well as control over their structures and act as bridge to fill the gap between purely synthetic materials such as Dacron and ePTFE (Figure 8.4). Endothelialization of an implanted graft can be done either by seeding the graft with autologous ECs ex vivo, or by creating surface features on the graft which induces in situ endothelialization. In the later method, graft surface is coated by heparin and/or albumin to migrate endothelial to the graft surface, as well as attachment of mitogens such as FGF and ECGF to the graft surface. It has not really shown enough promise. However, the first approach has gone to clinical trials [92,93]. Dacron seeded with of autologous ECs is under human trial, which has shown sufficient positive results in animals [94].

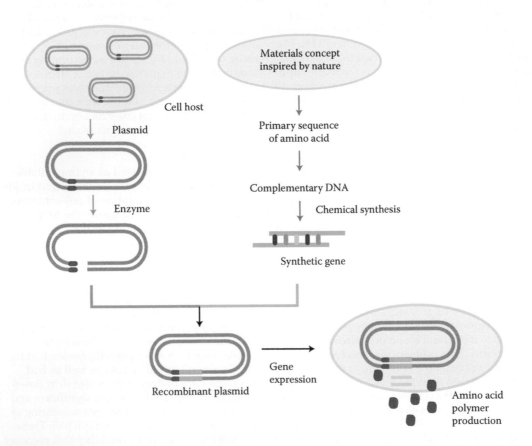

Figure 8.4 Schematic representation of the protein biosynthesis method.

8.4.3.2.6 Polyamides

Polyamides (PA), commonly called nylon, are thermoplastic materials that have molecular mass greater than 10,000 considered as "super polyester" fiber and applied in transparent tubings for cardiovascular applications, hemodialysis membranes, and also production of percutaneous transluminal coronary angioplasty (PTCA) catheters [95].

8.4.3.2.7 Polyolefin

Polyolefins (polyethylene and polypropylene) are polymers that contain repeated unit of olefin or alkene in their polymeric chain, and have been widely applied in medical application because of its better biocompatibility and chemical resistance [96]. Low-density and high-density polyethylene are used in cardiovascular arena in making tubings and housings for blood supply as well as in production of blood bags to store blood. Polypropylene is used for making heart valve structures [95,97].

8.4.4 Metals and Alloys

Metal and their alloys (stainless steel, cobalt chromium [CoCr] alloys and titanium [Ti] alloys) have been used in cardiovascular applications including heart valves, endovascular stents, and stent–graft combinations from last century due to their better stiffness, strength, corrosion resistance, and biocompatible nature [98–100]. Stents can be typically classified into three types based on their function and physical characters, namely, bare metal stents (BMS), drug-eluting stent (DES), and bio-absorbable stents. In early stage, vanadium-containing stainless steel was used for implants but incorporation of 18% Cr and 8% Ni alloy in lace of vanadium made it stronger, corrosion resistant, and blood compatible for applications. Therefore, stainless steel is widely used in heart valves, especially in making struts to support leaflets to avoid corrosion and provide mechanical strength to the valves.

Presently cobalt-based materials (MP35N or cobalt-nickel-chromium-molybdenum [CoNiCrMo] alloys with a nickel content of 35%) have gained much attention due to their better properties than stainless steel such as high strength, nonferromagnetic nature, and denser nature, and used for cardiovascular pacing leads, stylets, and catheters. Cobalt-based materials are highly preferred in coronary stent manufacturing because coronary interventionist demands for thinner struts, which can be easily achieved by using the Co alloys [101]. Since 1970 titanium-based materials (pure titanium [CP-Ti] and 5Ti-6Al-4 V [titanium-aluminium-vanadium]) are widely used in biomedical application due to their excellent tensile strength and pitting corrosion resistance, biocompatibility, shape memory effect, light weight, and low density than stainless steel and cobalt-based alloys. Bare metal stents possess good mechanical strength but lack in biocompatibility. This problem was resolve by development of DES. There are two types of DES: polymer-free stents, for example, Amazon Pax (MINVASYS) using Amazonia CroCo (L605) cobalt chromium (Co-Cr) stent with Paclitaxel as an antiproliferative agent, BioFreedom using stainless steel as base with modified abluminal coating as carrier surface for the antiproliferative drug Biolimus A9, YUKON choice (Translumina) used 316 L stainless steel as base for the drugs Sirolimus in combination with Probucol, etc.; and metallic stents with polymer carrier to hold and release the drug, for example, Cypheruses a 316 L stainless steel coated with polyethylenevinyl acetate (PEVA) and poly-butyl methacrylate (PBMA) for carrying the drug Sirolimus, Taxus (Boston Scientific) utilizes 316 L stainless-steel stents coated with styrene isoprene butadiene (SIBS) copolymer for carrying Paclitaxel, and Endeavour (Medtronic) uses a cobalt chrome driver stent for carrying zotarolimus with phosphorylcholine. DES basically consists of three parts: stent platform, coating, and drug [102–104].

Recently, Bio Matrix was developed as bioabsorbable DES that uses S-Stent (316 L) stainless steel as base with polylactic acid surface for carrying the antiproliferative drug Biolimus. Another advance bioabsorbable DES is ELIXIR-DES program developed by Elixir Medical Corp, which consists of cobalt–chromium (Co–Cr) alloy as base that is coated with both polyester and polylactide for delivery of drug Novolimus. JACTAX was developed by Boston Scientific Corp., which has coating of D-lactic polylactic acid (DLPLA) over the surface of (316 L) stainless steel and is used as stent to deliver Paclitaxel. NEVO is cobalt–chromium (Co–Cr) stent coated with polylactic-co-glycolic acid (PLGA) for delivery of drug Sirolimus that is developed by Cordis Corporation, Johnson & Johnson [99]. For a perfect cardiovascular application like stents, a wide varied biodegradable iron and magnesium alloys have been experimented with a reasonable degradation life of 12–24 months [105–108].

8.5 SURFACE MODIFICATION OF CARDIOVASCULAR BIOMATERIALS

Cardiovascular biomaterials are used in cardio system where they come in contact of blood. It is found that the major cause of failure of cardiovascular biomaterials is due to their poor compatibility with the blood. Therefore, it is required to modify the surface of materials to make it more blood compatible (Figure 8.5). Currently, three major strategies, that is, physical immobilization of biological material, chemical modification, and modification of materials using energy-possessing substances like plasma, ion implantation were adopted to modify the surface in order to improve the compatibility of the material. Physical immobilization of biological material technique uses coating of any biological substance (heparin, fibronectin, collagen, and vitronectin) as a simple coating material on the surface dictating the anticoagulation property of the implant without changing the structure of either. Heparinization is one of the commonly used biological materials for modifying the surface of cardiovascular implants made of 316 L SS, ePTFE, PET, and PU because it inhibits the active site of thrombin and thereby promoting blood compatibility [109–111]. Other anticoagulant molecules like thrombomodulin (TM) and NO have also been used for surface modification of cardiovascular biomaterials.

Chemical modification method uses coupling, grafting, and coating of various materials such as diamond, TiN, Ti–O, SiC, and polymers on the material surface, which not only decreases the platelet adhesion with less inflammatory reactions, but also provides higher hardness and smoothness, lower frictional coefficient, chemical inertness, biostability, and also good blood compatibility to materials. Diamond like carbon was used to coat the artificial heart valves (AHV) [112], ventricular assist devices (VAD), TiN coating for VAD, and Ti–O in metal stents [113]. Polyethylene oxide (PEO) and polyethylene glycol (PEG) are used in cardiovascular implants and show anticoagulation properties and display excellent blood compatibility, and providing adhesion resistance to small biomolecules like fibrinogen and cells such as platelets and leukocytes [114,115]. Modifications using energy-possessing substances such as air plasma modified, oxygen plasma modified, laser treatment, microwave treatment, ion implantation, and UV-exposure alter the surface of the implant and also facilitate the addition of coatings to improve the blood compatibility. Plasma surface modification is one of the widely utilized techniques to improve blood compatibility of cardiovascular implants [116]. Ion implantation utilizes precisely controlled ion species and doses to modify the surface. Recent investigations implied that ion implantation can improve the wettability and anticoagulant nature of polypropylene and polystyrene and thereby promoting EC adhesion [117,118].

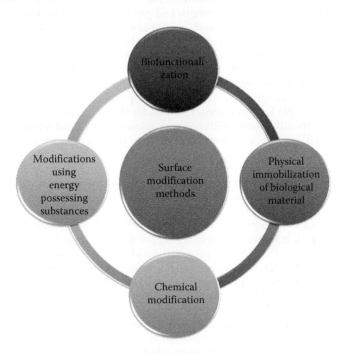

Figure 8.5 Cardiovascular biomaterials surface modification methods.

8.6 BIOFUNCTIONALIZATION OF CARDIOVASCULAR BIOMATERIALS

Endothelium is the layer which surrounds the entire vasculature ranging from heart to minute capillaries. Therefore, it is necessary to make endothelial surface on the cardiovascular implants to mimic the natural environment for better biocompatibility [119]. Several strategies such as impregnating the surface with active molecules such as VEGF, stromal derived factor-1 (SDF-1), nerve growth factor (NGF), and granulocyte-colony stimulating factor (G-CSF) were employed to promote anticoagulant nature of cardiovascular materials to induce neovascularization and repair the injury [120]. A recent study utilizing NGF-bound vascular grafts showed significant immobilization of endothelial progenitor cells (EPC) and a similar preparation using SDF-1/heparin found to recruit both EPCs and smooth muscle progenitor cells tackling the two important issues, namely, endothelization and remodeling of blood vessels [121,122]. One of the studies postulated that this EPC capture technology was feasible and safe for primary percutaneous coronary intervention for STEMI without the incidence of late stent restenosis [123].

Recently, DNA-aptamers with a high affinity to EPCs were identified as active molecule for bio functionalization of materials and grafted on the surface of polymer disk [124], stents [125], and Ti-implants [126] that promoted endothelial wound healing and also decreased the neointimal hyperplasia to a certain extent. Recent researches utilize human embryonic stem cells (h-ESC), mesenchymal stem cells, EPCs, and induced human pluripotent stem cells (ihPSCs), some of the cell sources explored for treatment of CVDs. It is found that human-iPSCs are better for cardiomyocytes differentiation used for autologous cardiomyocyte transplantation therapy than h-ESCs because they do not damage the human embryos and help to achieve a considerable quantity of patient-specific cardiomyocytes [127].

8.7 CURRENT CHALLENGES FOR CLINICAL TRIALS OF CARDIOVASCULAR MEDICAL DEVICES

The materials used for developing body implants or interfaces are commonly called biomaterials. Numerous medical devices are available that prolong survival, decrease morbidity, reduce symptoms, and improve functional status and/or health-related quality of life (HRQOL) in patients across the spectrum of CVD. Cardiovascular device therapy differs in important ways from cardiovascular drug therapy, and these differences often necessitate a modified approach to clinical trials. Several features of cardiovascular devices raise considerations for clinical trial conduct. Prospective, randomized, controlled trials remain the highest quality evidence for safety and effectiveness assessments, but, for instance, blinding may be challenging. The FDA provides three paths whereby medical devices can achieve market access: Demonstration of Substantial Equivalence to a "Pre-Amendment Device" product [510(k)], by Pre-Market Approval, and Humanitarian Device Exemption. For devices that present the highest level of risk to the patient in event of failure, the stringent requirements of a premarket approval process are generally necessary. A humanitarian device exemption reduces the level of benefit that must be demonstrated to permit use in a clearly defined plausible patient subset of no more than 4000 patients annually [128]. For many cardiovascular devices, adherence to standard practices of blinding and control groups is not possible. However, accurate assessment of risk and benefit is equally, if not perhaps more, important for a device that is often permanently implanted.

In order to avoid bias and not confound data interpretation, the use of objective endpoints and blinding patients, study staff, core labs, and clinical endpoint committees to treatment assignment are helpful approaches. Anticipation of potential bias should be considered and planned for prospectively in a cardiovascular device trial. No single research design will be appropriate for every cardiovascular device or target patient population. The type of trial, appropriate control group, optimal length of follow-up, and extent to which postmarket observational studies should be used will depend on the specific device, its potential benefits, the target patient population and the existence (or lack) of effective therapies, and its anticipated risks [129].

Issues that will affect medical industry's growth are as follows:

1. Changing sterilization technique and increased usage of disposable products due to infectious diseases

2. Changing FDA regulations with respect to emerging quality needs

3. Shift in healthcare payments from individual physicians and hospitals to a better defined centralized system

4. Trend toward defensive medicine, primarily due to lawsuits

5. Aging population

6. Advances in diagnostic imaging, laser surgery, and improved biocompatible materials

7. Continued drive toward industry cost containment

REFERENCES

1. Maitz MF, Tsyganov I, Pham MT, Wieser E. Institute of ion beam physics and materials research. *Annu Report* 2002, 11M, FZR 362.

2. Murray CJL, Richards MA, Newton JN, Fenton KA, Anderson HR, Atkinson C et al. UK health performance: Findings of the global burden of disease study 2010. *Lancet* 2013;381:997–1020.

3. Lloyd J. Heart disease and stroke statistics—2010 update: A report from the American Heart Association (vol. 121, p. e46, 2010). *Circulation* 2011;124:E425-E.

4. Tofield A. European cardiovascular disease statistics 4th edition 2012: Euro Heart II. *Eur Heart J* 2013;34:3007–3014.

5. http://www.who.int/entity/whr/2004/annex/topic/en/annex_2_en.pdf

6. Rufaihah AJ, Seliktar D. Hydrogels for therapeutic cardiovascular angiogenesis. *Adv Drug Deliv Rev* 2016;96:31–39.

7. International Standards Organization (ISO). *Biological Evaluation of Medical Devices, Part 1: Evaluation and Testing*. Document Number 10993. Geneva: ISO; 1997.

8. Weslowski SA. *Evaluation of Tissue and Prosthetic Vascular Grafts*. Springfield, IL: Charles C. Thomas; 1963.

9. Guidoin RC, Snyder RW, Awad JA, King MW. Biostability of vascular prostheses. In: Hastings GW, editor. *Cardiovascular Biomaterials*. New York: Springer-Verlag; 1991.

10. Greisler HP. *New Biologic and Synthetic Vascular Prostheses*. Austin, TX: R. G. Landes Co.; 1991.

11. Nicholson C, Paz JC. Total artificial heart and physical therapy management. *Cardiopulm Phys Ther J* 2009;21(2):13–21.

12. Roger WS, Michael NH. *Cardiovascular Biomaterials*. Digital Engineering Library Press; 2004.

13. Curtis MW, Russell B. Cardiac tissue engineering. *J Cardiovasc Nurs* 2009;24(2):87–92.

14. Biological evaluation of medical devices—Part 1: Evaluation and testing within a risk management process. http://www.fda.gov/downloads/MedicalDevices/DeviceRegulationandGuidance/GuidanceDocuments/UCM348890.pdf

15. Biological evaluation of medical devices—Part 12: Sample preparation and reference materials. ISO 10993-12:2012.

16. Vogler EA, Siedllecki CA. Contact activation of blood plasma coagulation. *Biomaterials* 2009;30:1857–1869.

17. Weng Y, Chen J, Tu Q, Li Q, Maitz MF, Huang N. Biomimetic modification of metallic cardiovascular biomaterials: From function mimicking to endothelialization *in vivo*. *Interface Focus* 2012;2:356–365.

18. Gorbet MB, Sefton MV. Biomaterial-associated thrombosis: Roles of coagulation factors, complement, platelets and leukocytes. *Biomaterials* 2004;25(26):5681–5703.

19. Pallister CJ, Watson MS. *Haematology*. Scion Publishing, UK; 2010.

20. Tegoulia VA, Rao WS, Kalambur AT, Rabolt JR, Cooper, SL. Surface properties, fibrinogen adsorption, and cellular interactions of a novel phosphorylcholine-containing self-assembled monolayer on gold. *Langmuir* 2001;17:4396–4404.

21. Lu JR, Murphy EF, Su TJ, Lewis AL, Stratford PW, Satija SK. Reduced protein adsorption on the surface of a chemically grafted phospholipid monolayer. *Langmuir* 2001;17:3382–3389.

22. Glasmastar K, Larsson C, Hook F, Kasemo B. Protein adsorption on supported phospholipid bilayers. *J Colloid Interface Sci* 2002;246:40–47.

23. Andersson AS, Glasmastar K, Sutherland D, Lidberg U, Kasemo B. Cell adhesion on supported lipid bilayers. *J Biomed Mater Res A* 2003;64A:622–629.

24. Jordan SW, Faucher KM, Caves JM, Apkarian RP, Rele SS, Sun XL et al. Fabrication of a phospholipid membrane-mimetic film on the luminal surface of an ePTFE vascular graft. *Biomaterials* 2006;27:3473–3481.

25. http://en.wikipedia.org/wiki/List_of_causes_of_death_by_rate. Accessed in July 2007.

26. Young JB, Mills RM. *Clinical Management of Heart Failure*. Caddo, OK: Professional Communications; 2004.

27. Chen FY, Cohn LH. The surgical treatment of heart failure. A new frontier: Nontransplant surgical alternatives in heart failure. *Cardiol Rev* 2002;10(6):326–333.

28. Loebe M, Soltero E, Thohan V, Lafuente JA, Noon GP. New surgical therapies for heart failure. *Curr Opin Cardiol* 2003;18(3):194–198.

29. Hawkins NM, Petrie MC, MacDonald MR, Hogg KJ, McMurray JJV. Selecting patients for cardiac resynchronization therapy: Electrical or mechanical dyssynchrony? *Eur Heart J* 2006;27(11):1270–1281.

30. Martinez C, Tzur A, Hrachian H, Zebede J, Lamas GA. Pacemakers and defibrillators: Recent and ongoing studies that impact the elderly. *Am J Geriat Cardiol* 2006;15(2):82–87.

31. Kohli SK, Elliott P. Cardiac resynchronization therapy: The procedure and progress so far. *Br J Hosp Med* 2005;66(8):469–473.

32. Packer M. The impossible task of developing a new treatment for heart failure. *J Card Fail* 2002;8(4):193–196.

33. Zammaretti P, Jaconi M. Cardiac tissue engineering: Regeneration of the wounded heart. *Curr Opin Biotechnol* 2004;15(5):430–434.

34. Miller BJ, Gibbon JH, Fineberg C. An improved mechanical heart and lung apparatus; its use during open cardiotomy in experimental animals. *Med Clin North Am* 1953;1:1603–1624.

35. Ross DN. Homograft replacement of the aortic valve. *Lancet* 1962;2:487.

36. Senning A. Fascia lata replacement of aortic valves. *J Thorac Cardiovasc Surg* 1967;54:465–470.

37. Walsh RG. Design and features of the Acorn CorCap Cardiac Support Device: The concept of passive mechanical diastolic support. *Heart Fail Rev* 2005;10(2):101–107.

38. Moainie SL, Gorman JH, Guy TS, Bowen FW, Jackson BM, Plappert T et al. Infarct restraint attenuates ischemic mitral regurgitation following posterolateral infarction. *Ann Thorac Surg* 2002;74(3):753–760.

39. Chachques JC, Berrebi A, Hernigou A, Cohen Solal A, Lavergne T, Marino JP et al. Study of muscular and ventricular function in dynamic cardiomyoplasty: A ten-year follow-up. *J Heart Lung Transpl* 1997;16(8):854–868.

40. Lorusso R, Milan E, Volterrani M, Giubbini R, vander Veen FH, Schreuder JJ et al. Cardiomyoplasty as an isolated procedure to treat refractory heart failure. *Eur J Cardio-Thorac Surg* 1997;11(2):363–372.

41. Kelley ST, Malekan R, Gorman JH, Jackson BM, Gorman RC, Suzuki Y et al. Restraining infarct expansion preserves left ventricular geometry and function after acute anteroapical infarction. *Circulation* 1999;99(1):135–142.

42. Enomoto Y, Gorman JH, Moainie SL, Jackson BM, Parish LM, Plappert T et al. Early ventricular restraint after myocardial infarction: Extent of the wrap determines the outcome of remodeling. *Ann Thorac Surg* 2005;79(3):881–887.

43. Jawad H, Lyon AR, Harding SE, Ali NN, Boccaccini AR. Myocardial tissue engineering. *Br Med Bull* 2008;87:31–47.

44. Yang J, Yamato M, Okano T. Cell-sheet engineering using intelligent surfaces. *MRS Bull* 2005;30(3):189–193.

45. Eschenhagen T, Fink C, Remmers U, Scholz H, Wattchow J, Weil J et al. Three-dimensional reconstitution of embryonic cardiomyocytes in a collagen matrix: A new heart muscle model system. *FASEB J* 1997;11(8):683–694.

46. Chen QZ, Harding SE, Ali NN, Boccaccini AR. Chap 16: Myocardial tissue engineering. In: Boccaccini AR, Gough J, editors. *Tissue Engineering Using Ceramics and Polymers*. Woodhead Publishing Limited; 2008.

47. Fujimoto KL, Tobita K, Merryman WD, Guan JJ, Momoi N, Stolz DB et al. An elastic, biodegradable cardiac patch induces contractile smooth muscle and improves cardiac remodeling and function in subacute myocardial infarction. *J Am Coll Cardiol* 2007;49(23):2292–2300.

48. Wall ST, Walker JC, Healy KE, Ratcliffe MB, Guccione JM. Theoretical impact of the injection of material into the myocardium: A finite element model simulation. *Circulation* 2006;114(24):2627–2635.

49. Nerem RM. The challenge of imitating nature. In: Lanza RP, Langer R, Vacanti JP, editors. *Principles of Tissue Engineering*, 2nd ed. California: Academic Press; 2000. p. 9–15.

50. Giraud MN, Armbuster C, Carrel T, Tevaearai HT. Current state of the art in myocardial tissue engineering. *Tissue Eng* 2007;138:1825–1836.

51. Opinion on the State of the Art Concerning Tissue Engineering, European Commission health and Consumer Protection, http://ec.europa.eu, 2001.

52. Rufaihah AJ, Seliktar D. Hydrogels for therapeutic cardiovascular angiogenesis. *Adv Drug Deliv Rev* 2016;96:31–39.

53. Nair LS, Laurencin CT. Biodegradable polymers as biomaterials. *Prog Polym Sci* 2007;32:762–798.

54. Omenetto FG, Kaplan DL. New opportunities for an ancient material. *Science* 2010;329:528–531.

55. Omenetto FG, Kaplan DL. A new route for silk. *Nat Photonics* 2008;2:641–643.

56. Hota MK, Bera MK, Kundu B, Kundu SC, Maiti CK. A natural silk fibroin protein-based transparent bio-memristor. *Adv Funct Mater* 2012;22:4493–4499.

57. Ayoub NA, Garb JE, Tinghitella RM, Collin MA, Hayashi CY. Blueprint for a high-performance biomaterial: Full-length spider dragline silk genes. *PLoS One* 2007;2:e514.

58. Vollrath F, Porter D. Spider silk as a model biomaterial. *Appl Phys A: Mater Sci Process* 2006;82:205–212.

59. Lefèvre T, Rousseau M-E, Pézolet M. Protein secondary structure and orientation in silk as revealed by Raman spectromicroscopy. *Biophys J* 2007;92:2885–2895.

60. Vollrath F, Knight DP. Liquid crystalline spinning of spider silk. *Nature* 2001;410:541–548.

61. Vollrath F. Strength and structure of spiders' silks. *J Biotechnol* 2000;74:67–83.

62. Causin F, Pascarella R, Pavesi G, Marasco R, Zambon G, Battaglia R et al. Acute endovascular treatment (48 hours) of uncoilable ruptured aneurysms at non-branching sites using silk flow-diverting devices. *Interv Neuroradiol* 2011;17(3):357–364.

63. Leonardi M, Cirillo L, Toni F, Dall'Olio M, Princiotta C, Stafa A et al. Treatment of intracranial aneurysms using flow-diverting silk stents (BALT): A single centre experience. *Interv Neuroradiol* 2011;17(3):306–315.

64. Yagi T, Sato M, Nakazawa Y, Tanaka K, Sata M, Itoh K et al. Preparation of double-raschel knitted silk vascular grafts and evaluation of short-term function in a rat abdominal aorta. *J Artif Organs* 2011;14:89–99.

65. Soffer L, Wang X, Zhang X, Kluge J, Dorfmann L, Kaplan DL et al. Silk-based electrospun tubular scaffolds for tissue-engineered vascular grafts. *J Biomater Sci Polym Ed* 2008;19:653–664.

66. Devine C, McCollum C. Heparin-bonded Dacron® or polytetrafluorethylene for femoropopliteal bypass: Five-year results of a prospective randomized multicenter clinical trial. *J Vasc Surg* 2004;40:924–931.

67. Niklason LE, Gao J, Abbott WM, Hirschi KK, Houser S, Marini R et al. Functional arteries grown *in vitro*. *Science* 1999;284:489–493.

68. Eiberg JP, Roder O, Stahl-Madsen M, Eldrup N, Qvarfordt P, Laursen A et al. Fluropolymer-coated Dacron® graft versus PTFE grafts for femorofemoral crossover by pass. *Eur J Vasc Endovasc Surg* 2006;32:431–438.

69. Parsson H, Jundzill W, Johansson K, Jonung T, Norgren L. Healing characteristics of polymer-coated or collagen-treated Dacron® grafts: An experimental porcine study. *Cardiovasc Surg* 1994;2:242–248.

70. Sreerekha PR, Krishnan LK. Cultivation of endothelial progenitor cells on fibrin matrix and layering on Dacron®/polytetrafluoroethylene vascular grafts. *Artif Organs* 2006;30:242–249.

71. van der Bas JM, Quax PH, Van Der Berg C, Visser MJ, van der Linden E, van Bockel JH. Ingrowth of aorta wall into stent grafts impregnated with basic fibroblast growth factor: A porcine *in vivo* study of blood vessel prosthesis healing. *J Vasc Surg* 2004;39:850–858.

72. Granke K, Ochsner JL, McClugage SG, Zdrahal P. Analysis of graft healing in a new elastomer-coated vascular prosthesis. *Cardiovasc Surg* 1993;1:254–261.

73. Grigioni AM, Daniele C, D'Avenio G, Barbaro V. Biomechanics and hemodynamics of grafting. In: Tura A, editor. *Vascular Grafts: Experiment and Modelling*. Boston: WIT Press; 2003. p. 41–82.

74. Lee JM, Wilson GJ. Anisotropic tensile viscoelastic properties of vascular graft materials at low strain rates. *Biomaterials* 1986;7:423–431.

75. Jensen LP, Lepäntalo M, Fossdal JE, Røder OC, Jensen BS, Madsen MS et al. Dacron® or PTFE for above-knee femoropopliteal bypass: A multicenter randomised study. *Eur J Endovasc Surg* 2007;34:44–49.

76. Akers DL, Du YH, Kempscinski RF. The effect of carbon coating and porosity on early patency of expanded polytetrafluoroethylene grafts: An experimental study. *J Vasc Surg* 1993;18:10–15.

77. Kohler TR, Stratton JR, Kirkman TR, Johansen KH, Zierler BK, Cloves AW. Conventional high porosity polytetrafluoroethylene grafts: Clinical evaluation. *Surgery* 1992;112:901–907.

78. Kapfer X, Meichelboeck W, Groegler FM. Comparison of carbon impregnated and standard ePTFE prostheses in extra-anatomical anterior tibial artery bypass: A prospective randomized multicenter study. *Eur J Vasc Endovasc Surg* 2006;32:155–168.

79. Bacourt F. Prospective randomized study of carbon-impregnate d-polytetrafluoroethylene grafts for below the knee popliteal and distal by pass: Results at 2 years. *Ann Vasc Surg* 1997;11:596–603.

80. Tanzi MC, Fare S, Petrini P. *In vitro* stability of polyether and polycarbonate urethanes. *J Biomater Appl* 2000;14:325–348.

81. Gilding DK, Reed AM, Askill IN, Briana SG. Biocompatible microporous polymeric materials and methods of making the same. *US Patent* 1987;4,704:310.

82. Martz H, Paynter R, Slimane SB, Beaudoin G, Guidoin R. Hydrophilic microporous polyurethane versus expanded PTFE grafts as substitutes in the carotid arteries of dogs: A limited study. *J Biomed Mater Res* 1988;22:63–69.

83. Teijeira FJ, Lamoureaux G, Tetreault J-P, Bauset R, Guidoin R, Marois Y et al. Hydrophilic polyurethane versus autologous femoral vein as substitutes in the femoral arteries of dogs: Quantification of platelets and fibrin deposits. *Biomaterials* 1989;10:80–84.

84. Kakkos SK, Haddad R, Haddad GK, Reddy DJ, Nypaver TJ, Lin JC et al. Results of aggressive graft surveillance and endovascular treatment on secondary patency rates of Vectra® Vascular Access Grafts. *J Vasc Surg* 2007;45:974–980.

85. Hess F, Jerusalem C, Braun B. Endothelialization process of a fibrous polyurethane microvascular prosthesis after implantation in the abdominal aorta of the rat—A scanning electron microscopic study. *J Cardiovasc Surg* 1983;24:516–524.

86. Gupta BS, Kasyanov VA. Biomechanics of human common carotid artery and design of novel hybrid textile compliant vascular grafts. *J Biomed Mater Res* 1997;34:341–349.

87. Gomez-Alonso A, Garcia-Criado FJ, Parreno-Manchado FC, Garcia-Sanchez JE, Garcia-Sanchez E, Parreno-Manchado A et al. Study of the efficacy of coated Vicryl Plus® antibacterial suture (coated polyglactin 910 suture with triclosan) in two animal models of general surgery. *J Infect* 2007;54:82–88.

88. Greisler HP, Dennis JW, Endean ED, Ellinger J, Friesel R, Burgess W. Macrophage/biomaterial interactions: The stimulation of endothelialization. *J Vasc Surg* 1989;9:588–593.

89. Zweep HP, Satoh S, vander Lei B, Hinrichs WL, Feijen J, Wildevuur CR. Degradation of a supporting prosthesis can optimize arterialization of autologous veins. *Ann Thorac Surg* 1993;56:1117–1122.

90. Greisler HP, Endean ED, Klosak JJ, Ellinger J, Dennis JW, Buttle K et al. Polyglactin 910/polydioxanonebi component totally resorbable vascular prostheses. *J Vasc Surg* 1988;7:697–705.

91. Hibino N, Imai Y, Shin-Oka T, Aoki M, Watanabe M, Kosaka Y et al. First successful clinical application of tissue-engineered blood vessel, Kyobugeka. *Jpn J Thorac Surg* 2002;55:368–373.

92. Gray JL, Kang SS, Zenni GC, Kim DU, Kim PI, Burgess WH et al. FGF-1 affixation stimulates ePTF endothelialization without intimal hyperplasia. *J Surg Res* 1994;57(5):596–612.

93. Doi K, Matsuda T. Enhanced vascularization in a microporous polyurethane graft impregnated with basic fibroblast growth factor and heparin. *J Biomed Mater Res* 1997;34:361–370.

94. Herring M, Baughman S, Glover J. Endothelium develops on seeded human arterial prosthesis: A brief clinical note. *J Vasc Surg* 1985;2:727–730.

95. Helmus MN, Hubbell JA. Chapter 6: Materials selection. *Cardiovascular Pathology* 1993;2(3):53–71.

96. http://biomerics.com/Polyolefin

97. Eberhart RC, Huo H, Nelson K. *Cardiovascular Materials, MRS Bulletin*. 17th edition, 1991.

98. Lane WA. Some remarks on the treatment of fractures. *Brit Med J* 1895;1:861.

99. Metals for Biomedical Applications, http://www.intechopen.com/download/get/type/pdfs/id/18658

100. Moravej M, Mantovani D. Biodegradable metals for cardiovascular stent application: Interests and new opportunities. *Int J Mol Sci* 2011;12(7):4250–4270.

101. BomBac D, Brojan M, FajFar P, Kosel F, Turk R. Review of materials in medical applications. *RMZ-Mater Geoenviron* 2007;54(4):471–499.

102. Abizaid A, Costa JR Jr. New drug-eluting stents an overview on biodegradable and polymer-free next-generation stent systems. *Circulation: Cardiovasc Interventions* 2010;3(4):384–393.

103. http://biomed.brown.edu/Courses/BI108/BI1082004Groups/Group05/Drug%20Eluting%20Stents/drug eluting stents.htm

104. http://www.everydayhealth.com/health-center/blood-clots-alate-hazard-for-drug-coated-stents.aspx

105. Saito S. New horizon of bioabsorbable stent. *Catheterization Cardiovasc Intervention* 2005;66(4):595–596.

106. Erne P, Schier M, Resink TJ. The road to bio absorbable stents: Reaching clinical reality? *Cardiovas Interven Radiol* 2006;29(1):11–16.

107. Peuster M, Wohlsein P, Brugmann M, Ehlerding M, Seidler K, Fink C et al. A novel approach to temporary stenting: Degradable cardio vascular stents produced from corrodible metal—Results 6–18 months after implantation into New Zealand white rabbits. *Heart* 2001;86(5):563–569.

108. Colombo A, Karvouni E. Biodegradable stents: Fulfilling the mission and stepping away. *Circulation* 2000;102(4):371–373.

109. Matthew D, Berceli SA, Bide MJ, Quist WG, LoGerfo FW. Diminished adhesion and activation of platelets and neutrophils with CD47 functionalized blood contacting surfaces. *Biomaterials* 1997;18:755.

110. Lei L, Li Q-L, Maitz MF, Chen J-L, Huang N. Immobilization of the direct thrombin inhibitor-bivalirudin on 316L stainless steel via polydopamine and the resulting effects on hemocompatibility *in vitro*. *J Biomed Mater Res A* 2012;100A(9):2421–2430.

111. Murugesan S, Xie J, Linhardt RJ. Immobilization of heparin: Approaches and applications. *Curr Topics Med Chem* 2008;8(2):80–100.

112. Hauert R. A review of modified DLC coatings for biological applications. *Diamond Related Mater* 2003;12(3–7):583–589.

113. Huang N, Yang P, Leng YX, Chen JY, Sun H, Wang J et al. Hemocompatibility of titanium oxide films. *Biomaterials* 2003;24(13):2177–2187.

114. Andrade JD, Nagaoka S, Cooper S, Okano T, Kim SW. Surfaces and blood compatibility. *ASAIO Transactions* 1987;10:75–84.

115. Hansson KM, Tosatti S, Isaksson J, Wettero J, Textor M, Lindahl TL et al. Whole blood coagulation on protein adsorption-resistant PEG and peptide functionalised PEG-coated titanium surfaces. *Biomaterials* 2005;26(8):861–872.

116. Kawamoto Y, Nakao A, Ito Y, Wada N, Kaibara M. Endothelial cells on plasma-treated segmented-polyurethane: Adhesion strength, antithrombogenicity and cultivation in tubes. *J Mater Sci: Mater Med* 1997;8(9):551–557.

117. Ion beam process polymer. In: *American Symposium on Strategies to Improve Biocompatibility of Blood Interacting Biomaterials*, Boston, MA, USA, 1995.

118. Suzuki Y, Iwata H, Nakao A, Iwaki M, Kaibara M, Sasabe H et al. Ion implantation into collagen for the substrate of small diameter artificial grafts. *Nucl Instruments Methods Phys Res B: Beam Int Mater Atoms* 1997;127–128:1019–1022.

119. Otsuka F, Finn AV, Yazdani SK, Nakano M, Kolodgie FD, Virmani R. The importance of the endothelium in atherothrombosis and coronary stenting. *Nat Rev Cardiol* 2012;9(8):439–453.

120. Melchiorr AJ, Hibino N, Fisher JP. Strategies and techniques to enhance the *in situ* endothelialization of small diameter biodegradable polymeric vascular grafts. *Tissue Eng B: Rev* 2012;19(4):292–307.

121. Zeng W, Yuan W, Li L, Mi J, Xu S, Wen C et al. The promotion of endothelial progenitor cells recruitment by nerve growth factors in tissue engineered blood vessels. *Biomaterials* 2010;31(7):1636–1645.

122. Yu J, Wang A, Tang Z, Henry J, Li-Ping Lee B, Zhu Y et al. The effect of stromal cell-derived factor-1α/heparin coating of biodegradable vascular grafts on the recruitment of both endothelial and smooth muscle progenitor cells for accelerated regeneration. *Biomaterials* 2012;33:8062–8074.

123. Co M, Tay E, Lee CH, Poh KK, Low A, Lim J et al. Use of endothelial progenitor cell capture stent (Genous Bio-Engineered R Stent) during primary percutaneous coronary intervention in acute myocardial infarction: Intermediate- to long-term clinical follow-up. *Am Heart J* 2008;155(1):128–132.

124. Hoffmann J, Paul A, Harwardt M, Groll J, Reeswinkel T, Klee D, Moeller M et al. Immobilized DNA aptamers used as potent attractors for porcine endothelial precursor cells. *J Biomed Mater Res A* 2008;84(3):614–621.

125. Sim DS, Jeong MH, Ahn Y, Kim YJ, Chae SC, Hong TJ, Seong IW et al. Effectiveness of drug eluting stents versus bare-metal stents in large coronary arteries in patients with acute myocardial infarction. *J Korean Med Sci* 2011;26(4):521–527.

126. Meng QH, Song YM, Zhao J, Yu CJ, Zhan QM. Optimization of transfection efficiency of small interfering RNA in purified human prolactinoma cells. *Chem J Chin Univ* 2011;124(12):1862–1869.

127. Ye L, Zhang S, Greder L, Dutton J, Keirstead SA, Lepley M et al. Effective cardiac myocyte differentiation of human induced pluripotent stem cells requires VEGF. *PLoS ONE* 2013;8(1).

128. Food Drug and Cosmetic Act Amendment. Federal Register (21U.S.C.396, Section 906). 1998;63(225):64617.

129. Zannad F, Stough WG, Piña IL, Mehrane R, Abraham WT, Anker SD et al. Current challenges for clinical trials of cardiovascular medical devices. *Int J Cardiol* 2014;175:30–33.

9 Market Scenario of Biomaterial-Based Devices

9.1 INTRODUCTION

Biomaterials have made a significant contribution in improving the outcomes of patients suffering from the issues associated with long-term chronic conditions as well as helping to resolve the problems of traumatic injury. It is anticipated that the use of medical biomaterials will continue to expand rapidly through the emergence of new and innovative technologies as well as the identification of new applications for products based on biomaterial technologies. Polymers play a central role both in the natural world and in modern industrial economies [1].

9.2 THE BIOMATERIALS MARKET

The "Biomaterials Market [By Products (Polymers, Metals, Ceramics, Natural Biomaterials) and Applications (Cardiovascular, Orthopedic, Dental, Plastic Surgery, Wound Healing, Tissue Engineering, Ophthalmology, Neurology Disorders)]—Global Forecasts to 2017" analyzes and studies the major market drivers, restraints, and opportunities in North America, Europe, Asia, and Rest of the World.

The global biomaterial market is broadly segmented into two categories, by type and by application. The global biomaterial market, by type, is broadly categorized into metals, ceramics, polymers, and natural biomaterials. The biomaterial applications market is broadly segmented into orthopedic, cardiovascular, neurological, dental, tissue engineering, wound healing, plastic surgery, ophthalmology, and other applications such as gastrointestinal, urinary, bariatric surgery, and drug delivery system. In 2012, the cardiovascular biomaterial segment contributed 34.5% to the global biomaterial market, followed by the orthopedic segment. Plastic surgery and wound-healing applications are expected to witness the highest growth in the coming years.

The biomaterial polymers market is expected to show the highest growth at a compounded annual growth rate (CAGR) of 22.1% (2012–2017) due to tremendous ongoing research for the development of biodegradable and biocompatible polymeric biomaterial and its use in a wide range of applications.

North America is the largest biomaterial market and is expected to grow at a high CAGR from the year 2012 to 2017 due to an increase in the aging population. Due to rising awareness of biomaterial products in Asia, and increased conferences and collaborations, the Asian market is expected to grow at a CAGR of 21.5% from 2012 to 2017.

9.2.1 Orthopedic Biomaterials Worldwide Market

The orthopedic devices market has been extensively analyzed on the basis of factors such as the technology used, success rate, reimbursement coverage, and geographical reach. Orthopedic devices report studies the global market for orthopedic devices from the perspective of various anatomical locations in the human body. An important factor for orthopedic devices manufacturers' success is their capability to innovate products with newer technologies such as introduction of biodegradable products along with making the products available at low cost, to competently encourage market growth.

The rise in aging population and sports and road injuries, coupled with increasing demand for minimally invasive surgeries has spurred the growth of the global orthopedic devices market, according to a new report published by Transparency Market Research. The report, titled "Orthopedic Devices Market—Global Industry Analysis, Size, Share, Growth, Trends and Forecast, 2013–2019," indicates that registering a 4.9% CAGR from 2013 to 2019, the worldwide market for orthopedic devices is likely to develop from US$29.2 billion in 2012 to US$41.2 billion by 2019. Each of the segments in the orthopedic devices market has been analyzed on the basis of its current and future market size for the period 2011–2019, in terms of revenue generation in USD million, considering 2011 and 2012 as the base years. The CAGR for each market segment of orthopedic devices have been provided for the forecast period 2013–2019 along with the estimations of market size. Orthopedic devices report also includes market overview section, which covers beneficial qualitative information regarding introduction of orthopedic devices, technological trends and future advances, reimbursement scenario. On the basis of anatomical location, the market for orthopedic devices is segmented into knee, hip, elbow, shoulder, spine, foot and ankle, craniomaxillofacial, and other extremities. Each of these locations is further fragmented into internal fixation devices, joint implants, and external fixation devices. By anatomical location, knees dominated the overall market in terms of revenue.

Orthopedic biomaterials market by region, worldwide

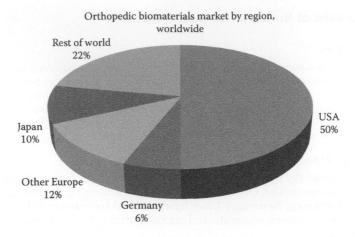

Figure 9.1 Orthopedic biomaterials market by region, worldwide.

However, this segment is predicted to witness a slight drop in market share by 2019 owing to frequent product recalls.

The orthopedic biomaterials field is like a cake that can be cut in various ways; for example, by the types of materials used, the different structures involved, and by the clinical uses to which they are put. And of course the business of orthopedic biomaterials can involve analysis of the market (actual and potential) and of the industry, which supplies these materials and the devices of which they are made [2]. In Figure 9.1, the segmentation of the global market by main regions and countries is shown [3].

Any ranking of the major players in the orthopedic biomaterials marketplace must take account of the fact that some companies have orthopedic product offerings other than biomaterials, and/or they are subsidiaries of larger concerns, which do not provide detailed breakdowns of revenues. For example, among industry leaders are Genzyme Biosurgery, DePuy, and Medtronic SofamorDanek all of which are subsidiaries, while Smith & Nephew has a range of orthopedic product offerings not including biomaterials.

9.2.1.1 Orthopedic Biomaterials Market Growth in the United States

Growth in the US market for orthopedic biomaterials is expected to be somewhat faster than in Europe and significantly greater than in the developing world, partly because new biomaterials are relatively expensive and their uptake is related, in general terms, to GDP. Newly emerging technologies such as bone morphogenetic proteins (BMPs) are expected to grow at rates up to

US orthopedic biomaterials market

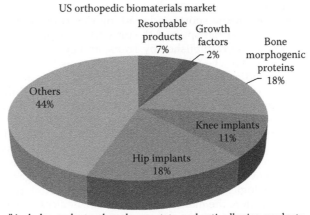

"Others" includes: sealants, glues, haemostats, and anti-adhesion products

Figure 9.2 US orthopedic biomaterials market.

30%–35% per annum during the forecast period (2007–2011), although their contribution to the overall orthopedic biomaterials market will be relatively modest, since they are starting from a small base. Overall, the US market for orthopedic biomaterials is expected to grow by approximately 12% per annum over the next 5 years. The US market is the best-documented of the world's regional markets for orthopedic biomaterials, and US-specific data are to be found later in this section, under discussions of the market by surgical procedures and classes of biomaterials (Figure 9.2) [4].

Although the "other" category is the largest category included in this overall market, and has been included because of both "biomaterials" aspect of these technologies and their clinical utility in orthopedic applications, these products are part of the larger market for sealing, adhesion, hemostasis, and prevention of postsurgical adhesions [5].

9.2.2 Tissue Engineering and Cell Therapy Global Market Development

Tissue engineering and cell therapy comprise a market for regenerative products that is expected to grow worldwide to almost $32 billion by 2018 (Figures 9.3 and 9.4). This market spans many specialties, the biggest of which is therapies for degenerative and traumatic orthopedic and spine applications. Other disorders that will benefit from cell therapies include cardiac and vascular disease, a wide range of neurological disorders, diabetes, inflammatory diseases, and dental decay and/or injury.

Key factors expected to influence the market for regenerative medicine are continued political actions, government funding, clinical trials results, industry investments, and an increasing awareness among both physicians and the general public of the accessibility of cell therapies for medical applications [6].

On a country-by-country basis, there is considerable variation in the forces impacting the clinical practice and industry of cell therapy especially, along with tissue engineering, and these forces are fluid over time. Certainly among the most significant was President Bush's Presidential

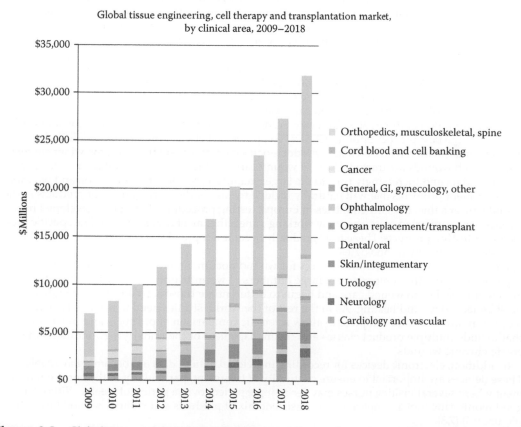

Figure 9.3 Global tissue engineering, cell therapy, and transplantation market.

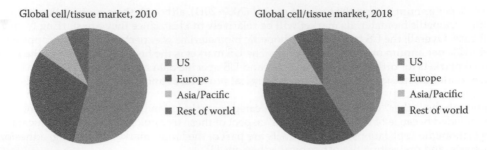

Global cell/tissue market, 2010 Global cell/tissue market, 2018

- US
- Europe
- Asia/Pacific
- Rest of world

Figure 9.4 Global cell and tissue market, 2010–2018.

Executive Order in 2001 banning federal funds for embryonic cell therapy other than for existing cell lines, an order that President Obama promptly rescinded after the 2008 election. The 2001–2008 hiatus impeded development of embryonic cell therapy solutions, while shifting the emphasis of development toward adult stem cell technology. Now, in 2012, development is moving rapidly on both fronts [6].

9.2.3 The Global Wound Management Market

The global wound management market is comprised of very diverse products spanning many different wound dressing types, growth factors, tissue engineering, and a growing portfolio of physical therapies. Growth in wound management product revenues varies considerably, and will result in different market distribution.

Clinical protocols for the treatment of specific wounds can vary considerably from country to country. Venous stasis ulcers, which account for approximately 4% of wounds and 75% of leg ulcers, are treated with short stretch compression bandages in Germany, elastic adhesive bandages in Italy, high-compression bandages in France, and multilayer compression systems in the United Kingdom. As in the United States, the routine use of strong antiseptics is discouraged in the United Kingdom and Germany but still prevalent in East European countries as well as the Netherlands and Italy.

The quest for standardized modern approaches to wound healing is aided by groups such as the European Wound Management Association and European Tissue Repair Society, which encourage pan-European dialog on issues pertaining to wound care. Such organizations have had significant effect on the development of US wound care policy and practices.

The proliferation of different wound care products and strategies leads to confusion and uncertainty over the best practice options. Clinical comparisons between treatment modalities have been minimal, with reliance on small, product-focused studies that often omit the wider context under which wounds are treated. Users of wound care products rely on manufacturers for performance data and increasingly turn to the larger manufacturers for staff education and wound care treatment protocols that will naturally include the use of the large number of products in the manufacturer's line. In many countries in Europe, testing procedures have been developed by government-supported cross-company working panels that meet regularly to define specific protocols for testing products. These tests gradually become adopted by manufacturers as first lines of evaluation for new technologies.

The emerging use of electronic devices for wound documentation and assessment is expected to allow the comparison of large numbers of wounds undergoing different integrated approaches to wound care and begin to differentiate those activities that provide the most benefit to wound healing. As in the rest of the world, studies need to become larger, more standardized, and complete to allow scientific comparison of products and practices that include multiple product classes and the management of the underlying conditions that create chronic wounds.

In addition, electronic devices for recording individual patient data are becoming available. These devices are important to ensure continuity of treatment, particularly in the home environment where several visiting nurses may see a single patient over a period of weeks. Without a good monitoring tool a complex and inconsistent mix of products and strategies could be applied (Figure 9.5) [7,8].

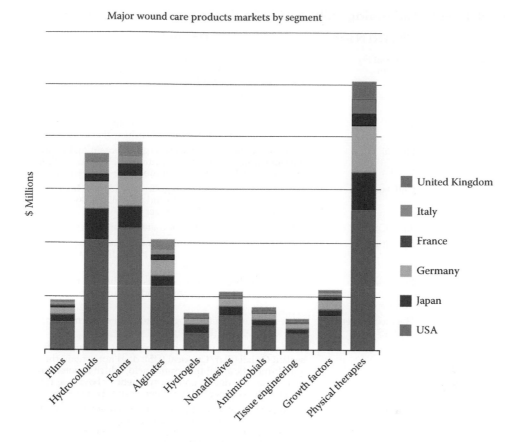

Figure 9.5 Major wound care products markets.

9.2.3.1 Bioactive Agents in Wound Sealing and Closure

Biologically active sealants typically contain various formulations of fibrin and/or thrombin, either of human or animal origin, which mimic or facilitate the final stages of the coagulation cascade. The most common consist of a liquid fibrin sealant product in which fibrinogen and thrombin are stored separately as a frozen liquid or lyophilized powder (Table 9.1). Before use, both components need to be reconstituted or thawed and loaded into a two-compartment applicator device that allows mixing of the two components just prior to delivery to the wound. Because of the laborious preparation process, these products are not easy to use. However, manufacturers have been developing some new formulations designed to make the process more user friendly (Figure 9.6) [9,10].

The emergence and rapid adoption of growth factors in wound management is testimony to the expectation that they will hasten wound healing and result in better outcomes, lowered cost, or both. While the market for growth factors in wound management is largely represented by the US market (as with most advanced medical technologies), economics, technology diffusion, and other forces will lead to more rapid growth in the use of these products in Asia Pacific (in particular, China will see strong growth, given that powerhouse country's propensity to bypass progressive development in favor of very rapid adoption of new technologies) (Figure 9.7) [11].

9.2.4 The Global Dental Market

■ The "Oral Care Products and Other Dental Consumables Market (Dental Biomaterials, Specialty Products, and Restoratives) Current Trends, Opportunities and Global Forecasts to 2016" analyzes and studies the major market drivers, restraints, and opportunities in Americas, Europe, Asia, and rest of the world.

Table 9.1: Selected Biologically Active Sealants, Glues, and Hemostats

Company	Product Name	Description/(Status)
Asahi Kasei Medical	CryoSeal FS System	Fibrin sealant system comprising an automated device and sterile blood processing disposables that enable autologous fibrin sealant to be prepared from a patient's own blood plasma in about an hour
Baxter	Artiss	Fibrin sealant spray
Baxter	Tisseel	Biodegradable fibrin sealant made of human fibrinogen and human thrombin; for oozing and diffuse bleeding
Baxter	FloSeal	Hemostatic bioresorbable sealant/glue containing human thrombin and bovine-derived, glutaraldehyde-cross-linked proprietary gelatin matrix. For moderate-to-severe bleeding
Baxter	GelFoam Plus	Hemostatic sponge comprising Pfizer's Gelfoam hemostatic sponge, made of porcine skin and gelatin, packaged with human plasma-derived thrombin powder
Behring/Nycomed	TachoComb	Fleece-type collagen hemostat coated with fibrin glue components
Bristol-Myers	Recothrom	First recombinant, plasma-free thrombin hemostat; Squibb/ZymoGenetics (sold by The Medicines Company in the United States and Canada)
CSL Behring	Beriplast P/ Beriplast P Combi-Set	Freeze-dried fibrin sealant; comprised of human fibrinogen-factor XIII and thrombin in aprotinin and calcium chloride solution
CSL Behring	Haemocomplettan P, RiaSTAP	Freeze-dried human fibrinogen concentrate; Haemocomplettan (US) and RiaSTAP (Europe)
J&J/Ethicon	Evicel	Evicel is a new formulation of the previously available fibrin sealant Quixil (EU)/Crosseal (US); does not contain the antifibrinolytic agent tranexamic acid, which is potentially neurotoxic, nor does it contain synthetic or bovine aprotinin, which reduces potential for hypersensitivity reactions
J&J/Ethicon	Evarrest	Absorbable fibrin sealant patch comprised of flexible matrix of oxidized, regenerated cellulose backing under a layer of polyglactin 910 nonwoven fibers and coated on one side with human fibrinogen and thrombin
J&J/Ethicon	BIOSEAL Fibrin Sealant	Low-cost porcine-derived surgical sealant manufactured in China by J&J company Bioseal Biotechnology and targeted to emerging markets
J&J/Ethicon	Evithrom	Human thrombin for topical use as hemostat; made of pooled human blood
Pfizer/King Pharmaceuticals	Thrombin JMI	Bovine-derived topical thrombin hemostat
Stryker/Orthovita	Vitagel Surgical	Bovine collagen and thrombin hemostat
Takeda/Nycomed	TachoSil	Absorbable surgical patch made of collagen sponge matrix combined with human fibrinogen and thrombin
Teijin Pharma Ltd./Teijin Group (Tokyo, Japan)	KTF-374	Company is working with Chemo-Sero-Therapeutic Research Institute (KAKETSUKEN) to develop a sheet-type surgical fibrin sealant; product combines KAKETSUKEN's recombinant thrombin and fibrinogen technology with Teijin's high-performance fiber technology to create the world's first recombinant fibrin sealant on a bioabsorbable, flexible, nonwoven electrospun fiber sheet
The Medicines Company (TMC)	Raplixa (formerly Fibrocaps)	Sprayable dry-powder formulation of fibrinogen and thrombin to aid in hemostasis during surgery to control mild or moderate bleeding
The Medicines Company (TMC)	In development: Fibropad patch	FDA accepted company's BLA application for Fibrocaps in April 2014 and set an action date (PDUFA) in 2015; in November 2013, the European Medicines Agency agreed to review the firm's EU marketing authorization application. Status update in report #S192
Vascular Solutions	D-Stat Flowable	Thick, but flowable, thrombin-based mixture to prevent bleeding in the subcutaneous pectoral pockets created during pacemaker and ICD implantations
Stryker/Orthovita	Vitagel Surgical	Bovine collagen and thrombin hemostat

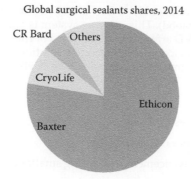

Figure 9.6 Worldwide surgical sealants.

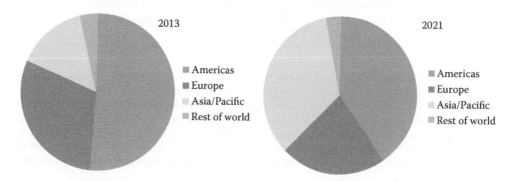

Figure 9.7 Distribution of wound growth factor markets, 2013 and 2021.

- This report studies the global diagnostic oral care products market over the forecast period 2011–2016.

- The oral care products market (or dental consumables) includes the small tools and products used to deliver dental care, such as biomaterials, prostheses, endodontic, orthodontic and periodontic products, restoratives, alloys, cements, bonding agents, impression materials, preventives, disposables, and other products.

- The increasing aging population across the globe and a concurrent increase in demand for enhanced oral care offers huge opportunities for product innovation and differentiation to dental care providers. Most providers practice direct customer interaction to improve sales and increase awareness toward their products as well as overall oral health. Moreover, increasing awareness in the developing nations about oral hygiene and new product developments has also given a boost to the dental consumables market. Rising demand for esthetic dentistry and growing dental tourism further ensures growth of this market in coming years.

Introduction of CAD/CAM technology has considerably reduced the designing time for dental prostheses like crowns and bridges and 3D imaging techniques have improved patient diagnosis and procedure planning. While lack of consumer awareness in developing economies may hinder market growth, industry players still have immense growth opportunities due to less stringent regulations with respect to introduction of new and advanced products and also their pricing. Increasing insurance coverage in the developed countries and rising income levels in developing nations like India and China are also expected to contribute significantly to the growth of this market [12].

9.2.5 The Cardiovascular Market

Cardiovascular disease (CVD) encompasses numerous heart and blood vessel conditions that can affect the cardiac electrical system (which controls heart rhythm and rate), cardiac muscle with the circulation system (needed for blood flow and distribution), and heart valves (required for one-way directional flow of blood). This complex system is addressed by the largest medical device market segment as CVD affects about one-third of the population. QiG is committed to developing technology and devices that will provide solutions for the cardiovascular system whose medical device market segment has expanded over $55B worldwide and is expected to grow due to

- An aging population
- Improved treatment capabilities in developing countries
- Increased worldwide prevalence of chronic CVD
- Innovation and technology advancements (including smaller devices, extended product life, and surgical improvements)
- Increased risk factors (diabetes, smoking, obesity, and hypertension)

9.2.5.1 Asia Driving Diagnostic Cardiology Device Market

"Cardiovascular disease (CVD) is the biggest cause of deaths worldwide, accounting for 17 million fatalities in 2008, according to the World Health Organization," said Nicola Goatman, analyst for HIS (Figure 9.8).

Owing to the increased prominence of cardiac diseases in the country, exploring the cardiovascular device sector would show the trend, pitfall, and the growth of innovation in this area. Worldwide market revenue for diagnostic cardiology devices is projected to rise to $882 million in 2016, up from $786 million in 2011. Asia will lead in global growth, with revenue climbing 57% during the 5-year period. North America is the world's largest region for diagnostic cardiology devices, but the region has reached market saturation. Growth has now shifted to emerging regions, particularly Asia. Within Asia, growth is being generated by China, India, and the Asian countries including Indonesia, Malaysia, Singapore, and the Philippines [13].

"The cost of this cardiac crisis is straining already overburdened healthcare services, compelling medical providers to seek preventative care measures to cut down on expensive procedures, such as coronary artery bypass surgery. Diagnostic cardiology devices, particularly portable systems, play a key role in reducing healthcare costs."

9.2.5.2 Key Players in the Cardiovascular Medical Device Industry

"The Cardiovascular Medical Device Sector: A Patent Landscape Report" summarizes that foreign companies like Koninklijke Philips Electronics and Sunshine Heart Company Pvt. Ltd. are the key players in cardiovascular medical device in India.

These companies have involved in intellectual gains of their devices through patents. Cardiovascular medical devices by Koninklijke Philips Electronics includes stents (two granted patents), monitoring device (four published applications), magnetic resonance imaging involved in cardiac

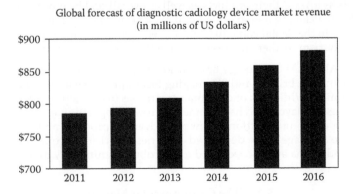

Figure 9.8 Global forecast of diagnostic cardiology device market.

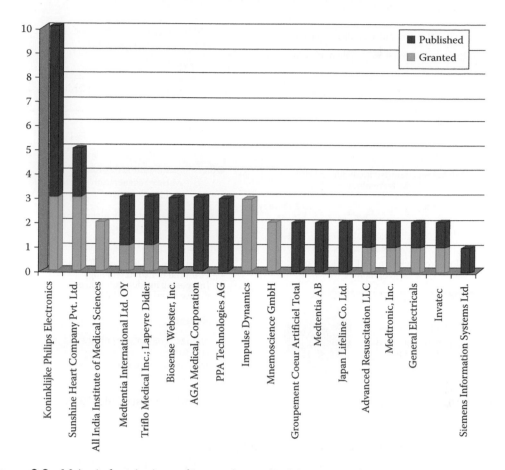

Figure 9.9 Major industries in cardiovascular medical device in India.

disease diagnosis (one in granted patents and one published application), and computed topography (two granted patents). This data reveals that Philips is actively involved in patenting their cardiovascular device innovation and marketing in India. Sunshine Heart Company Pvt. Ltd., a US–Australia-based medical device company, is engaged in the design and development of C-Pulse heart assist devices. The Company has only one operating segment, which is the research and development of heart assist devices and keenly involved in innovation of cardiac assist devices. All India Institute of Medical Science is the only Indian player in this field. Medtronic Inc. (US) is the world's leading medical technology company specializing in implantable and invasive therapies. Medtronics in India have two granted patents in heart valve sector and two granted patents in other cardiac medical device (Figure 9.9) [13].

9.3 GLOBAL OPHTHALMOLOGY DEVICES MARKET

Increasing incidence of degenerative diseases of eyes, increasing baby boomer population, increase in R&D activities in ophthalmology key players, and extensive use of high-end technologies involving use of software and computer-aided devices and platforms in ophthalmology drive the market of ophthalmology devices. Lack of ophthalmologists, economic slowdown, and saturation of the market in developed countries are the factors hampering the market growth.

North America accounts for the highest market share followed by Europe. Steep rise in aging population, increase in minimally invasive surgeries, and favorable government policies make the United States the leader of ophthalmology devices market. However, Asian countries, especially India and China, are the fast growing regions with its growing demand for ophthalmology devices and increasing research investments [14].

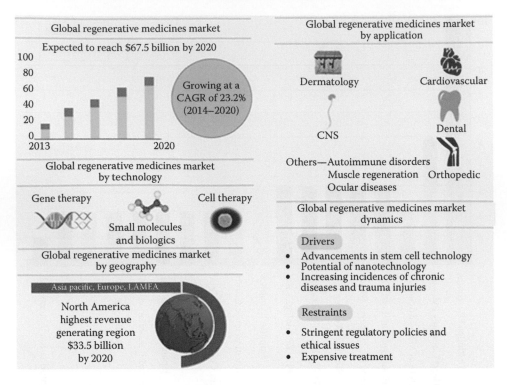

Figure 9.10 Global regenerative medicines market—size and forecasts, 2013–2020.

9.4 GLOBAL REGENERATIVE MEDICINES MARKET

Regenerative medicines have the unique ability to repair, replace, and regenerate tissues and organs, affected due to some injury, disease, or due to natural aging process. These medicines are capable of restoring the functionality of cells and tissues.

Based on its applications, this market can be classified into dermatology, cardiovascular, orthopedic, central nervous system (CNS), dental, and others. Researchers are engaged in developing technologies based on biologics, genes, somatic, as well as stem cells. The cardiovascular applications have commercialized products as well as ongoing trials. Therefore, this is the largest revenue-regenerating application market. However, due to immense focus on clinical studies in CNS disorders, this market is expected to gain momentum by 2020 (Figure 9.10). The market for CNS is the fastest growing application segment at a CAGR of 30.8% during 2014–2020. This is due to recent approvals for a regenerative product intended to treat multiple sclerosis and increasing number of clinical trials for neurodegenerative disorders [15].

9.5 CONCLUSIONS

Medical devices are now a pervasive part of modern medical care. The medical device industry includes a wide range of products for various kinds of therapeutic area and diseases. It is comprised of the companies that are involved in developing, manufacturing, and marketing medical apparatuses, instruments, equipment, devices, and supplies. The medical device sector comprises of different types of products ranging from simple bandages to life-sustaining implantable devices. Medical devices in Indian market have made enormous growth in last 5 years and the growth rate of technological convergence in medical device will become deeper over time. There is considerable work being done at the interface between mechanical and electronic engineering, with bioscience, in developing sophisticated biomaterial-based devices such as life-sustaining stents, prosthetic heart valves, sophisticated operational tools, imaging technologies and ultra-modern diagnostic kits, and many more on the list. The number of granted patents and applications are increasing every year in way giving enough space for the innovators to apply their technical skills by innovating new equipments in the field of cardiovascular medical devices.

Indian market of medical supplies and disposables is dominated by the domestic manufacturers, whereas importers dominate the costly and high-end medical equipment market. Thus, the report emphasizes that India is emerging as the biggest market for the medical giant to invest their intellectuals in the Indian patent pool.

REFERENCES

1. Ige OO, Umoru LE, Aribo S. *Nat Prod Minefield Biomater* 2012;2012:1–20.

2. Orthopedic Devices Market (Hip, Knee, Spine, Shoulder, Elbow, Foot and Ankle, Craniomaxillofacial and Other Extremities)—Global Industry Analysis, Size, Share, Growth, Trends and Forecast, 2013–2019.

3. Emerging Trends, Technologies and Opportunities in the Markets for Orthopedic Biomaterials, Worldwide.

4. Source: Report #S625MedMarket Diligence. http://www.mediligence.com/rpt/rpt-m625.htm.

5. Source: Report #S175MedMarket Diligence "Worldwide Sealants, Glues and Wound Closure, 2009–2013."

6. Source: Report #S520 (MedMarket Diligence, LLC).

7. Worldwide Wound Management, 2008–2017: Established and Emerging Products, Technologies and Markets in the U.S., Europe, Japan and Rest of World.

8. Source: Report #S247. MedMarket Diligence, LLC.

9. Source: Worldwide Surgical Sealants, Glues, and Wound Closure 2013–2018.

10. Source: Report #S192. MedMarket Diligence, LLC.

11. Source: Report #S249. MedMarket Diligence, LLC.

12. Oral Care Products and Other Dental Consumables Market (Dental Biomaterials, Specialty Products and Restoratives) Current Trends, Opportunities and Global Forecasts to 2016.

13. Global Forecast of Diagnostic Cardiology Device Market (IHSinmedica Research February 2013).

14. http://www.researchandmarkets.com/research/t5t8lk/ophthalmology "Ophthalmology Devices Global Market—Forecast To 2021."

15. World Regenerative Medicines Market—Opportunities and Forecasts, 2013–2020.

Index

A

Acetabular cup, 44; *see also* Bone
2-Acrylamido-2-methylpropane sulfonic acid
(AMPS), 115
Adherent dressings, 107
Aerogel-based drug delivery systems, 75, 81; *see also*
Polymer-based nanocarrier systems
Agarose, 144
Age-related macular degeneration (AMD), 163
AHV, *see* Rtificial heart valves (AHV)
Albumin, 138, 140
Alginate, 111, 144–146
dressings, 108, 109
fabricating procedures of alginate-based
sponge, 145
issues in, 145
Allen implants, 167
AMC, *see* Amphiphilically modified chitosan (AMC)
AMD, *see* Age-related macular degeneration (AMD)
Amphiphilically modified chitosan (AMC), 69;
see also Polymer-based nanocarrier systems
biomedical applications, 79
with sites for hydrophilic and hydrophobic
modifications, 78
Amphiphilic block polymer with redox-responsive
linkage, 79
AMPS, *see* 2-Acrylamido-2-methylpropane sulfonic
acid (AMPS)
Ang-1, *see* Angiopoietin-1 (Ang-1)
Angiogenesis, 189
Angiopoietin-1 (Ang-1), 189
Arteriovenous (AV), 16
AV, *see* Arteriovenous (AV)

B

Bare metal stents (BMS), 195
Basic fibroblast growth factor (bFGF), 189
bFGF, *see* Basic fibroblast growth factor (bFGF)
Bio-absorbable stents, 195
Bioactive agents, 211, 212
Bioceramics, 31
Biocompatibility, 1–2, 27
of cardiovascular biomaterials, 186
Biodegradable polymers, 76; *see also* Polymer-based
nanocarrier systems
Biodegradation, 2
Biofunctionalization, 197
Bio-inspired materials, 194
Biologic dressing, 107
Biomaterial, 1, 25, 132, 185, 207; *see also* Polymers;
Smart biomaterials; Tissue-engineering
advance, 56–57
advantages of nanoengineering on biomedical
implants, 57
biodegradable, 54
to deliver growth factors, 190
development of, 130
mechanical properties of, 52

physical characteristics of, 138
polymeric biomaterials for tissue
engineering, 137
Biomedical implants; *see also* Cardiovascular
implants; Dental implants; Ocular
implants; Orthopedic devices
advantages of nanoengineering on, 57
BIS-GMA, *see* Bisphenol A-glycidyl methacrylate
(BIS-GMA)
Bisphenol A-glycidyl methacrylate (BIS-GMA), 33
Blade implants, *see* Endodontic implants
Blending, 114
Blood–biomaterial interfacial interaction
mechanism, 185
coagulation cascade, 186
BMPs, *see* Bone morphogenetic proteins (BMPs)
BMS, *see* Bare metal stents (BMS)
Bone, 43; *see also* Human tissue; Orthopedic devices
-bonding polymer, 51
defects, 43
fixation devices, 49
formation, 54
graft materials, 43
implants, 56
replacement materials, 57–58
synthetic substitutes, 44
trauma, 45
types of, 44
Bone morphogenetic proteins (BMPs), 208
Bridges, 31

C

CAGR, *see* Compounded annual growth rate (CAGR)
Capillarity, 58
Carbon-based materials, 88; *see also* Polymer-based
nanocarrier systems
drug and applications of graphene-based
composites, 91
graphene applications, 89
graphene-based materials, 88
graphene oxide, 91–92
loading of drugs on graphene sheets, 90
Carbon-fiber reinforced (CFR), 57
Carboxymethylcellulose (CMC), 111, 112, 115
Carboxymethyl chitosan (CMCS), 66, 147–148
route followed by different CMCS-based
formulations, 77
Cardiovascular biomaterials, 187
biofunctionalization of, 197
bio-inspired materials, 194
challenges in clinical trials, 197–198
chemical modification method, 196
classification of, 189
cobalt-based materials, 195
ePTFE grafts, 192–193
hydrogel-based cardiovascular biomaterials, 189
hydrogel for angiogenesis, 190
materials selection criteria, 187
metals and alloys, 195

Printed and bound by CPI Group (UK) Ltd, Croydon, CR0 4YY

01/11/2024

01782603-0003